Injury & Trauma Sourcebook

Learning Disabilities Sourcebook, 2nd Edition

Leukemia Sourcebook

Liver Disorders Sourcebook

Lung Disorders Sourcebook

Medical Tests Sourcebook, 3rd Edition

Men's Health Concerns Sourcebook, 2nd
Edition

Mental Health Disorders Sourcebook, 3rd
Edition

Mental Retardation Sourcebook

Movement Disorders Sourcebook

Multiple Sclerosis Sourcebook

Muscular Dystrophy Sourcebook

Obesity Sourcebook

Osteoporosis Sourcebook

Pain Sourcebook, 3rd Edition

Pediatric Cancer Sourcebook

Physical & Mental Issues in Aging
Sourcebook

Podiatry Sourcebook, 2nd Edition

Pregnancy & Birth Sourcebook, 2nd
Edition

Prostate Cancer Sourcebook

Prostate & Urological Disorders Sourcebook

Reconstructive & Cosmetic Surgery
Sourcebook

Rehabilitation Sourcebook

Respiratory Disorders Sourcebook, 2nd
Edition

Sexually Transmitted Diseases Sourcebook,
3rd Edition

Sleep Disorders Sourcebook, 2nd Edition

Smoking Concerns Sourcebook

Sports Injuries Sourcebook, 3rd Edition

Stress-Related Disorders Sourcebook, 2nd
Edition

Stroke Sourcebook, 2nd Edition

Surgery Sourcebook, 2nd Edition

Thyroid Disorders Sourcebook

Transplantation Sourcebook

Traveler'

Urinary
Disorders Sourcebook, 2nd Edition

Vegetarian Sourcebook

Women's Health Concerns Sourcebook, 2nd
Edition

Workplace Health & Safety Sourcebook

Worldwide Health Sourcebook

Teen Health Series

Abuse and Violence Information for
Teens

Alcohol Information for Teens

Allergy Information for Teens

Asthma Information for Teens

Body Information for Teens

Cancer Information for Teens

Complementary & Alternative
Medicine Information for Teens

Diabetes Information for Teens

Diet Information for Teens, 2nd Edition

Drug Information for Teens, 2nd Edition

Eating Disorders Information for Teens

Fitness Information for Teens, 2nd
Edition

Learning Disabilities Information for
Teens

Mental Health Information for Teens,
2nd Edition

Pregnancy Information for Teens

Sexual Health Information for Teens,
2nd Edition

Skin Health Information for Teens

Sleep Information for Teens

Sports Injuries Information for Teens,
2nd Edition

Stress Information for Teens

Suicide Information for Teens

Tobacco Information for Teens

Stroke
SOURCEBOOK
Second Edition

Health Reference Series

Second Edition

Stroke
SOURCEBOOK

Basic Consumer Health Information about Stroke, Including Ischemic, Hemorrhagic, and Mini Strokes, as Well as Risk Factors, Prevention Guidelines, Diagnostic Tests, Medications and Surgical Treatments, and Complications of Stroke

Along with Rehabilitation Techniques and Innovations, Tips on Staying Healthy and Maintaining Independence after Stroke, a Glossary of Related Terms, and a Directory of Resources for Stroke Survivors and Their Families

Edited by
Amy L. Sutton

Omnigraphics

P.O. Box 31-1640, Detroit, MI 48231

Bibliographic Note

Because this page cannot legibly accommodate all the copyright notices, the Bibliographic Note portion of the Preface constitutes an extension of the copyright notice.

Edited by Amy L. Sutton

Health Reference Series

Karen Bellenir, *Managing Editor*
David A. Cooke, M.D., *Medical Consultant*
Elizabeth Collins, *Research and Permissions Coordinator*
Cherry Stockdale, *Permissions Assistant*
EdIndex, Services for Publishers, *Indexers*

* * *

Omnigraphics, Inc.
Matthew P. Barbour, *Senior Vice President*
Kevin M. Hayes, *Operations Manager*

* * *

Peter E. Ruffner, *Publisher*

Copyright © 2008 Omnigraphics, Inc.

ISBN 978-0-7808-1035-8

Library of Congress Cataloging-in-Publication Data

Stroke sourcebook : basic consumer health information about stroke, including ischemic, hemorrhagic, and mini strokes, as well as risk factors, prevention guidelines, diagnostic tests, medications and surgical treatments, and complications of stroke; along with rehabilitation techniques and innovations, tips on staying healthy and maintaining independence after stroke, a glossary of related terms, and a directory of resources for stroke survivors and their families / edited by Amy L. Sutton. -- 2nd ed.
   p. cm.
 Includes bibliographical references and index.
 ISBN 978-0-7808-1035-8 (hardcover : alk. paper) 1. Cerebrovascular disease--Popular works. I. Sutton, Amy L.
  RC388.5.S8566 2008
  616.8'1--dc22

                                                          2008025775

This book is printed on acid-free paper meeting the ANSI Z39.48 Standard. The infinity symbol that appears above indicates that the paper in this book meets that standard.

Printed in the United States

Table of Contents

Visit www.healthreferenceseries.com to view *A Contents Guide to the Health Reference Series*, a listing of more than 14,000 topics and the volumes in which they are covered.

Part II: Stroke Risk Factors and Prevention

Part III: Diagnosing and Treating Stroke

Part IV: Stroke Complications

Part V: Life after Stroke: Rehabilitation and Daily Living Concerns

Part VI: Additional Help and Information

Preface

About This Book

Strokes—also known as brain attacks—occur when a part of the brain is unable to get the blood and oxygen it needs to function. As a result of this interruption, stroke victims may lose control of their speech, movement, and memory, and without emergency medical treatment, they may suffer mild to severe brain damage and even death. Although strokes happen quickly, the effects of stroke often require long-term rehabilitation and medical care. Strokes are the leading cause of serious long-term disability in the United States, but there is hope: Experts estimate that up to 80% of strokes can be prevented with lifestyle changes and medication.

Stroke Sourcebook, Second Edition, provides updated information about stroke, its causes, risk factors, diagnosis, acute and long-term treatment, and recent innovations in poststroke care. Readers will learn about the types of strokes, including ischemic, hemorrhagic, and mini strokes, as well as common poststroke complications, such as loss of muscle control and balance, thinking and cognitive disabilities, and emotional and sleep problems. Information on rehabilitation therapies, prevention strategies, and tips on caring for a stroke survivor is also included, along with a glossary of related terms and a directory of organizations that offer additional information to stroke survivors and their families.

How to Use This Book

This book is divided into parts and chapters. Parts focus on broad areas of interest. Chapters are devoted to single topics within a part.

Part I: Understanding Stroke (Brain Attack) and Its Causes provides general information about brain attacks and highlights statistics on the incidence and projected costs of stroke in the United States. This part also offers specific facts about strokes caused by clots, such as ischemic strokes and transient ischemic attacks (mini strokes), as well as information on strokes caused by ruptured blood vessels, including brain aneurysms and hemorrhages.

Part II: Stroke Risk Factors and Prevention offers detailed information on both modifiable and unmodifiable factors that influence a person's risk of stroke. Information is also included about prescription medication use and stroke risk, as well as personal and community prevention strategies that may reduce the burden of stroke in the United States.

Part III: Diagnosing and Treating Stroke notes the warning signs of brain attacks and offers readers information about the neurological tests and procedures used to diagnose stroke. Because rapid action is a critical component of successful stroke treatment, this part also details commonly used stroke medications and identifies early treatment measures that may save patients' lives and reduce stroke-related disability. The part concludes with information about surgical procedures that may prevent initial or recurrent strokes—such as stents, carotid endarterectomy, and angioplasty—and innovations in stroke treatment.

Part IV: Stroke Complications provides detailed facts on the wide variety of impairments that may occur after stroke, including pain, cognitive problems and dementia, communication difficulties, emotional disorders, motor and muscle control problems, bowel and bladder disorders, and sleep difficulties.

Part V: Life after Stroke: Rehabilitation and Daily Living Concerns highlights specific therapies—including physical, occupational, speech-language, and psychological therapy—used to help patients overcome common stroke-related complications and regain independence in daily life. Included in this part are tips for patients and families when choosing stroke rehabilitation or assisted-living facilities, as well as advice on employment, financial, and legal concerns during the post-stroke period.

Part VI: Additional Help and Information includes a glossary of important terms and a directory of organizations for stroke patients and their families.

Bibliographic Note

This volume contains documents and excerpts from publications issued by the following U.S. government agencies: Administration on Aging (AOA); Centers for Disease Control and Prevention (CDC); National Heart, Lung, and Blood Institute (NHLBI); National Institute of Biomedical Imaging and Bioengineering (NIBIB); National Institute of Neurological Disorders and Stroke (NINDS); National Institute on Aging (NIA); National Institute on Drug Abuse (NIDA); National Institutes of Health (NIH); National Women's Health Information Center (NWHIC); Social Security Administration (SSA); U.S. Department of Energy (DOE); U.S. Department of Health and Human Services (HHS); and the U.S. Food and Drug Administration (FDA).

In addition, this volume contains copyrighted documents from the following organizations: A.D.A.M., Inc.; American Academy of Neurology; American College of Physicians; American Health Care Association; American Heart Association; Assisted Living Federation of America; Baylor College of Medicine; CMP Healthcare Media; Columbia University Medical Center Department of Psychiatry; Internet Stroke Center at Washington University in St. Louis; Join Together; Medical College of Wisconsin; National Stroke Association; The Nemours Foundation; North Carolina Stroke Association; Quackwatch; Quadrant HealthCom Inc.; The *Star-Ledger*; Rehabilitation Institute of Chicago; State of Victoria (Australia); The Stroke Association; *Therapy Times;* University of Connecticut Health Center; The University of Iowa; University of Maryland Medical Center; and the University of Pittsburgh Department of Neurological Surgery.

Full citation information is provided on the first page of each chapter or section. Every effort has been made to secure all necessary rights to reprint the copyrighted material. If any omissions have been made, please contact Omnigraphics to make corrections for future editions.

Acknowledgements

Thanks go to the many organizations, agencies, and individuals who have contributed materials for this *Sourcebook* and to medical consultant Dr. David Cooke and document engineer Bruce Bellenir. Special thanks go to managing editor Karen Bellenir and research and permissions coordinator Liz Collins for their help and support.

About the Health Reference Series

The *Health Reference Series* is designed to provide basic medical information for patients, families, caregivers, and the general public. Each volume takes a particular topic and provides comprehensive coverage. This is especially important for people who may be dealing with a newly diagnosed disease or a chronic disorder in themselves or in a family member. People looking for preventive guidance, information about disease warning signs, medical statistics, and risk factors for health problems will also find answers to their questions in the *Health Reference Series*. The *Series*, however, is not intended to serve as a tool for diagnosing illness, in prescribing treatments, or as a substitute for the physician/patient relationship. All people concerned about medical symptoms or the possibility of disease are encouraged to seek professional care from an appropriate health care provider.

A Note about Spelling and Style

Health Reference Series editors use *Stedman's Medical Dictionary* as an authority for questions related to the spelling of medical terms and the *Chicago Manual of Style* for questions related to grammatical structures, punctuation, and other editorial concerns. Consistent adherence is not always possible, however, because the individual volumes within the *Series* include many documents from a wide variety of different producers and copyright holders, and the editor's primary goal is to present material from each source as accurately as is possible following the terms specified by each document's producer. This sometimes means that information in different chapters or sections may follow other guidelines and alternate spelling authorities. For example, occasionally a copyright holder may require that eponymous terms be shown in possessive forms (Crohn's disease *vs.* Crohn disease) or that British spelling norms be retained (leukaemia *vs.* leukemia).

Locating Information within the Health Reference Series

The *Health Reference Series* contains a wealth of information about a wide variety of medical topics. Ensuring easy access to all the fact sheets, research reports, in-depth discussions, and other material contained within the individual books of the *Series* remains one of our highest priorities. As the *Series* continues to grow in size and scope, however, locating the precise information needed by a reader may become more challenging.

A Contents Guide to the Health Reference Series was developed to direct readers to the specific volumes that address their concerns. It presents an extensive list of diseases, treatments, and other topics of general interest compiled from the Tables of Contents and major index headings. To access *A Contents Guide to the Health Reference Series*, visit www.healthreferenceseries.com.

Medical Consultant

Medical consultation services are provided to the *Health Reference Series* editors by David A. Cooke, M.D. Dr. Cooke is a graduate of Brandeis University, and he received his M.D. degree from the University of Michigan. He completed residency training at the University of Wisconsin Hospital and Clinics. He is board-certified in Internal Medicine. Dr. Cooke currently works as part of the University of Michigan Health System and practices in Ann Arbor, MI. In his free time, he enjoys writing, science fiction, and spending time with his family.

Our Advisory Board

We would like to thank the following board members for providing guidance to the development of this *Series*:

- Dr. Lynda Baker,
  Associate Professor of Library and Information Science,
  Wayne State University, Detroit, MI

- Nancy Bulgarelli,
  William Beaumont Hospital Library, Royal Oak, MI

- Karen Imarisio,
  Bloomfield Township Public Library, Bloomfield Township, MI

- Karen Morgan,
  Mardigian Library, University of Michigan-Dearborn,
  Dearborn, MI

- Rosemary Orlando,
  St. Clair Shores Public Library, St. Clair Shores, MI

Health Reference Series *Update Policy*

The inaugural book in the *Health Reference Series* was the first edition of *Cancer Sourcebook* published in 1989. Since then, the *Series* has been enthusiastically received by librarians and in the medical community. In order to maintain the standard of providing high-quality health information for the layperson the editorial staff at Omnigraphics felt it was necessary to implement a policy of updating volumes when warranted.

Medical researchers have been making tremendous strides, and it is the purpose of the *Health Reference Series* to stay current with the most recent advances. Each decision to update a volume is made on an individual basis. Some of the considerations include how much new information is available and the feedback we receive from people who use the books. If there is a topic you would like to see added to the update list, or an area of medical concern you feel has not been adequately addressed, please write to:

Editor
Health Reference Series
Omnigraphics, Inc.
P.O. Box 31-1640
Detroit, MI 48231
E-mail: editorial@omnigraphics.com

Part One

Understanding Stroke
(Brain Attack) and Its Causes

Chapter 1

All about Stroke

Introduction

More than 2,400 years ago the father of medicine, Hippocrates, recognized and described stroke—the sudden onset of paralysis. Until recently, modern medicine has had very little power over this disease, but the world of stroke medicine is changing and new and better therapies are being developed every day. Today, some people who have a stroke can walk away from the attack with no or few disabilities if they are treated promptly. Doctors can finally offer stroke patients and their families the one thing that until now has been so hard to give: hope.

In ancient times stroke was called apoplexy, a general term that physicians applied to anyone suddenly struck down with paralysis. Because many conditions can lead to sudden paralysis, the term apoplexy did not indicate a specific diagnosis or cause. Physicians knew very little about the cause of stroke and the only established therapy was to feed and care for the patient until the attack ran its course.

The first person to investigate the pathological signs of apoplexy was Johann Jacob Wepfer. Born in Schaffhausen, Switzerland, in 1620, Wepfer studied medicine and was the first to identify postmortem signs of bleeding in the brains of patients who died of apoplexy. From

Excerpted from "Stroke: Hope Through Research," by the National Institute of Neurological Disorders and Stroke (NINDS, www.ninds.nih.gov), part of the National Institutes of Health, September 11, 2007.

autopsy studies he gained knowledge of the carotid and vertebral arteries that supply the brain with blood. He also was the first person to suggest that apoplexy, in addition to being caused by bleeding in the brain, could be caused by a blockage of one of the main arteries supplying blood to the brain; thus stroke became known as a cerebrovascular disease ("cerebro" refers to a part of the brain; "vascular" refers to the blood vessels and arteries).

Medical science would eventually confirm Wepfer's hypotheses, but until very recently doctors could offer little in the area of therapy. Over the last two decades basic and clinical investigators, many of them sponsored and funded in part by the National Institute of Neurological Disorders and Stroke (NINDS), have learned a great deal about stroke. They have identified major risk factors for the disease and have developed surgical techniques and drug treatments for the prevention of stroke. But perhaps the most exciting new development in the field of stroke research is the recent approval of a drug treatment that can reverse the course of stroke if given during the first few hours after the onset of symptoms.

Studies with animals have shown that brain injury occurs within minutes of a stroke and can become irreversible within as little as an hour. In humans, brain damage begins from the moment the stroke starts and often continues for days afterward. Scientists now know that there is a very short window of opportunity for treatment of the most common form of stroke. Because of these and other advances in the field of cerebrovascular disease stroke patients now have a chance for survival and recovery.

Cost of stroke to the United States:

- Total cost of stroke to the United States: estimated at about $43 billion/year

- Direct costs for medical care and therapy: estimated at about $28 billion/year

- Indirect costs from lost productivity and other factors: estimated at about $15 million/year

- Average cost of care for a patient up to 90 days after a stroke: $15,000*

- For 10% of patients, cost of care for the first 90 days after a stroke: $35,000*

- Percentage of direct cost of care for the first 90 days*:
  - Initial hospitalization = 43%

- Rehabilitation = 16%
- Physician costs = 14%
- Hospital readmission = 14%
- Medications and other expenses = 13%

*Note: From *The Stroke/Brain Attack Reporter's Handbook,* National Stroke Association, Englewood, CO, 1997

What Is Stroke?

A stroke occurs when the blood supply to part of the brain is suddenly interrupted or when a blood vessel in the brain bursts, spilling blood into the spaces surrounding brain cells. In the same way that a person suffering a loss of blood flow to the heart is said to be having a heart attack, a person with a loss of blood flow to the brain or sudden bleeding in the brain can be said to be having a "brain attack."

Brain cells die when they no longer receive oxygen and nutrients from the blood or when they are damaged by sudden bleeding into or around the brain. Ischemia is the term used to describe the loss of oxygen and nutrients for brain cells when there is inadequate blood flow. Ischemia ultimately leads to infarction, the death of brain cells which are eventually replaced by a fluid-filled cavity (or infarct) in the injured brain.

When blood flow to the brain is interrupted, some brain cells die immediately, while others remain at risk for death. These damaged cells make up the ischemic penumbra and can linger in a compromised state for several hours. With timely treatment these cells can be saved. Even though a stroke occurs in the unseen reaches of the brain, the symptoms of a stroke are easy to spot. They include sudden numbness or weakness, especially on one side of the body; sudden confusion or trouble speaking or understanding speech; sudden trouble seeing in one or both eyes; sudden trouble walking, dizziness, or loss of balance or coordination; or sudden severe headache with no known cause. All of the symptoms of stroke appear suddenly, and often there is more than one symptom at the same time. Therefore stroke can usually be distinguished from other causes of dizziness or headache. These symptoms may indicate that a stroke has occurred and that medical attention is needed immediately.

There are two forms of stroke: ischemic—blockage of a blood vessel supplying the brain, and hemorrhagic—bleeding into or around the brain. The following sections describe these forms in detail.

Ischemic Stroke

An ischemic stroke occurs when an artery supplying the brain with blood becomes blocked, suddenly decreasing or stopping blood flow and ultimately causing a brain infarction. This type of stroke accounts for approximately 80 percent of all strokes. Blood clots are the most common cause of artery blockage and brain infarction. The process of clotting is necessary and beneficial throughout the body because it stops bleeding and allows repair of damaged areas of arteries or veins. However, when blood clots develop in the wrong place within an artery they can cause devastating injury by interfering with the normal flow of blood.

Problems with clotting become more frequent as people age. Blood clots can cause ischemia and infarction in two ways. A clot that forms in a part of the body other than the brain can travel through blood vessels and become wedged in a brain artery. This free-roaming clot is called an embolus and often forms in the heart. A stroke caused by an embolus is called an embolic stroke. The second kind of ischemic stroke, called a thrombotic stroke, is caused by thrombosis, the formation of a blood clot in one of the cerebral arteries that stays attached to the artery wall until it grows large enough to block blood flow.

Ischemic strokes can also be caused by stenosis, or a narrowing of the artery due to the buildup of plaque (a mixture of fatty substances, including cholesterol and other lipids) and blood clots along the artery wall. Stenosis can occur in large arteries and small arteries and is therefore called large vessel disease or small vessel disease, respectively. When a stroke occurs due to small vessel disease, a very small infarction results, sometimes called a lacunar infarction, from the French word "lacune" meaning "gap" or "cavity."

The most common blood vessel disease that causes stenosis is atherosclerosis. In atherosclerosis, deposits of plaque build up along the inner walls of large and medium-sized arteries, causing thickening, hardening, and loss of elasticity of artery walls and decreased blood flow. The role of cholesterol and blood lipids with respect to stroke risk is discussed in the section on cholesterol under "Who is at Risk for Stroke?"

Hemorrhagic Stroke

In a healthy, functioning brain, neurons do not come into direct contact with blood. The vital oxygen and nutrients the neurons need from the blood come to the neurons across the thin walls of the cerebral capillaries. The glia (nervous system cells that support and protect neurons) form a blood-brain barrier, an elaborate meshwork that surrounds blood vessels and capillaries and regulates which elements of the blood can pass through to the neurons.

When an artery in the brain bursts, blood spews out into the surrounding tissue and upsets not only the blood supply but the delicate chemical balance neurons require to function. This is called a hemorrhagic stroke. Such strokes account for approximately 20 percent of all strokes.

Hemorrhage can occur in several ways. One common cause is a bleeding aneurysm, a weak or thin spot on an artery wall. Over time, these weak spots stretch or balloon out under high arterial pressure. The thin walls of these ballooning aneurysms can rupture and spill blood into the space surrounding brain cells.

Hemorrhage also occurs when arterial walls break open. Plaque-encrusted artery walls eventually lose their elasticity and become brittle and thin, prone to cracking. Hypertension, or high blood pressure, increases the risk that a brittle artery wall will give way and release blood into the surrounding brain tissue.

A person with an arteriovenous malformation (AVM) also has an increased risk of hemorrhagic stroke. AVMs are a tangle of defective blood vessels and capillaries within the brain that have thin walls and can therefore rupture.

Bleeding from ruptured brain arteries can either go into the substance of the brain or into the various spaces surrounding the brain. **Intracerebral hemorrhage** occurs when a vessel within the brain leaks blood into the brain itself. **Subarachnoid hemorrhage** is bleeding under the meninges, or outer membranes, of the brain into the thin fluid-filled space that surrounds the brain.

The subarachnoid space separates the arachnoid membrane from the underlying pia mater membrane. It contains a clear fluid (cerebrospinal fluid or CSF) as well as the small blood vessels that supply the outer surface of the brain. In a subarachnoid hemorrhage, one of the small arteries within the subarachnoid space bursts, flooding the area with blood and contaminating the cerebrospinal fluid. Since the CSF flows throughout the cranium, within the spaces of the brain, subarachnoid hemorrhage can lead to extensive damage throughout the brain. In fact, subarachnoid hemorrhage is the most deadly of all strokes.

Transient Ischemic Attacks

A transient ischemic attack (TIA), sometimes called a mini-stroke, starts just like a stroke but then resolves leaving no noticeable symptoms or deficits. The occurrence of a TIA is a warning that the person is at risk for a more serious and debilitating stroke. Of the approximately 50,000 Americans who have a TIA each year, about one-third will have an acute stroke sometime in the future. The addition of other risk factors compounds a person's risk for a recurrent stroke. The average duration of a TIA is a few minutes. For almost all TIAs, the symptoms go away within an hour. There is no way to tell whether symptoms will be just a TIA or persist and lead to death or disability. The patient should assume that all stroke symptoms signal an emergency and should not wait to see if they go away.

Recurrent Stroke

Recurrent stroke is frequent; about 25 percent of people who recover from their first stroke will have another stroke within 5 years. Recurrent stroke is a major contributor to stroke disability and death, with the risk of severe disability or death from stroke increasing with each stroke recurrence. The risk of a recurrent stroke is greatest right after a stroke, with the risk decreasing with time. About 3 percent of stroke patients will have another stroke within 30 days of their first stroke and one-third of recurrent strokes take place within 2 years of the first stroke.

How Do You Recognize Stroke?

Symptoms of stroke appear suddenly. Watch for these symptoms and be prepared to act quickly for yourself or on behalf of someone you are with:

- Sudden numbness or weakness of the face, arm, or leg, especially on one side of the body.
- Sudden confusion, trouble talking, or understanding speech.
- Sudden trouble seeing in one or both eyes.
- Sudden trouble walking, dizziness, or loss of balance or coordination.
- Sudden severe headache with no known cause.

If you suspect you or someone you know is experiencing any of these symptoms indicative of a stroke, do not wait. Call 911 emergency immediately. There are now effective therapies for stroke that must be administered at a hospital, but they lose their effectiveness if not given within the first 3 hours after stroke symptoms appear. Every minute counts!

How Is the Cause of Stroke Determined?

Physicians have several diagnostic techniques and imaging tools to help diagnose the cause of stroke quickly and accurately. The first step in diagnosis is a short neurological examination. When a possible stroke patient arrives at a hospital, a health care professional, usually a doctor or nurse, will ask the patient or a companion what happened and when the symptoms began. Blood tests, an electrocardiogram, and a brain scan, such CT or MRI, will often be done. One test that helps doctors judge the severity of a stroke is the standardized NIH Stroke Scale, developed by the NINDS. Health care professionals use the NIH Stroke Scale to measure a patient's neurological deficits by asking the patient to answer questions and to perform several physical and mental tests. Other scales include the Glasgow Coma Scale, the Hunt and Hess Scale, the Modified Rankin Scale, and the Barthel Index.

Imaging for the Diagnosis of Acute Stroke

Health care professionals also use a variety of imaging devices to evaluate stroke patients. The most widely used imaging procedure is the computed tomography (CT) scan. Also known as a CAT scan or computed axial tomography, CT creates a series of cross-sectional images of the head and brain. Because it is readily available at all hours at most major hospitals and produces images quickly, CT is the most commonly used diagnostic technique for acute stroke. CT also has unique diagnostic benefits. It will quickly rule out a hemorrhage, can occasionally show a tumor that might mimic a stroke, and may even show evidence of early infarction. Infarctions generally show up on a CT scan about 6 to 8 hours after the start of stroke symptoms.

If a stroke is caused by hemorrhage, a CT can show evidence of bleeding into the brain almost immediately after stroke symptoms appear. Hemorrhage is the primary reason for avoiding certain drug treatments for stroke, such as thrombolytic therapy, the only proven acute stroke therapy for ischemic stroke. Thrombolytic therapy cannot be used until the doctor can confidently diagnose the patient as suffering from an ischemic stroke because this treatment might increase bleeding and could make a hemorrhagic stroke worse.

Another imaging device used for stroke patients is the magnetic resonance imaging (MRI) scan. MRI uses magnetic fields to detect subtle changes in brain tissue content. One effect of stroke is the slowing of water movement, called diffusion, through the damaged brain tissue. MRI can show this type of damage within the first hour after the stroke symptoms start. The benefit of MRI over a CT scan is more accurate and earlier diagnosis of infarction, especially for smaller strokes, while showing equivalent accuracy in determining when hemorrhage is present. MRI is more sensitive than CT for other types of brain disease, such as brain tumor, that might mimic a stroke. MRI cannot be performed in patients with certain types of metallic or electronic implants, such as pacemakers for the heart.

Although increasingly used in the emergency diagnosis of stroke, MRI is not immediately available at all hours in most hospitals, where CT is used for acute stroke diagnosis. Also, MRI takes longer to perform than CT, and may not be performed if it would significantly delay treatment.

Other types of MRI scans, often used for the diagnosis of cerebrovascular disease and to predict the risk of stroke, are magnetic resonance angiography (MRA) and functional magnetic resonance imaging (fMRI). Neurosurgeons use MRA to detect stenosis (blockage) of the brain arteries inside the skull by mapping flowing blood. Functional MRI uses a magnet to pick up signals from oxygenated blood and can show brain activity through increases in local blood flow. Duplex Doppler ultrasound and arteriography are two diagnostic imaging techniques used to decide if an individual would benefit from a surgical procedure called carotid endarterectomy. This surgery is used to remove fatty deposits from the carotid arteries and can help prevent stroke.

Doppler ultrasound is a painless, noninvasive test in which sound waves above the range of human hearing are sent into the neck. Echoes bounce off the moving blood and the tissue in the artery and can be formed into an image. Ultrasound is fast, painless, risk-free, and relatively inexpensive compared to MRA and arteriography, but it is not considered to be as accurate as arteriography. Arteriography is an X-ray of the carotid artery taken when a special dye is injected into the artery. The procedure carries its own small risk of causing a stroke and is costly to perform. The benefits of arteriography over MR techniques and ultrasound are that it is extremely reliable and still the best way to measure stenosis of the carotid arteries. Even so, significant advances are being made every day involving noninvasive imaging techniques such as fMRI.

Who Is at Risk for Stroke?

Some people are at a higher risk for stroke than others. Unmodifiable risk factors include age, gender, race/ethnicity, and stroke family history. In contrast, other risk factors for stroke, like high blood pressure or cigarette smoking, can be changed or controlled by the person at risk.

Unmodifiable Risk Factors

It is a myth that stroke occurs only in elderly adults. In actuality, stroke strikes all age groups, from fetuses still in the womb to centenarians. It is true, however, that older people have a higher risk for stroke than the general population and that the risk for stroke increases with age. For every decade after the age of 55, the risk of stroke doubles, and two-thirds of all strokes occur in people over 65 years old. People over 65 also have a seven-fold greater risk of dying from stroke than the general population. And the incidence of stroke is increasing proportionately with the increase in the elderly population. When the baby boomers move into the over-65 age group, stroke and other diseases will take on even greater significance in the health care field.

Gender also plays a role in risk for stroke. Men have a higher risk for stroke, but more women die from stroke. The stroke risk for men is 1.25 times that for women. But men do not live as long as women, so men are usually younger when they have their strokes and therefore have a higher rate of survival than women. In other words, even though women have fewer strokes than men, women are generally older when they have their strokes and are more likely to die from them.

Stroke seems to run in some families. Several factors might contribute to familial stroke risk. Members of a family might have a genetic tendency for stroke risk factors, such as an inherited predisposition for hypertension or diabetes. The influence of a common lifestyle among family members could also contribute to familial stroke.

The risk for stroke varies among different ethnic and racial groups. The incidence of stroke among African Americans is almost double that of white Americans, and twice as many African Americans who have a stroke die from the event compared to white Americans. African Americans between the ages of 45 and 55 have four to five times the stroke death rate of whites. After age 55 the stroke mortality rate for whites increases and is equal to that of African Americans.

Compared to white Americans, African Americans have a higher incidence of stroke risk factors, including high blood pressure and cigarette smoking. African Americans also have a higher incidence and prevalence of some genetic diseases, such as diabetes and sickle cell anemia, that predispose them to stroke.

Hispanics and Native Americans have stroke incidence and mortality rates more similar to those of white Americans. In Asian Americans stroke incidence and mortality rates are also similar to those in white Americans, even though Asians in Japan, China, and other countries of the Far East have significantly higher stroke incidence and mortality rates than white Americans. This suggests that environment and lifestyle factors play a large role in stroke risk.

The "Stroke Belt"

Several decades ago, scientists and statisticians noticed that people in the southeastern United States had the highest stroke mortality rate in the country. They named this region the stroke belt. For many years, researchers believed that the increased risk was due to the higher percentage of African Americans and an overall lower socioeconomic status (SES) in the southern states. A low SES is associated with an overall lower standard of living, leading to a lower standard of health care and therefore an increased risk of stroke. But researchers now know that the higher percentage of African Americans and the overall lower SES in the southern states does not adequately account for the higher incidence of, and mortality from, stroke in those states. This means that other factors must be contributing to the higher incidence of and mortality from stroke in this region.

Recent studies have also shown that there is a stroke buckle in the stroke belt. Three southeastern states, North Carolina, South Carolina, and Georgia, have an extremely high stroke mortality rate, higher than the rate in other stroke belt states and up to two times the stroke mortality rate of the United States overall. The increased risk could be due to geographic or environmental factors or to regional differences in lifestyle, including higher rates of cigarette smoking and a regional preference for salty, high-fat foods.

Other Risk Factors

The most important risk factors for stroke are hypertension, heart disease, diabetes, and cigarette smoking. Others include heavy alcohol consumption, high blood cholesterol levels, illicit drug use, and genetic or congenital conditions, particularly vascular abnormalities. People with more than one risk factor have what is called "amplification of risk." This means that the multiple risk factors compound their destructive effects and create an overall risk greater than the simple cumulative effect of the individual risk factors.

Hypertension

Of all the risk factors that contribute to stroke, the most powerful is hypertension, or high blood pressure. People with hypertension have a risk for stroke that is four to six times higher than the risk for those without hypertension. One third of the adult U.S. population, about 50 million people (including 40 to 70 percent of those over age 65) have high blood pressure. Forty to 90 percent of stroke patients have high blood pressure before their stroke event.

A systolic pressure of 120 mm of Hg over a diastolic pressure of 80 mm of Hg is generally considered normal. Persistently high blood pressure greater than 140 over 90 leads to the diagnosis of the disease called hypertension. The impact of hypertension on the total risk for stroke decreases with increasing age, therefore factors other than hypertension play a greater role in the overall stroke risk in elderly adults. For people without hypertension, the absolute risk of stroke increases over time until around the age of 90, when the absolute risk becomes the same as that for people with hypertension.

Like stroke, there is a gender difference in the prevalence of hypertension. In younger people, hypertension is more common among men than among women. With increasing age, however, more women than men have hypertension. This hypertension gender-age difference probably has an impact on the incidence and prevalence of stroke in these populations.

Antihypertensive medication can decrease a person's risk for stroke. Recent studies suggest that treatment can decrease the stroke incidence rate by 38 percent and decrease the stroke fatality rate by 40 percent. Common hypertensive agents include adrenergic agents, beta-blockers, angiotensin-converting enzyme inhibitors, calcium channel blockers, diuretics, and vasodilators.

Heart Disease

After hypertension, the second most powerful risk factor for stroke is heart disease, especially a condition known as atrial fibrillation. Atrial fibrillation is irregular beating of the left atrium, or left upper chamber, of the heart. In people with atrial fibrillation, the left atrium beats up to four times faster than the rest of the heart. This leads to an irregular flow of blood and the occasional formation of blood clots that can leave the heart and travel to the brain, causing a stroke.

Atrial fibrillation, which affects as many as 2.2 million Americans, increases an individual's risk of stroke by 4 to 6 percent, and about 15 percent of stroke patients have atrial fibrillation before they experience a stroke. The condition is more prevalent in the upper age groups, which means that the prevalence of atrial fibrillation in the United States will increase proportionately with the growth of the elderly population. Unlike hypertension and other risk factors that have a lesser impact on the ever-rising absolute risk of stroke that comes with advancing age, the influence of atrial fibrillation on total risk for stroke increases powerfully with age. In people over 80 years old, atrial fibrillation is the direct cause of one in four strokes.

Other forms of heart disease that increase stroke risk include malformations of the heart valves or the heart muscle. Some valve diseases, like mitral valve stenosis or mitral annular calcification, can double the risk for stroke, independent of other risk factors.

Heart muscle malformations can also increase the risk for stroke. Patent foramen ovale (PFO) is a passage or a hole (sometimes called a "shunt") in the heart wall separating the two atria, or upper chambers, of the heart. Clots in the blood are usually filtered out by the lungs, but PFO could allow emboli or blood clots to bypass the lungs and go directly through the arteries to the brain, potentially causing a stroke. Research is currently under way to determine how important PFO is as a cause for stroke. Atrial septal aneurysm (ASA), a congenital (present from birth) malformation of the heart tissue, is a bulging of the septum or heart wall into one of the atria of the heart. Researchers do not know why this malformation increases the risk for stroke. PFO and ASA frequently occur together and therefore amplify the risk for stroke. Two other heart malformations that work to increase the risk for stroke for unknown reasons are left atrial enlargement and left ventricular hypertrophy. People with left atrial enlargement have a larger than normal left atrium of the heart; those with left ventricular hypertrophy have a thickening of the wall of the left ventricle.

Another risk factor for stroke is cardiac surgery to correct malformations or reverse the effects of heart disease. Strokes that occur in this situation are usually the result of surgically dislodged plaques from the aorta that travel through the bloodstream to arteries in the neck and head, causing stroke. Cardiac surgery increases a person's risk of stroke by about 1 percent. Other kinds of surgery can also increase the risk of stroke.

Blood Cholesterol Levels

Most people know that high cholesterol levels contribute to heart disease. But many don't realize that a high cholesterol level also contributes to stroke risk. Cholesterol, a waxy substance produced by the liver, is a vital body product. It contributes to the production of hormones and vitamin D and is an integral component of cell membranes. The liver makes enough cholesterol to fuel the body's needs and this natural production of cholesterol alone is not a large contributing factor to atherosclerosis, heart disease, and stroke. Research has shown that the danger from cholesterol comes from a dietary intake of foods that contain high levels of cholesterol. Foods high in saturated fat and cholesterol, like meats, eggs, and dairy products, can increase the amount of total cholesterol in the body to alarming levels, contributing to the risk of atherosclerosis and thickening of the arteries.

Cholesterol is classified as a lipid, meaning that it is fat-soluble rather than water-soluble. Other lipids include fatty acids, glycerides, alcohol, waxes, steroids, and fat-soluble vitamins A, D, and E. Lipids and water, like oil and water, do not mix. Blood is a water-based liquid, therefore cholesterol does not mix with blood. In order to travel through the blood without clumping together, cholesterol needs to be covered by a layer of protein. The cholesterol and protein together are called a lipoprotein.

There are two kinds of cholesterol, commonly called the "good" and the "bad." Good cholesterol is high-density lipoprotein, or HDL; bad cholesterol is low-density lipoprotein, or LDL. Together, these two forms of cholesterol make up a person's total serum cholesterol level. Most cholesterol tests measure the level of total cholesterol in the blood and don't distinguish between good and bad cholesterol. For these total serum cholesterol tests, a level of less than 200 mg/dL is considered safe, while a level of more than 240 is considered dangerous and places a person at risk for heart disease and stroke.

Most cholesterol in the body is in the form of LDL. LDLs circulate through the bloodstream, picking up excess cholesterol and depositing cholesterol where it is needed (for example, for the production and maintenance of cell membranes). But when too much cholesterol starts circulating in the blood, the body cannot handle the excessive LDLs, which build up along the inside of the arterial walls. The buildup of LDL coating on the inside of the artery walls hardens and turns into arterial plaque, leading to stenosis and atherosclerosis. This plaque blocks blood vessels and contributes to the formation of blood clots. A person's LDL level should be less than 130 mg/dL to be safe. LDL levels between

15

130 and 159 put a person at a slightly higher risk for atherosclerosis, heart disease, and stroke. A score over 160 puts a person at great risk for a heart attack or stroke.

The other form of cholesterol, HDL, is beneficial and contributes to stroke prevention. HDL carries a small percentage of the cholesterol in the blood, but instead of depositing its cholesterol on the inside of artery walls, HDL returns to the liver to unload its cholesterol. The liver then eliminates the excess cholesterol by passing it along to the kidneys. Currently, any HDL score higher than 35 is considered desirable. Recent studies have shown that high levels of HDL are associated with a reduced risk for heart disease and stroke and that low levels (less than 35 mg/dL), even in people with normal levels of LDL, lead to an increased risk for heart disease and stroke.

A person may lower his risk for atherosclerosis and stroke by improving his cholesterol levels. A healthy diet and regular exercise are the best ways to lower total cholesterol levels. In some cases, physicians may prescribe cholesterol-lowering medication, and recent studies have shown that the newest types of these drugs, called reductase inhibitors or statin drugs, significantly reduce the risk for stroke in most patients with high cholesterol. Scientists believe that statins may work by reducing the amount of bad cholesterol the body produces and by reducing the body's inflammatory immune reaction to cholesterol plaque associated with atherosclerosis and stroke.

Diabetes

Diabetes is another disease that increases a person's risk for stroke. People with diabetes have three times the risk of stroke compared to people without diabetes. The relative risk of stroke from diabetes is highest in the fifth and sixth decades of life and decreases after that. Like hypertension, the relative risk of stroke from diabetes is highest for men at an earlier age and highest for women at an older age. People with diabetes may also have other contributing risk factors that can amplify the overall risk for stroke. For example, the prevalence of hypertension is 40 percent higher in the diabetic population compared to the general population.

Modifiable Lifestyle Risk Factors

Cigarette smoking is the most powerful modifiable stroke risk factor. Smoking almost doubles a person's risk for ischemic stroke, independent of other risk factors, and it increases a person's risk for subarachnoid hemorrhage by up to 3.5 percent. Smoking is directly responsible for a greater percentage of the total number of strokes in young adults than in older adults. Risk factors other than smoking—like hypertension, heart disease, and diabetes—account for more of the total number of strokes in older adults.

Heavy smokers are at greater risk for stroke than light smokers. The relative risk of stroke decreases immediately after quitting smoking, with a major reduction of risk seen after 2 to 4 years. Unfortunately, it may take several decades for a former smoker's risk to drop to the level of someone who never smoked.

Smoking increases the risk of stroke by promoting atherosclerosis and increasing the levels of blood-clotting factors, such as fibrinogen. In addition to promoting conditions linked to stroke, smoking also increases the damage that results from stroke by weakening the endothelial wall of the cerebrovascular system. This leads to greater damage to the brain from events that occur in the secondary stage of stroke.

High alcohol consumption is another modifiable risk factor for stroke. Generally, an increase in alcohol consumption leads to an increase in blood pressure. While scientists agree that heavy drinking is a risk for both hemorrhagic and ischemic stroke, in several research studies daily consumption of smaller amounts of alcohol has been found to provide a protective influence against ischemic stroke, perhaps because alcohol decreases the clotting ability of platelets in the blood. Moderate alcohol consumption may act in the same way as aspirin to decrease blood clotting and prevent ischemic stroke. Heavy alcohol consumption, though, may seriously deplete platelet numbers and compromise blood clotting and blood viscosity, leading to hemorrhage. In addition, heavy drinking or binge drinking can lead to a rebound effect after the alcohol is purged from the body. The consequences of this rebound effect are that blood viscosity (thickness) and platelet levels skyrocket after heavy drinking, increasing the risk for ischemic stroke.

The use of illicit drugs, such as cocaine and crack cocaine, can cause stroke. Cocaine may act on other risk factors, such as hypertension, heart disease, and vascular disease, to trigger a stroke. It decreases relative cerebrovascular blood flow by up to 30 percent, causes vascular constriction, and inhibits vascular relaxation, leading to narrowing of the arteries. Cocaine also affects the heart, causing arrhythmias and rapid heart rate that can lead to the formation of blood clots.

Marijuana smoking may also be a risk factor for stroke. Marijuana decreases blood pressure and may interact with other risk factors, such as hypertension and cigarette smoking, to cause rapidly fluctuating blood pressure levels, damaging blood vessels.

Other drugs of abuse, such as amphetamines, heroin, and anabolic steroids (and even some common, legal drugs, such as caffeine and L-asparaginase and pseudoephedrine found in over-the-counter decongestants), have been suspected of increasing stroke risk. Many of these drugs are vasoconstrictors, meaning that they cause blood vessels to constrict and blood pressure to rise.

Head and Neck Injuries

Injuries to the head or neck may damage the cerebrovascular system and cause a small number of strokes. Head injury or traumatic brain injury may cause bleeding within the brain leading to damage akin to that caused by a hemorrhagic stroke. Neck injury, when associated with spontaneous tearing of the vertebral or carotid arteries caused by sudden and severe extension of the neck, neck rotation, or pressure on the artery, is a contributing cause of stroke, especially in young adults. This type of stroke is often called "beauty-parlor syndrome," which refers to the practice of extending the neck backwards over a sink for hair-washing in beauty parlors. Neck calisthenics, "bottoms-up" drinking, and improperly performed chiropractic manipulation of the neck can also put strain on the vertebral and carotid arteries, possibly leading to ischemic stroke.

Infections

Recent viral and bacterial infections may act with other risk factors to add a small risk for stroke. The immune system responds to infection by increasing inflammation and increasing the infection-fighting properties of the blood. Unfortunately, this immune response increases the number of clotting factors in the blood, leading to an increased risk of embolic-ischemic stroke.

Genetic Risk Factors

Although there may not be a single genetic factor associated with stroke, genes do play a large role in the expression of stroke risk factors such as hypertension, heart disease, diabetes, and vascular malformations. It is also possible that an increased risk for stroke within a family is due to environmental factors, such as a common sedentary lifestyle or poor eating habits, rather than hereditary factors.

Vascular malformations that cause stroke may have the strongest genetic link of all stroke risk factors. A vascular malformation is an abnormally formed blood vessel or group of blood vessels. One genetic

18

vascular disease called CADASIL, which stands for cerebral autosomal dominant arteriopathy with subcortical infarcts and leukoencephalopathy. CADASIL is a rare, genetically inherited, congenital vascular disease of the brain that causes strokes, subcortical dementia, migraine-like headaches, and psychiatric disturbances. CADASIL is very debilitating and symptoms usually surface around the age of 45. Although CADASIL can be treated with surgery to repair the defective blood vessels, patients often die by the age of 65. The exact incidence of CADASIL in the United States is unknown.

What Stroke Therapies Are Available?

Physicians have a wide range of therapies to choose from when determining a stroke patient's best therapeutic plan. The type of stroke therapy a patient should receive depends upon the stage of disease. Generally there are three treatment stages for stroke: prevention, therapy immediately after stroke, and poststroke rehabilitation. Therapies to prevent a first or recurrent stroke are based on treating an individual's underlying risk factors for stroke, such as hypertension, atrial fibrillation, and diabetes, or preventing the widespread formation of blood clots that can cause ischemic stroke in everyone, whether or not risk factors are present. Acute stroke therapies try to stop a stroke while it is happening by quickly dissolving a blood clot causing the stroke or by stopping the bleeding of a hemorrhagic stroke. The purpose of poststroke rehabilitation is to overcome disabilities that result from stroke damage.

Therapies for stroke include medications, surgery, or rehabilitation.

Medications

Medication or drug therapy is the most common treatment for stroke. The most popular classes of drugs used to prevent or treat stroke are antithrombotics (antiplatelet agents and anticoagulants) and thrombolytics.

Antithrombotics prevent the formation of blood clots that can become lodged in a cerebral artery and cause strokes. Antiplatelet drugs prevent clotting by decreasing the activity of platelets, blood cells that contribute to the clotting property of blood. These drugs reduce the risk of blood-clot formation, thus reducing the risk of ischemic stroke. In the context of stroke, physicians prescribe antiplatelet drugs mainly for prevention. The most widely known and used antiplatelet drug is aspirin. Other antiplatelet drugs include clopidogrel, ticlopidine, and dipyridamole. The NINDS sponsors a wide range of clinical trials to determine the effectiveness of antiplatelet drugs for stroke prevention.

Anticoagulants reduce stroke risk by reducing the clotting property of the blood. The most commonly used anticoagulants include warfarin (also known as Coumadin®), heparin, and enoxaparin (also known as Lovenox). The NINDS has sponsored several trials to test the efficacy of anticoagulants versus antiplatelet drugs. The Stroke Prevention in Atrial Fibrillation (SPAF) trial found that, although aspirin is an effective therapy for the prevention of a second stroke in most patients with atrial fibrillation, some patients with additional risk factors do better on warfarin therapy. Another study, the Trial of Org 10127 in Acute Stroke Treatment (TOAST), tested the effectiveness of low-molecular weight heparin (Org 10172) in stroke prevention. TOAST showed that heparin anticoagulants are not generally effective in preventing recurrent stroke or improving outcome.

Thrombolytic agents are used to treat an ongoing, acute ischemic stroke caused by an artery blockage. These drugs halt the stroke by dissolving the blood clot that is blocking blood flow to the brain. Recombinant tissue plasminogen activator (rtPA) is a genetically engineered form of tPA, a thrombolytic substance made naturally by the body. It can be effective if given intravenously within 3 hours of stroke symptom onset, but it should be used only after a physician has confirmed that the patient has suffered an ischemic stroke. Thrombolytic agents can increase bleeding and therefore must be used only after careful patient screening. The NINDS rtPA Stroke Study showed the efficacy of tPA and in 1996 led to the first FDA [U.S. Food and Drug Administration]-approved treatment for acute ischemic stroke. Other thrombolytics are currently being tested in clinical trials.

Neuroprotectants are medications that protect the brain from secondary injury caused by stroke. Although no neuroprotectants are FDA-approved for use in stroke at this time, many are in clinical trials. There are several different classes of neuroprotectants that show promise for future therapy, including glutamate antagonists, antioxidants, apoptosis inhibitors, and many others.

Surgery

Surgery can be used to prevent stroke, to treat acute stroke, or to repair vascular damage or malformations in and around the brain. There are two prominent types of surgery for stroke prevention and treatment: carotid endarterectomy and extracranial/intracranial (EC/IC) bypass.

Carotid endarterectomy is a surgical procedure in which a doctor removes fatty deposits (plaque) from the inside of one of the carotid arteries, which are located in the neck and are the main suppliers of blood to the brain. As mentioned earlier, the disease atherosclerosis is characterized by the buildup of plaque on the inside of large arteries, and the blockage of an artery by this fatty material is called stenosis. The NINDS has sponsored two large clinical trials to test the efficacy of carotid endarterectomy: the North American Symptomatic Carotid Endarterectomy Trial (NASCET) and the Asymptomatic Carotid Atherosclerosis Trial (ACAS). These trials showed that carotid endarterectomy is a safe and effective stroke prevention therapy for most people with greater than 50 percent stenosis of the carotid arteries when performed by a qualified and experienced neurosurgeon or vascular surgeon.

Currently, the NINDS is sponsoring the Carotid Revascularization Endarterectomy vs. Stenting Trial (CREST), a large clinical trial designed to test the effectiveness of carotid endarterectomy versus a newer surgical procedure for carotid stenosis called stenting. The procedure involves inserting a long, thin catheter tube into an artery in the leg and threading the catheter through the vascular system into the narrow stenosis of the carotid artery in the neck. Once the catheter is in place in the carotid artery, the radiologist expands the stent with a balloon on the tip of the catheter. The CREST trial will test the effectiveness of the new surgical technique versus the established standard technique of carotid endarterectomy surgery.

EC/IC bypass surgery is a procedure that restores blood flow to a blood-deprived area of brain tissue by rerouting a healthy artery in the scalp to the area of brain tissue affected by a blocked artery. The NINDS-sponsored EC/IC Bypass Study tested the ability of this surgery to prevent recurrent strokes in stroke patients with atherosclerosis. The study showed that, in the long run, EC/IC does not seem to benefit these patients. The surgery is still performed occasionally for patients with aneurysms, some types of small artery disease, and certain vascular abnormalities.

One useful surgical procedure for treatment of brain aneurysms that cause subarachnoid hemorrhage is a technique called "clipping." Clipping involves clamping off the aneurysm from the blood vessel, which reduces the chance that it will burst and bleed.

A new therapy that is gaining wide attention is the detachable coil technique for the treatment of high-risk intracranial aneurysms. A small platinum coil is inserted through an artery in the thigh and threaded through the arteries to the site of the aneurysm. The coil is then released into the aneurysm, where it evokes an immune response from the body. The body produces a blood clot inside the aneurysm, strengthening the artery walls and reducing the risk of rupture. Once the aneurysm is stabilized, a neurosurgeon can clip the aneurysm with less risk of hemorrhage and death to the patient.

Table 1.1. Types and Goals of Poststroke Rehabilitation

Type	Goal
Physical Therapy (PT)	Relearn walking, sitting, lying down, switching from one type of movement to another
Occupational Therapy (OT)	Relearn eating, drinking, dressing, bathing, cooking, reading, writing, toileting
Speech Therapy	Relearn language and communications skills, including swallowing
Psychological/Psychiatric Therapy	Alleviate some mental and emotional problems

Rehabilitation Therapy

Stroke is the number one cause of serious adult disability in the United States. Stroke disability is devastating to the stroke patient and family, but therapies are available to help rehabilitate poststroke patients.

For most stroke patients, physical therapy (PT) is the cornerstone of the rehabilitation process. A physical therapist uses training, exercises, and physical manipulation of the stroke patient's body with the intent of restoring movement, balance, and coordination. The aim of PT is to have the stroke patient relearn simple motor activities such as walking, sitting, standing, lying down, and the process of switching from one type of movement to another.

Another type of therapy involving relearning daily activities is occupational therapy (OT). OT also involves exercise and training to help the stroke patient relearn everyday activities such as eating, drinking, dressing, bathing, cooking, reading and writing, and toileting. The goal of OT is to help the patient become independent or semi-independent.

Speech and language problems arise when brain damage occurs in the language centers of the brain. Due to the brain's great ability to learn and change (called brain plasticity), other areas can adapt to take over some of the lost functions. Speech language pathologists help stroke patients relearn language and speaking skills, including swallowing, or learn other forms of communication. Speech therapy is appropriate for any patients with problems understanding speech or written words, or problems forming speech. A speech therapist helps stroke patients help themselves by working to improve language skills, develop alternative ways of communicating, and develop coping skills to deal with the frustration of not being able to communicate fully. With time and patience, a stroke survivor should be able to regain some, and sometimes all, language and speaking abilities.

Many stroke patients require psychological or psychiatric help after a stroke. Psychological problems, such as depression, anxiety, frustration, and anger, are common poststroke disabilities. Talk therapy, along with appropriate medication, can help alleviate some of the mental and emotional problems that result from stroke. Sometimes it is also beneficial for family members of the stroke patient to seek psychological help as well.

What Disabilities Can Result from a Stroke?

Although stroke is a disease of the brain, it can affect the entire body. Some of the disabilities that can result from a stroke include paralysis, cognitive deficits, speech problems, emotional difficulties, daily living problems, and pain.

Paralysis: A common disability that results from stroke is complete paralysis on one side of the body, called hemiplegia. A related disability that is not as debilitating as paralysis is one-sided weakness or hemiparesis. The paralysis or weakness may affect only the face, an arm, or a leg or may affect one entire side of the body and face. A person who suffers a stroke in the left hemisphere of the brain will show right-sided paralysis or paresis. Conversely, a person with a stroke in the right hemisphere of the brain will show deficits on the left side of the body. A stroke patient may have problems with the simplest of daily activities, such as walking, dressing, eating, and using the bathroom. Motor deficits can result from damage to the motor cortex in the frontal lobes of the brain or from damage to the lower parts of the brain, such as the cerebellum, which controls balance and coordination. Some stroke patients also have trouble swallowing, called dysphagia.

Cognitive deficits: Stroke may cause problems with thinking, awareness, attention, learning, judgment, and memory. In some cases of stroke, the patient suffers a "neglect" syndrome. The neglect means that a stroke patient has no knowledge of one side of his or her body,

23

or one side of the visual field, or is unaware of the deficit. A stroke patient may be unaware of his or her surroundings, or may be unaware of the mental deficits that resulted from the stroke.

Language deficits: Stroke victims often have problems understanding or forming speech. A deficit in understanding or forming speech is called aphasia. Aphasia usually occurs along with similar problems in reading or writing. In most people, language problems result from damage to the left hemisphere of the brain. Slurred speech due to weakness or incoordination of the muscles involved in speaking is called dysarthria, and is not a problem with language. Because it can result from any weakness or incoordination of the speech muscles, dysarthria can arise from damage to either side of the brain.

Emotional deficits: A stroke can lead to emotional problems. Stroke patients may have difficulty controlling their emotions or may express inappropriate emotions in certain situations. One common disability that occurs with many stroke patients is depression. Poststroke depression may be more than a general sadness resulting from the stroke incident. It is a clinical behavioral problem that can hamper recovery and rehabilitation and may even lead to suicide. Poststroke depression is treated as any depression is treated, with antidepressant medications and therapy.

Pain: Stroke patients may experience pain, uncomfortable numbness, or strange sensations after a stroke. These sensations may be due to many factors including damage to the sensory regions of the brain, stiff joints, or a disabled limb. An uncommon type of pain resulting from stroke is called central stroke pain or central pain syndrome (CPS). CPS results from damage to an area in the mid-brain called the thalamus. The pain is a mixture of sensations, including heat and cold, burning, tingling, numbness, and sharp stabbing and underlying aching pain. The pain is often worse in the extremities—the hands and feet—and is made worse by movement and temperature changes, especially cold temperatures. Unfortunately, since most pain medications provide little relief from these sensations, very few treatments or therapies exist to combat CPS.

What Special Risks Do Women Face?

Some risk factors for stroke apply only to women. Primary among these are pregnancy, childbirth, and menopause. These risk factors are tied to hormonal fluctuations and changes that affect a woman in different stages of life. Research in the past few decades has shown that high-dose oral contraceptives, the kind used in the 1960s and 1970s, can increase the risk of stroke in women. Fortunately, oral contraceptives with high doses of estrogen are no longer used and have been replaced with safer and more effective oral contraceptives with lower doses of estrogen. Some studies have shown the newer low-dose oral contraceptives may not significantly increase the risk of stroke in women.

Other studies have demonstrated that pregnancy and childbirth can put a woman at an increased risk for stroke. Pregnancy increases the risk of stroke as much as three to 13 times. Of course, the risk of stroke in young women of childbearing years is very small to begin with, so a moderate increase in risk during pregnancy is still a relatively small risk. Pregnancy and childbirth cause strokes in approximately eight in 100,000 women. Unfortunately, 25 percent of strokes during pregnancy end in death, and hemorrhagic strokes, although rare, are still the leading cause of maternal death in the United States. Subarachnoid hemorrhage, in particular, causes one to five maternal deaths per 10,000 pregnancies.

A study sponsored by the NINDS showed that the risk of stroke during pregnancy is greatest in the postpartum period—the 6 weeks following childbirth. The risk of ischemic stroke after pregnancy is about nine times higher and the risk of hemorrhagic stroke is more than 28 times higher for postpartum women than for women who are not pregnant or postpartum. The cause is unknown.

In the same way that the hormonal changes during pregnancy and childbirth are associated with increased risk of stroke, hormonal changes at the end of the childbearing years can increase the risk of stroke. Several studies have shown that menopause, the end of a woman's reproductive ability marked by the termination of her menstrual cycle, can increase a woman's risk of stroke. Fortunately, some studies have suggested that hormone replacement therapy can reduce some of the effects of menopause and decrease stroke risk. Currently, the NINDS is sponsoring the Women's Estrogen for Stroke Trial (WEST), a randomized, placebo-controlled, double-blind trial, to determine whether estrogen therapy can reduce the risk of death or recurrent stroke in postmenopausal women who have a history of a recent TIA or non-disabling stroke. The mechanism by which estrogen can prove beneficial to postmenopausal women could include its role in cholesterol control. Studies have shown that estrogen acts to increase levels of HDL while decreasing LDL levels.

Are Children at Risk for Stroke?

The young have several risk factors unique to them. Young people seem to suffer from hemorrhagic strokes more than ischemic strokes, a significant difference from older age groups where ischemic strokes make up the majority of stroke cases. Hemorrhagic strokes represent 20 percent of all strokes in the United States and young people account for many of these.

Clinicians often separate the "young" into two categories: those younger than 15 years of age, and those 15 to 44 years of age. People 15 to 44 years of age are generally considered young adults and have many of the risk factors mentioned above, such as drug use, alcohol abuse, pregnancy, head and neck injuries, heart disease or heart malformations, and infections. Some other causes of stroke in the young are linked to genetic diseases.

Medical complications that can lead to stroke in children include intracranial infection, brain injury, vascular malformations such as moyamoya syndrome, occlusive vascular disease, and genetic disorders such as sickle cell anemia, tuberous sclerosis, and Marfan syndrome.

The symptoms of stroke in children are different from those in adults and young adults. A child experiencing a stroke may have seizures, a sudden loss of speech, a loss of expressive language (including body language and gestures), hemiparesis (weakness on one side of the body), hemiplegia (paralysis on one side of the body), dysarthria (impairment of speech), convulsions, headache, or fever. It is a medical emergency when a child shows any of these symptoms.

In children with stroke the underlying conditions that led to the stroke should be determined and managed to prevent future strokes. For example, a recent clinical study sponsored by the National Heart, Lung, and Blood Institute found that giving blood transfusions to young children with sickle cell anemia greatly reduces the risk of stroke. The Institute even suggests attempting to prevent stroke in high-risk children by giving them blood transfusions before they experience a stroke.

Most children who experience a stroke will do better than most adults after treatment and rehabilitation. This is due in part to the immature brain's great plasticity, the ability to adapt to deficits and injury. Children who experience seizures along with stroke do not recover as well as children who do not have seizures. Some children may experience residual hemiplegia, though most will eventually learn how to walk.

What Research Is Being Done by the NINDS?

The NINDS is the leading supporter of stroke research in the United States and sponsors a wide range of experimental research studies, from investigations of basic biological mechanisms to studies with animal models and clinical trials.

Currently, NINDS researchers are studying the mechanisms of stroke risk factors and the process of brain damage that results from stroke. Some of this brain damage may be secondary to the initial death of brain cells caused by the lack of blood flow to the brain tissue. This secondary wave of brain injury is a result of a toxic reaction to the primary damage and mainly involves the excitatory neurochemical, glutamate. Glutamate in the normal brain functions as a chemical messenger between brain cells, allowing them to communicate. But an excess amount of glutamate in the brain causes too much activity and brain cells quickly "burn out" from too much excitement, releasing more toxic chemicals, such as caspases, cytokines, monocytes, and oxygen-free radicals. These substances poison the chemical environment of surrounding cells, initiating a cascade of degeneration and programmed cell death, called apoptosis. NINDS researchers are studying the mechanisms underlying this secondary insult, which consists mainly of inflammation, toxicity, and a breakdown of the blood vessels that provide blood to the brain. Researchers are also looking for ways to prevent secondary injury to the brain by providing different types of neuroprotection for salvageable cells that prevent inflammation and block some of the toxic chemicals created by dying brain cells. From this research, scientists hope to develop neuroprotective agents to prevent secondary damage.

Basic research has also focused on the genetics of stroke and stroke risk factors. One area of research involving genetics is gene therapy. Gene therapy involves putting a gene for a desired protein in certain cells of the body. The inserted gene will then "program" the cell to produce the desired protein. If enough cells in the right areas produce enough protein, then the protein could be therapeutic. Scientists must find ways to deliver the therapeutic DNA to the appropriate cells and must learn how to deliver enough DNA to enough cells so that the tissues produce a therapeutic amount of protein. Gene therapy is in the very early stages of development and there are many problems to overcome, including learning how to penetrate the highly impermeable blood-brain barrier and how to halt the host's immune reaction to the virus that carries the gene to the cells. Some of the proteins used for stroke therapy could include neuroprotective proteins, anti-inflammatory proteins, and DNA/cellular repair proteins, among others.

The NINDS supports and conducts a wide variety of studies in animals, from genetics research on zebra fish to rehabilitation research on primates. Much of the Institute's animal research involves rodents, specifically mice and rats. For example, one study of hypertension and stroke uses rats that have been bred to be hypertensive and therefore stroke-prone. By studying stroke in rats, scientists hope to get a better picture of what might be happening in human stroke patients. Scientists can also use animal models to test promising therapeutic interventions for stroke. If a therapy proves to be beneficial to animals, then scientists can consider testing the therapy in human subjects.

One promising area of stroke animal research involves hibernation. The dramatic decrease of blood flow to the brain in hibernating animals is extensive—extensive enough that it would kill a non-hibernating animal. During hibernation, an animal's metabolism slows down, body temperature drops, and energy and oxygen requirements of brain cells decrease. If scientists can discover how animals hibernate without experiencing brain damage, then maybe they can discover ways to stop the brain damage associated with decreased blood flow in stroke patients. Other studies are looking at the role of hypothermia, or decreased body temperature, on metabolism and neuroprotection.

Both hibernation and hypothermia have a relationship to hypoxia and edema. Hypoxia, or anoxia, occurs when there is not enough oxygen available for brain cells to function properly. Since brain cells require large amounts of oxygen for energy requirements, they are especially vulnerable to hypoxia. Edema occurs when the chemical balance of brain tissue is disturbed and water or fluids flow into the brain cells, making them swell and burst, releasing their toxic contents into the surrounding tissues. Edema is one cause of general brain tissue swelling and contributes to the secondary injury associated with stroke.

The basic and animal studies discussed above do not involve people and fall under the category of preclinical research; clinical research involves people. One area of investigation that has made the transition from animal models to clinical research is the study of the mechanisms underlying brain plasticity and the neuronal rewiring that occurs after a stroke.

New advances in imaging and rehabilitation have shown that the brain can compensate for function lost as a result of stroke. When cells in an area of the brain responsible for a particular function die after a stroke, the patient becomes unable to perform that function. For example, a stroke patient with an infarct in the area of the brain responsible for facial recognition becomes unable to recognize faces, a syndrome called facial agnosia. But, in time, the person may come to recognize faces again, even though the area of the brain originally programmed to perform that function remains dead. The plasticity of the brain and the rewiring of the neural connections make it possible for one part of the brain to change functions and take up the more important functions of a disabled part. This rewiring of the brain and restoration of function, which the brain tries to do automatically, can be helped with therapy. Scientists are working to develop new and better ways to help the brain repair itself to restore important functions to the stroke patient.

One example of a therapy resulting from this research is the use of transcranial magnetic stimulation (TMS) in stroke rehabilitation. Some evidence suggests that TMS, in which a small magnetic current is delivered to an area of the brain, may possibly increase brain plasticity and speed up recovery of function after a stroke. The TMS device is a small coil which is held outside of the head, over the part of the brain needing stimulation. Currently, several studies at the NINDS are testing whether TMS has any value in increasing motor function and improving functional recovery.

Chapter 2

Strokes Caused by Clots

Chapter Contents

Section 2.1

Ischemic Stroke

What is it?

Ischemic ("is-skeem-ic") stroke occurs when an artery to the brain
is blocked. The brain depends on its arteries to bring fresh blood from
the heart and lungs. The blood carries oxygen and nutrients to the
brain, and takes away carbon dioxide and cellular waste. If an artery
is blocked, the brain cells (neurons) cannot make enough energy and
will eventually stop working. If the artery remains blocked for more
than a few minutes, the brain cells may die. This is why immediate
medical treatment is absolutely critical.

What causes it?

Ischemic stroke can be caused by several different kinds of diseases.
The most common problem is narrowing of the arteries in the neck
or head. This is most often caused by atherosclerosis, or gradual cholesterol deposition. If the arteries become too narrow, blood cells may
collect and form blood clots. These blood clots can block the artery
where they are formed (thrombosis), or can dislodge and become
trapped in arteries closer to the brain (embolism). Another cause of
stroke is blood clots in the heart, which can occur as a result of irregular heartbeat (for example, atrial fibrillation), heart attack, or
abnormalities of the heart valves. While these are the most common
causes of ischemic stroke, there are many other possible causes. Examples include use of street drugs, traumatic injury to the blood vessels of the neck, or disorders of blood clotting.

Are there different kinds of ischemic stroke?

Yes. Ischemic stroke can further be divided into two main types:
thrombotic and embolic.

A thrombotic stroke occurs when diseased or damaged cerebral arteries become blocked by the formation of a blood clot within the brain. Clinically referred to as cerebral thrombosis or cerebral infarction, this type of event is responsible for almost 50% of all strokes. Cerebral thrombosis can also be divided into an additional two categories that correlate to the location of the blockage within the brain: large-vessel thrombosis and small-vessel thrombosis. Large-vessel thrombosis is the term used when the blockage is in one of the brain's larger blood-supplying arteries such as the carotid or middle cerebral, while small-vessel thrombosis involves one (or more) of the brain's smaller, yet deeper penetrating arteries. This latter type of stroke is also called a lacunar stroke.

An embolic stroke is also caused by a clot within an artery, but in this case the clot (or emboli) was formed somewhere other than in the brain itself. Often from the heart, these emboli will travel the bloodstream until they become lodged and can not travel any further. This naturally restricts the flow of blood to the brain and results in almost immediate physical and neurological deficits. Deprived of oxygen and other nutrients, the brain suffers damage as a result of the stroke.

Who gets it?

Ischemic stroke is by far the most common kind of stroke, accounting for about 88% of all strokes. Stroke can affect people of all ages, including children. Many people with ischemic strokes are older (60 or more years old), and the risk of stroke increases with older ages. At each age, stroke is more common in men than women, and it is more common among African Americans than white Americans. Many people with stroke have other problems or conditions which put them at higher risk for stroke, such as high blood pressure (hypertension), heart disease, smoking, or diabetes.

Section 2.2

Transient Ischemic Attack (Mini Strokes)

From "Transient Ischemic Attack Information Page," by the National Institute of Neurological Disorders and Stroke (NINDS, www.ninds.nih.gov), part of the National Institutes of Health, October 2, 2007.

What is transient ischemic attack?

A transient ischemic attack (TIA) is a transient stroke that lasts only a few minutes. It occurs when the blood supply to part of the brain is briefly interrupted. TIA symptoms, which usually occur suddenly, are similar to those of stroke but do not last as long. Most symptoms of a TIA disappear within an hour, although they may persist for up to 24 hours. Symptoms can include: numbness or weakness in the face, arm, or leg, especially on one side of the body; confusion or difficulty in talking or understanding speech; trouble seeing in one or both eyes; and difficulty with walking, dizziness, or loss of balance and coordination.

Is there any treatment?

Because there is no way to tell whether symptoms are from a TIA or an acute stroke, patients should assume that all stroke-like symptoms signal an emergency and should not wait to see if they go away. A prompt evaluation (within 60 minutes) is necessary to identify the cause of the TIA and determine appropriate therapy. Depending on a patient's medical history and the results of a medical examination, the doctor may recommend drug therapy or surgery to reduce the risk of stroke in people who have had a TIA. The use of antiplatelet agents, particularly aspirin, is a standard treatment for patients at risk for stroke. People with atrial fibrillation (irregular beating of the heart) may be prescribed anticoagulants.

What is the prognosis?

TIAs are often warning signs that a person is at risk for a more serious and debilitating stroke. About one third of those who have a TIA will have an acute stroke some time in the future. Many strokes can be prevented by heeding the warning signs of TIAs and treating underlying risk factors. The most important treatable factors linked to TIAs and stroke are high blood pressure, cigarette smoking, heart disease, carotid artery disease, diabetes, and heavy use of alcohol. Medical help is available to reduce and eliminate these factors. Lifestyle changes such as eating a balanced diet, maintaining healthy weight, exercising, and enrolling in smoking and alcohol cessation programs can also reduce these factors.

What research is being done?

NINDS is the leading supporter of research on stroke and TIA in the United States and sponsors studies ranging from clinical trials to investigations of basic biological mechanisms as well as studies with animals.

Chapter 3

Strokes Caused by Ruptured Blood Vessels

Chapter Contents

Section 3.1

Brain Aneurysms

From "Aneurysm," by the National Heart, Lung, and
Blood Institute (NHLBI, www.nhlbi.nih.gov), part of the
National Institutes of Health, August 2006.

What Is an Aneurysm?

An aneurysm is an abnormal bulge or "ballooning" in the wall of
an artery. Arteries are blood vessels that carry oxygen-rich blood from
the heart to other parts of the body. An aneurysm that grows and becomes large enough can burst, causing dangerous, often fatal, bleeding inside the body.

Most aneurysms occur in the aorta. The aorta is the main artery
that carries blood from the heart to the rest of the body. The aorta
comes out from the left ventricle of the heart and travels through
the chest and abdomen. An aneurysm that occurs in the aorta in
the chest is called a thoracic aortic aneurysm. An aneurysm that
occurs in the aorta in the abdomen is called an abdominal aortic
aneurysm.

Aneurysms also can occur in arteries in the brain, heart, intestine,
neck, spleen, back of the knees and thighs, and in other parts of the
body. If an aneurysm in the brain bursts, it causes a stroke.

About 15,000 Americans die each year from ruptured aortic aneurysms. Ruptured aortic aneurysm is the 10th leading cause of death
in men over age 50 in the United States.

Many cases of ruptured aneurysm can be prevented with early diagnosis and medical treatment. Because aneurysms can develop and
become large before causing any symptoms, it is important to look for
them in people who are at the highest risk. Experts recommend that
men who are 65 to 75 years old and have ever smoked (at least 100
cigarettes in their lifetime) should be checked for abdominal aortic
aneurysms.

When found in time, aneurysms can usually be treated successfully with medicines or surgery. If an aortic aneurysm is found, the

doctor may prescribe medicine to reduce the heart rate and blood pressure. This can reduce the risk of rupture.

Large aortic aneurysms, if found in time, can often be repaired with surgery to replace the diseased portion of the aorta. The outlook is usually excellent.

Types of Aneurysm

Types of aneurysm include aortic aneurysms, cerebral aneurysms, and peripheral aneurysms.

Aortic Aneurysm

Most aneurysms occur in the aorta. The aorta is the main artery that carries blood from the heart to the rest of the body. The aorta comes out from the left ventricle of the heart and travels through the chest and abdomen. The two types of aortic aneurysm are thoracic aortic aneurysm (TAA) and abdominal aortic aneurysm (AAA).

Thoracic Aortic Aneurysm

An aortic aneurysm that occurs in the part of the aorta running through the thorax (chest) is a thoracic aortic aneurysm. One in four aortic aneurysms is a TAA.

Most TAAs do not produce symptoms, even when they are large. Only half of all people with TAAs notice any symptoms. TAAs are identified more often now than in the past because of chest computed tomography (CT) scans performed for other medical problems.

In a common type of TAA, the walls of the aorta become weak and a section nearest to the heart enlarges. Then the valve between the heart and the aorta cannot close properly and blood leaks backward into the heart. Less commonly, a TAA can develop in the upper back away from the heart. A TAA in this location can result from an injury to the chest such as from an auto crash.

Abdominal Aortic Aneurysm

An aortic aneurysm that occurs in the part of the aorta running through the abdomen is an abdominal aortic aneurysm. Three in four aortic aneurysms are AAAs.

An AAA can grow very large without producing symptoms. About 1 in 5 AAAs rupture.

Cerebral Aneurysm

Aneurysms that occur in an artery in the brain are called cerebral aneurysms. They are sometimes called berry aneurysms because they are often the size of a small berry. Most cerebral aneurysms produce no symptoms until they become large, begin to leak blood, or rupture.

A ruptured cerebral aneurysm causes a stroke. Signs and symptoms can include a sudden, extremely severe headache, nausea, vomiting, stiff neck, sudden weakness in an area of the body, sudden difficulty speaking, and even loss of consciousness, coma, or death. The danger of a cerebral aneurysm depends on its size and location in the brain, whether it leaks or ruptures, and the person's age and overall health.

Peripheral Aneurysm

Aneurysms that occur in arteries other than the aorta (and not in the brain) are called peripheral aneurysms. Common locations for peripheral aneurysms include the artery that runs down the back of the thigh behind the knee (popliteal artery), the main artery in the groin (femoral artery), and the main artery in the neck (carotid artery).

Peripheral aneurysms are not as likely to rupture as aortic aneurysms, but blood clots can form in peripheral aneurysms. If a blood clot breaks away from the aneurysm, it can block blood flow through the artery. If a peripheral aneurysm is large, it can press on a nearby nerve or vein and cause pain, numbness, or swelling.

Other Names for Aneurysm

- Aortic aneurysm
- Abdominal aortic aneurysm, or AAA
- Thoracic aortic aneurysm, or TAA
- Cerebral aneurysm
- Peripheral aneurysm

What Causes an Aneurysm?

An aneurysm can result from atherosclerosis (hardening and narrowing of the inside of arteries). As atherosclerosis develops, the artery walls become thick and damaged and lose their normal inner lining. This damaged area of artery can stretch or "balloon" from the pressure of blood flow inside the artery, resulting in an aneurysm.

An aneurysm also can develop from constant high blood pressure inside an artery.

A thoracic aortic aneurysm can result from an injury to the chest (for example, an injury that occurs from an auto crash). Certain medical conditions, such as Marfan syndrome, that weaken the body's connective tissues, also can cause aneurysms.

In rare cases, infections such as untreated syphilis (a sexually transmitted infection) can cause aortic aneurysms. Aortic aneurysms also can occur as a result of diseases that cause inflammation of blood vessels, such as vasculitis.

Who Is at Risk for an Aneurysm?

Populations Affected

Men are 5 to 10 times more likely than women to have an abdominal aortic aneurysm (AAA)—the most common type of aneurysm.

The risk of AAA increases as you get older, and it is more likely to occur in people between the ages of 60 to 80. A peripheral aneurysm also is more likely to affect people ages 60 to 80. Cerebral (brain) aneurysms, though rare, are more likely to occur in people ages 35 to 60.

Risk Factors

Factors that increase your risk for aneurysm include:

- Atherosclerosis, a buildup of fatty deposits in the arteries.

- Smoking. You are eight times more likely to develop an aneurysm if you smoke.

- Overweight or obesity.

- A family history of aortic aneurysm, heart disease, or other diseases of the arteries.

- Certain diseases that can weaken the wall of the aorta, such as:

  - Marfan syndrome (an inherited disease in which tissues don't develop normally)

  - Untreated syphilis (a very rare cause today)

  - Tuberculosis (also a very rare cause today)

- Trauma such as a blow to the chest in a car accident.

41

- Severe and persistent high blood pressure between the ages of 35 and 60. This increases the risk for a cerebral aneurysm.

- Use of stimulant drugs such as cocaine.

What Are the Signs and Symptoms of an Aneurysm?

The signs and symptoms of an aneurysm depend on its type, location, and whether it has ruptured or is interfering with other structures in the body. Aneurysms can develop and grow for years without causing any signs or symptoms. It is often not until an aneurysm ruptures or grows large enough to press on nearby parts of the body or block blood flow that it produces any signs or symptoms.

Abdominal Aortic Aneurysm

Most abdominal aortic aneurysms (AAAs) develop slowly over years and have no signs or symptoms until (or if) they rupture. Sometimes, a doctor can feel a pulsating mass while examining a patient's abdomen. When symptoms are present, they can include:

- Deep penetrating pain in your back or the side of your abdomen

- Steady gnawing pain in your abdomen that lasts for hours or days at a time

- Coldness, numbness, or tingling in your feet due to blocked blood flow in your legs

If an AAA ruptures, symptoms can include sudden, severe pain in your lower abdomen and back; nausea and vomiting; clammy, sweaty skin; lightheadedness; and a rapid heart rate when standing up. Internal bleeding from a ruptured AAA can send you into shock. Shock is a life-threatening condition in which the organs of the body do not get enough blood flow.

Thoracic Aortic Aneurysm

A thoracic (chest) aortic aneurysm may have no symptoms until the aneurysm begins to leak or grow. Signs or symptoms may include:

- pain in your jaw, neck, upper back (or other part of your back), or chest; or

- coughing, hoarseness, or trouble breathing.

Cerebral Aneurysm

If a cerebral (brain) aneurysm presses on nerves in your brain, it can cause signs and symptoms. These can include:

- a droopy eyelid;
- double vision or other changes in vision;
- pain above or behind the eye;
- a dilated pupil; and
- numbness or weakness on one side of the face or body.

If a cerebral aneurysm ruptures, symptoms can include a sudden, severe headache, nausea and vomiting, stiff neck, loss of consciousness, and signs of a stroke. Signs of a stroke are similar to those listed above for cerebral aneurysm, but they usually come on suddenly and are more severe. Any of these symptoms require immediate medical attention.

Peripheral Aneurysm

Signs and symptoms of peripheral aneurysm may include:

- a pulsating lump that can be felt in your neck, arm, or leg;
- leg or arm pain, or cramping with exercise;
- painful sores on toes or fingers; and
- gangrene (tissue death) from severely blocked blood flow in your limbs.

An aneurysm in the popliteal artery (behind the knee) can compress nerves and cause pain, weakness, and numbness in your knee and leg.

Blood clots can form in peripheral aneurysms. If a clot breaks loose and travels through the bloodstream, it can lodge in your arm, leg, or brain and block the artery. An aneurysm in your neck can block the artery to the brain and cause a stroke.

How Is an Aneurysm Diagnosed?

An aneurysm may be found by chance during a routine physical exam. More often, an aneurysm is found by chance during an x-ray, ultrasound, or computed tomography (CT) scan performed for another reason, such as chest or abdominal pain.

If you have an abdominal aortic aneurysm (AAA), the doctor may feel a pulsating mass in your abdomen. A rapidly growing aneurysm about to rupture can be tender and very painful when pressed. If you are overweight or obese, it may be difficult for your doctor to feel even a large abdominal aneurysm.

If you have an AAA, your doctor may hear rushing blood flow instead of the normal whooshing sound when listening to your abdomen with a stethoscope.

Specialists Involved

You may be referred to a cardiothoracic surgeon, vascular surgeon, or neurosurgeon for diagnosis and treatment of an aneurysm. A cardiothoracic surgeon performs surgery on the heart, lungs, and other organs and structures in the chest, including the aorta. A vascular surgeon performs surgery on the abdominal aorta and on the peripheral arteries. A neurosurgeon performs surgery on the brain, including the arteries in the head, and on the spine and nerves.

Diagnostic Tests and Procedures

To diagnose and evaluate an aneurysm, one or more of the following tests or procedures may be performed:

- **Chest x ray.** A chest x-ray provides a picture of the organs and structures inside the chest, including the heart, lungs, and blood vessels.

- **Ultrasound.** This simple and painless test uses sound waves to create a picture of the inside of the body. It shows the size of an aneurysm, if one is detected. The ultrasound scan may be repeated every few months to see how quickly an aneurysm is growing.

- **CT scan.** A CT scan provides computer-generated, x-ray images of the internal organs. A CT scan may be performed if the doctor suspects a TAA or AAA. A liquid dye that can be seen on an x-ray is injected into an arm vein to outline the aorta or artery on the CT scan. The CT scan images can be used to determine the size and shape of an abdominal aneurysm more accurately than an ultrasound.

- **MRI.** MRI uses magnets and radio waves to create images of the inside of the body. It is very accurate in detecting aneurysms and determining their size and exact location.

- **Angiography.** Angiography also uses a special dye injected into the bloodstream to make the insides of arteries show up on x-ray pictures. An angiogram shows the amount of damage and blockage in blood vessels.

- **Aortogram.** An aortogram is an angiogram of the aorta. It may show the location and size of an aortic aneurysm, and the arteries of the aorta that are involved.

How Is an Aneurysm Treated?

Goals of Treatment

Some aneurysms, mainly small ones that are not causing pain, can be treated with "watchful waiting." Others need to be treated to prevent growth and complications. The goals of treatment are to prevent the aneurysm from growing, prevent or reverse damage to other body structures, prevent or treat a rupture, and to allow you to continue to participate in normal daily activities.

Treatment Options

Medicine and surgery are the two types of treatment for an aneurysm. Medicines may be prescribed before surgery or instead of surgery. Medicines are used to reduce pressure, relax blood vessels, and reduce the risk of rupture. Beta blockers and calcium channel blockers are the medicines most commonly used.

Surgery may be recommended if an aneurysm is large and likely to rupture.

Treatment by Type of Aneurysm

Aortic Aneurysm

Experts recommend that men who have ever smoked (at least 100 cigarettes in their lifetime) and are between the ages of 65 and 75 should have an ultrasound screening to check for abdominal aortic aneurysms.

Treatment recommendations for aortic aneurysms are based on the size of the aneurysm. Small aneurysms found early can be treated with "watchful waiting."

- If the diameter of the aorta is small—less than 3 centimeters (cm)—and there are no symptoms, "watchful waiting" and a followup screening in 5 to 10 years may be all that is needed, as determined by the doctor.

- If the aorta is between 3 and 4 cm in diameter, the patient should return to the doctor every year for an ultrasound to see if the aneurysm has grown.

- If the aorta is between 4 and 4.5 cm, testing should be repeated every 6 months.

- If the aorta is larger than 5 cm (2 inches around or about the size of a lemon) or growing more than 1 cm per year, surgery should be considered as soon as possible.

Two main types of surgery to repair aortic aneurysms are open abdominal or open chest repair and endovascular repair.

The traditional and most common type of surgery for aortic aneurysms is open abdominal or open chest repair. It involves a major incision in the abdomen or chest. General anesthesia is needed with this procedure.

The aneurysm is removed and the section of aorta is replaced with an artificial graft made of material such as Dacron® or Teflon®. The surgery takes 3 to 6 hours, and the patient remains in the hospital for 5 to 8 days. It often takes a month to recover from open abdominal or open chest surgery and return to full activity. Open abdominal and chest surgeries have been performed for 50 years. More than 90 percent of patients make a full recovery.

In endovascular repair, the aneurysm is not removed, but a graft is inserted into the aorta to strengthen it. This type of surgery is performed through catheters (tubes) inserted into the arteries; it does not require surgically opening the chest or abdomen.

To perform endovascular repair, the doctor first inserts a catheter into an artery in the groin (upper thigh) and threads it up to the area of the aneurysm. Then, watching on x-ray, the surgeon threads the graft (also called a stent graft) into the aorta to the aneurysm. The graft is then expanded inside the aorta and fastened in place to form a stable channel for blood flow. The graft reinforces the weakened section of the aorta to prevent the aneurysm from rupturing.

Endovascular repair surgery reduces recovery time to a few days and greatly reduces time in the hospital. The procedure has been used since 1999. Not all aortic aneurysms can be repaired with this procedure. The exact location or size of the aneurysm may prevent the stent graft from being safely or reliably positioned inside the aneurysm.

Cerebral Aneurysm

Treatment for cerebral (brain) aneurysms depends on the size and location of the aneurysm, whether it is infected, and whether it has ruptured. A small cerebral aneurysm that hasn't burst may not need treatment. A large cerebral aneurysm may press against brain tissue, causing a severe headache or impaired vision, and is likely to burst. If the aneurysm ruptures, there will be bleeding into the brain which will cause a stroke. If a cerebral aneurysm becomes infected, it requires immediate medical treatment. Treatment of many cerebral aneurysms, especially large or growing ones, involves surgery, which can be risky depending on the location of the aneurysm.

Peripheral Aneurysm

Most peripheral aneurysms have no symptoms, especially if they are small. They seldom rupture.

Treatment of peripheral aneurysms depends on the presence of symptoms, the location of the aneurysm, and whether the blood flow through the artery is blocked. Blood clots can form in a peripheral aneurysm, break loose, and block the artery.

An aneurysm in the back of the knee that is larger than 1 inch in diameter usually requires surgery. An aneurysm in the thigh also is usually repaired with surgery.

How Can an Aneurysm Be Prevented?

The best way to prevent an aneurysm is to avoid the risk factors that increase the changes of developing one. To do this, you can:

- Quit smoking.
- Eat a low-fat, low-cholesterol diet to reduce the buildup of plaque in the arteries. Plaque is a fatty buildup that narrows the arteries.
- Control high blood pressure (eating a low-salt diet helps).
- Control high cholesterol.
- Get regular physical activity.

Section 3.2

Intracerebral Hemorrhage

What is it?

Intracerebral hemorrhage occurs when a diseased blood vessel within the brain bursts, allowing blood to leak inside the brain. (The name means within the cerebrum, or brain). The sudden increase in pressure within the brain can cause damage to the brain cells surrounding the blood. If the amount of blood increases rapidly, the sudden buildup in pressure can lead to unconsciousness or death. Intracerebral hemorrhage usually occurs in selected parts of the brain, including the basal ganglia, cerebellum, brainstem, or cortex.

What causes it?

The most common cause of intracerebral hemorrhage is high blood pressure (hypertension). Since high blood pressure by itself often causes no symptoms, many people with intracranial hemorrhage are not aware that they have high blood pressure, or that it needs to be treated. Less common causes of intracerebral hemorrhage include trauma, infections, tumors, blood clotting deficiencies, and abnormalities in blood vessels (such as arteriovenous malformations). A ruptured blood vessel will leak blood into the brain, eventually causing the brain to compress due to the added amount of fluid.

Who gets it?

Intracerebral hemorrhage occurs at all ages. The average age is lower than for ischemic stroke. Less common than ischemic strokes, hemorrhagic strokes make up about 12% of all strokes.

Section 3.3

Subarachnoid Hemorrhage

"Subarachnoid Hemorrhage," © 2007 Internet Stroke Center at Washington University in St. Louis. Reprinted with permission.

What is it?

Subarachnoid hemorrhage occurs when a blood vessel just outside the brain ruptures. The area of the skull surrounding the brain (the subarachnoid space) rapidly fills with blood. A patient with subarachnoid hemorrhage may have a sudden, intense headache, neck pain, and nausea or vomiting. Sometimes this is described as the worst headache of one's life. The sudden buildup of pressure outside the brain may also cause rapid loss of consciousness or death.

What causes it?

Subarachnoid hemorrhage is most often caused by abnormalities of the arteries at the base of the brain, called cerebral aneurysms. These are small areas of rounded or irregular swellings in the arteries. Where the swelling is most severe, the blood vessel wall becomes weak and prone to rupture.

Who gets it?

The cause of cerebral aneurysms is not known. They may develop from birth or in childhood and grow very slowly. Some people have not one, but several aneurysms. Subarachnoid hemorrhage can occur at any age, including in teenagers and young adults. Subarachnoid hemorrhage is slightly more common in women than men.

49

Chapter 4

Strokes Caused by Carotid Dissection

Definition

A stroke secondary to carotid dissection is a type of stroke due to a tear in the lining of a major neck artery, called the carotid artery.

Causes

A stroke is an interruption of the blood supply to any part of the brain. When a tear in the lining of the carotid artery occurs (carotid dissection), blood flows in between layers of the blood vessel. This causes narrowing of the vessel, which makes it hard for blood to travel properly.

Stroke secondary to carotid dissection, unlike many other forms of stroke, may occur in young people, usually under 40 years old. Dissection accounts for less than 5% of strokes.

The risks for stroke secondary to carotid dissection include a history of disorders that cause weakness of the blood vessels, such as Marfan syndrome and fibromuscular dysplasia. Injury to the neck and certain medical procedures involving the carotid artery (such as an arteriogram) also raises your risk.

Symptoms

* Pain in the neck, which may travel to the eye

- Pulsing in the ears (pulsatile tinnitus)
- Weakness or total inability to move a body part
- Numbness, loss of sensation, or tingling
- Horner's syndrome
  - Eyelid drooping (ptosis)
  - Abnormal pupils
  - Abnormal facial sweating
- Trouble seeing, may occur in one or both eyes
- Problems talking or understanding speech
- Inability to recognize or identify sensory stimuli (agnosia)
- Loss of memory
- Vertigo (abnormal sensation of movement)
- Loss of coordination
- Swallowing difficulties
- Personality changes
- Mood and emotion changes
- Change in consciousness such as sleepiness, stupor, or lethargy
- Loss of consciousness
- Coma

Exams and Tests

A complete physical and neurological exam should be performed. This includes testing of all neurological functions, including vision, ability to feel sensations, movement, and mental function. The exam may reveal problems with vision, movement, sensation, reflexes, and speaking. The signs depend on how much blood flow is blocked at the time of the exam.

The doctor may hear an abnormal sound called a bruit when placing a stethoscope over the neck arteries. Blood pressure may be high. Some patients show signs of Horner's syndrome, such as drooping of one eyelid, lack of sweating on one side of the forehead, and a sunken appearance to one eye.

Tests may include:

- MRI or CT of the head
- Cerebral angiography
- MRA or a vascular ultrasound
- Blood tests to check for problems with connective tissue or certain genes

Treatment

Stroke is a serious condition. The sooner treatment is received, the better the person will do, and the lower the chance of permanent disability or death.

Treatment depends on the severity of symptoms.

Medicine may be needed to control high blood pressure. Blood thinning drugs, such as Coumadin or aspirin, may be needed for 3 to 6 months. Surgery to repair the carotid dissection may be required. Other therapies may be needed if there are any underlying disorders of the blood vessels.

Outlook (Prognosis)

The outcome for stroke secondary to carotid dissection may be better than for stroke from many other causes, especially if the dissection is discovered and treated promptly.

When to Contact a Medical Professional

Stroke is a medical emergency. Immediately go to the emergency room or call the local emergency number (911 in the United States) if signs of a stroke occur.

Prevention

Care should be taken to protect the neck from injury, especially if you have any conditions that increase your risk for this type of stroke. Wearing seat belts while riding in a vehicle and helmets for various activities may somewhat reduce the risk for a stroke secondary to carotid dissection.

Aspirin therapy (81 mg a day or 100 mg every other day) is now recommended for stroke prevention in women under 65 as long as the benefits outweigh the risks. It should be considered for women over age 65 only if their blood pressure is controlled and the benefit is greater than the risk of gastrointestinal bleeding and brain hemorrhage.

Chapter 5

Other Types of Stroke

Chapter Contents

Section 5.1

Spinal Cord Infarction: A Stroke in the Spine

"Spinal Cord Infarction Information Page" is from the National Institute of Neurological Disorders and Stroke (NINDS, www.ninds.nih.gov), part of the National Institutes of Health, September 11, 2007.

What is spinal cord infarction?

Spinal cord infarction is a stroke either within the spinal cord or the arteries that supply it. It is caused by arteriosclerosis or a thickening or closing of the major arteries to the spinal cord. Frequently spinal cord infarction is caused by a specific form of arteriosclerosis called atheromatosis, in which a deposit or accumulation of lipid-containing matter forms within the arteries.

Symptoms, which generally appear within minutes or a few hours of the infarction, may include intermittent sharp or burning back pain, aching pain down through the legs, weakness in the legs, paralysis, loss of deep tendon reflexes, loss of pain and temperature sensation, and incontinence.

Is there any treatment?

Treatment is symptomatic. Physical and occupational therapy may help individuals recover from weakness or paralysis. A catheter may be necessary for patients with urinary incontinence.

What is the prognosis?

Recovery depends upon how quickly treatment is received and how severely the body is compromised. Paralysis may persist for many weeks or be permanent. Most individuals have a good chance of recovery.

What research is being done?

NINDS conducts and supports research on disorders of the spinal cord such as spinal cord infarction, aimed at learning more about these disorders and finding ways to prevent and treat them.

Section 5.2

Wallenberg Syndrome

"Wallenberg's Syndrome Information Page" is from the National Institute of Neurological Disorders and Stroke (NINDS, www.ninds.nih.gov), part of the National Institutes of Health, February 15, 2007.

What is Wallenberg syndrome?

Wallenberg syndrome is a neurological condition caused by a stroke in the vertebral or posterior inferior cerebellar artery of the brain stem. Symptoms include difficulties with swallowing, hoarseness, dizziness, nausea and vomiting, rapid involuntary movements of the eyes (nystagmus), and problems with balance and gait coordination. Some individuals will experience a lack of pain and temperature sensation on only one side of the face, or a pattern of symptoms on opposite sides of the body—such as paralysis or numbness in the right side of the face, with weak or numb limbs on the left side. Uncontrollable hiccups may also occur, and some individuals will lose their sense of taste on one side of the tongue, while preserving taste sensations on the other side. Some people with Wallenberg syndrome report that the world seems to be tilted in an unsettling way, which makes it difficult to keep their balance when they walk.

Is there any treatment?

Treatment for Wallenberg syndrome is symptomatic. A feeding tube may be necessary if swallowing is very difficult. Speech/swallowing therapy may be beneficial. In some cases, medication may be used to reduce or eliminate pain.

Some doctors report that the antiepileptic drug gabapentin appears to be an effective medication for individuals with chronic pain.

What is the prognosis?

The outlook for someone with Wallenberg syndrome depends upon the size and location of the area of the brain stem damaged by the stroke. Some individuals may see a decrease in their symptoms within weeks or months. Others may be left with significant neurological disabilities for years after the initial symptoms appeared.

What research is being done?

The National Institute of Neurological Disorders and Stroke (NINDS) conducts research related to Wallenberg syndrome in its laboratories at the National Institutes of Health (NIH), and also supports additional research through grants to major medical institutions across the country. Much of this research focuses on finding better ways to prevent, treat, and ultimately cure disorders such as Wallenberg syndrome.

Chapter 6

The Effects of Stroke

The ability to define the world and our place in it distinguishes our humanity. Stroke or brain attack forever alters this world-making capacity. The stroke patient's world, once comprehensible and manageable, is transformed into a confusing, intimidating and hostile environment. The skills of intellect, sensation, perception and movement, which are honed over the course of a lifetime and which so characterize our humanity are the very abilities most compromised by stroke. Stroke can rob people of the most basic methods of interacting with the world.

The specific abilities that will be lost or affected by stroke depend on the extent of the brain damage and most importantly where in the brain the stroke occurred. The brain is an incredibly complex organ, and each area within the brain has responsibility for a particular function or ability. The brain is divided into four primary parts: the right hemisphere (or half), the left hemisphere, the cerebellum, and the brain stem.

Right-Hemisphere Stroke

The right hemisphere of the brain controls the movement of the left side of the body. It also controls analytical and perceptual tasks, such as judging distance, size, speed, or position and seeing how parts are connected to wholes.

A stroke in the right hemisphere often causes paralysis in the left side of the body. This is known as left hemiplegia. Survivors of right-hemisphere strokes may also have problems with their spatial and perceptual abilities. This may cause them to misjudge distances (leading to a fall) or be unable to guide their hands to pick up an object, button a shirt, or tie their shoes. They may even be unable to tell right-side up from upside-down when trying to read.

Along with their impaired ability to judge spatial relationships, survivors of right-hemisphere strokes often have judgment difficulties that show up in their behavioral styles. These patients often develop an impulsive style unaware of their impairments and certain of their ability to perform the same tasks as before the stroke. This behavioral style can be extremely dangerous. It may lead the left hemiplegic stroke survivor to try to walk without aid. Or it may lead the survivor with spatial and perceptual impairments to try to drive a car.

Survivors of right-hemisphere strokes may also experience left-sided neglect. Stemming from visual field impairments, left-sided neglect causes the survivor of a right-hemisphere stroke to "forget" or "ignore" objects or people on their left side.

Finally, some survivors of right-hemisphere strokes will experience problems with short-term memory. Although they may be able to recount a visit to the seashore that took place 30 years ago, they may be unable to remember what they ate for breakfast that morning.

Left-Hemisphere Stroke

The left hemisphere of the brain controls the movement of the right side of the body. It also controls speech and language abilities for most people. A left-hemisphere stroke often causes paralysis of the right side of the body. This is known as right hemiplegia.

Someone who has had a left-hemisphere stroke may also develop aphasia. Aphasia is a catch-all term used to describe a wide range of speech and language problems. These problems can be highly specific, affecting only one component of the patient's ability to communicate, such as the ability to move their speech-related muscles to talk properly. The same patient may be completely unimpaired when it comes to writing, reading, or understanding speech.

In contrast to survivors of right-hemisphere stroke, patients who have had a left-hemisphere stroke often develop a slow and cautious behavioral style. They may need frequent instruction and feedback to complete tasks.

Finally, patients with left-hemisphere stroke may develop memory problems similar to those of right-hemisphere stroke survivors. These problems can include shortened retention spans, difficulty in learning new information, and problems in conceptualizing and generalizing.

Cerebellar Stroke

The cerebellum controls many of our reflexes and much of our balance and coordination. A stroke that takes place in the cerebellum can cause abnormal reflexes of the head and torso, coordination and balance problems, dizziness, nausea, and vomiting.

Brain Stem Stroke

Strokes that occur in the brain stem are especially devastating. The brain stem is the area of the brain that controls all of our involuntary, "life-support" functions, such as breathing rate, blood pressure, and heartbeat. The brain stem also controls abilities such as eye movements, hearing, speech, and swallowing. Since impulses generated in the brain's hemispheres must travel through the brain stem on their way to the arms and legs, patients with a brain stem stroke may also develop paralysis in one or both sides of the body.

Chapter 7

Stroke: The Scope of the Problem

Chapter Contents

Section 7.1

The Burden of Heart Disease and Stroke in the United States

From "Heart Disease and Stroke: The Scope of the Problem," by the Centers for Disease Control and Prevention (CDC), Division for Heart Disease and Stroke Prevention (www.cdc.gov/dhdsp), January 2007.

We often describe death as untimely when it claims the lives of men, women, and children who die before their time on our highways, or from work-related injuries, overdoses, violent rampages, terrorist acts, or in war. Death from heart disease or stroke is often untimely—and often preventable.

Every 33 seconds, one American dies of some form of heart disease or of stroke. Every day, heart disease or stroke kills more than 2,600 Americans. And every year, these diseases claim the lives of 1.9 million men and women in this nation—a number so high it could fill the Rose Bowl nearly 20 times, Arlington National Cemetery nearly 8 times, and one third of the Pentagon's 6.5 million square feet. That number is nearly twice the number of lives claimed by cancer or collectively by World War II and the Korean and Vietnam conflicts. That number can be reduced, not just by keeping people with heart disease alive longer, but by preventing heart disease in the first place.

Who lives with heart disease or the consequences of stroke in America?

58,800,000 Americans, or 1 in 5 men and women, have one or more types of heart disease or live with the devastating impact of stroke. One in three men can expect to develop heart disease or have a stroke before age 60. For women, the odds are 1 in 10, although more than half of all deaths due to heart disease each year occur among women, and heart disease is the number one cause of death among women in this country. Further, the rate of premature deaths due to heart disease or stroke is greater among blacks than among whites. Heart disease disables and kills and often can strike both women and men in the prime of their lives.

How big is the problem of stroke in the United States?

Stroke is the third leading cause of death in the United States. In 1996, it killed nearly 160,000 individuals—accounting for 7 percent of all deaths in the United States that year. With its devastating effects including partial or full paralysis, stroke is the leading cause of serious, long-term disability. Here are some other facts you should know:

- In the United States, there are more than 4 million stroke survivors, most of whom are either moderately or severely impaired.

- Stroke accounts for more than half the patients hospitalized for acute neurological diseases.

- Stroke is a major factor in late-life dementia that affects more than 40 percent of Americans older than 80.

- The estimated combined cost of health care and lost productivity due to stroke in the United States was estimated at $45.3 billion during 1999 alone.

- The estimated lifetime cost of a mild stroke in an older individual is $100,000. The estimated lifetime cost of a severe stroke in a younger individual is $500,000.

- Stroke risk factors that can be changed or controlled include high blood pressure, diabetes, atrial fibrillation, smoking, high blood cholesterol, obesity, and physical inactivity.

What states carry the highest death rates due to stroke?

- The "Stroke Belt" is usually defined as an 8 to 12 state region (typically including Alabama, Georgia, Mississippi, North Carolina, South Carolina, Kentucky, Tennessee, Florida, Indiana, Arkansas, Louisiana, Virginia, and Washington, D.C.) where stroke death rates are substantially higher than in the rest of the country.

- Within the Stroke Belt, the highest death rates are clustered in the coastal plains regions of Georgia, North Carolina, and South Carolina. This region has been called the "Stroke Buckle."

- The stroke death rate in the Stroke Buckle is 2 times greater than that in the rest of the nation.

- The excess risk of stroke death in the Stroke Buckle impacts men and women, African Americans, and whites.

- The pattern of excess stroke death rates in the Stroke Buckle has existed for at least 50 years.

- The causes of the excess stroke death rates in the Stroke Buckle are not known. Causes that have been suggested include a higher prevalence of stroke risk factors, lack of access to health care, or factors associated with the geography of the region (such as water content).

Section 7.2

Projected Costs of Stroke in the United States Top $2 Trillion

"Projected Costs of Stroke in the United States Top $2 Trillion Dollars," © 2006 American Academy of Neurology (www.aan.com). Reprinted with permission.

Estimated costs of ischemic stroke in the United States in the next half century will exceed $2.2 trillion dollars. The findings are published in the online [August 2006] edition of *Neurology*, the scientific journal of the American Academy of Neurology. The study found the total cost of stroke from 2005–2050, in 2005 dollars, is projected to be $1.52 trillion for non-Hispanic whites, $379 billion for African Americans, and $313 billion for Hispanics.

The estimated per capita cost of stroke is highest in African Americans ($25,782), followed by Hispanics ($17,201), and non-Hispanic whites ($15,597).

"The economic burden of stroke in African Americans and Hispanics will be enormous over the next several decades," said the study's lead author Devin Brown, M.D., of the Stroke Program at the University of Michigan Medical School in Ann Arbor. "Further efforts to improve stroke prevention and treatment in these high stroke risk groups are necessary."

Brown says the ethnic disparities in stroke-related health care are a critical issue since Hispanics and African Americans are less likely to be insured, have limited access to quality health care, and have a higher incidence of ischemic stroke than non-Hispanic whites.

"As these two minority groups age, the impact of inequalities in stroke risk and stroke-related health care will result in mounting economic consequences," she said. "We hope the study's findings help public health planners in prioritizing resources and setting research agendas." In determining cost estimates, researchers considered ambulance services, initial hospitalization, nursing home costs, rehabilitation, outpatient clinic visits, drugs, informal care giving, and potential lost earnings.

Stroke is the third leading cause of death in the United States and the leading cause of adult disability.

The study was supported by the National Institute of Neurological Disorders and Stroke and the National Institutes of Health.

Part Two

Stroke Risk Factors and Prevention

Chapter 8

Do You Know Your Risk of Stroke?

Risk Factors for Stroke

Brain Basics: Preventing Stroke

If you're like most Americans, you plan for your future. When you take a job, you examine its benefit plan. When you buy a home, you consider its location and condition so that your investment is safe. Today, more and more Americans are protecting their most important asset—their health. Are you?

Stroke ranks as the third leading killer in the United States. A stroke can be devastating to individuals and their families, robbing them of their independence. It is the most common cause of adult disability. Each year more than 700,000 Americans have a stroke, with about 160,000 dying from stroke-related causes. Officials at the National Institute of Neurological Disorders and Stroke (NINDS) are committed to reducing that burden through biomedical research.

What Is a Stroke?

A stroke, or "brain attack," occurs when blood circulation to the brain fails. Brain cells can die from decreased blood flow and the resulting

This chapter includes text from "Brain Basics: Preventing Stroke," by the National Institute of Neurological Disorders and Stroke (NINDS, www.ninds.nih.gov), part of the National Institutes of Health, July 20, 2007; and "Stroke Risk Scorecard," Copyright © 2007 National Stroke Association. Reprinted with permission.

lack of oxygen. There are two broad categories of stroke: those caused by a blockage of blood flow and those caused by bleeding. While not usually fatal, a blockage of a blood vessel in the brain or neck, called an ischemic stroke, is the most frequent cause of stroke and is responsible for about 80 percent of strokes. These blockages stem from three conditions: the formation of a clot within a blood vessel of the brain or neck, called thrombosis; the movement of a clot from another part of the body such as the heart to the neck or brain, called embolism; or a severe narrowing of an artery in or leading to the brain, called stenosis. Bleeding into the brain or the spaces surrounding the brain causes the second type of stroke, called hemorrhagic stroke.

Two key steps you can take will lower your risk of death or disability from stroke: know stroke's warning signs and control stroke's risk factors. Scientific research conducted by the NINDS has identified warning signs and a large number of risk factors.

What Are Warning Signs of a Stroke?

Warning signs are clues your body sends that your brain is not receiving enough oxygen. If you observe one or more of these signs of a stroke or "brain attack," don't wait, call a doctor or 911 right away!

- Sudden numbness or weakness of face, arm or leg, especially on one side of the body
- Sudden confusion, trouble speaking, or understanding
- Sudden trouble seeing in one or both eyes
- Sudden trouble walking, dizziness, loss of balance or coordination
- Sudden severe headache with no known cause

Other danger signs that may occur include double vision, drowsiness, and nausea or vomiting. Sometimes the warning signs may last only a few moments and then disappear. These brief episodes, known as transient ischemic attacks or TIAs, are sometimes called "mini-strokes." Although brief, they identify an underlying serious condition that isn't going away without medical help. Unfortunately, since they clear up, many people ignore them. Don't. Heeding them can save your life.

What Are Risk Factors for a Stroke?

A risk factor is a condition or behavior that occurs more frequently in those who have, or are at greater risk of getting, a disease than in those who don't. Having a risk factor for stroke doesn't mean you'll have a stroke. On the other hand, not having a risk factor doesn't mean you'll avoid a stroke. But your risk of stroke grows as the number and severity of risk factors increases.

Stroke occurs in all age groups, in both sexes, and in all races in every country. It can even occur before birth, when the fetus is still in the womb. In African Americans, stroke is more common and more deadly—even in young and middle-aged adults—than for any ethnic or other racial group in the United States. Scientists have found more and more severe risk factors in some minority groups and continue to look for patterns of stroke in these groups.

What Are the Treatable Risk Factors?

Some of the most important treatable risk factors for stroke are:

- **High blood pressure.** Also called hypertension, this is by far the most potent risk factor for stroke. If your blood pressure is high, you and your doctor need to work out an individual strategy to bring it down to the normal range. Some ways that work: Maintain proper weight. Avoid drugs known to raise blood pressure. Cut down on salt. Eat fruits and vegetables to increase potassium in your diet. Exercise more. Your doctor may prescribe medicines that help lower blood pressure. Controlling blood pressure will also help you avoid heart disease, diabetes, and kidney failure.

- **Cigarette smoking.** Cigarette smoking has been linked to the buildup of fatty substances in the carotid artery, the main neck artery supplying blood to the brain. Blockage of this artery is the leading cause of stroke in Americans. Also, nicotine raises blood pressure; carbon monoxide reduces the amount of oxygen your blood can carry to the brain; and cigarette smoke makes your blood thicker and more likely to clot. Your doctor can recommend programs and medications that may help you quit smoking. By quitting, at any age, you also reduce your risk of lung disease, heart disease, and a number of cancers including lung cancer.

- **Heart disease.** Common heart disorders such as coronary artery disease, valve defects, irregular heart beat, and enlargement of one of the heart's chambers can result in blood clots that may break loose and block vessels in or leading to the brain. The most common blood vessel disease, caused by the buildup of fatty deposits in the arteries, is called atherosclerosis. Your doctor will treat your heart disease and may also prescribe medication, such as aspirin, to help prevent the formation of clots. Your doctor may recommend surgery to clean out a clogged neck artery if you match a particular risk profile. If you are over 50, NINDS scientists believe you and your doctor should make a decision about aspirin therapy. A doctor can evaluate your risk factors and help you decide if you will benefit from aspirin or other blood-thinning therapy.

- **Warning signs or history of stroke.** If you experience a TIA, get help at once. Many communities encourage those with stroke's warning signs to dial 911 for emergency medical assistance. If you have had a stroke in the past, it's important to reduce your risk of a second stroke. Your brain helps you recover from a stroke by drawing on body systems that now do double duty. That means a second stroke can be twice as bad.

- **Diabetes.** You may think this disorder affects only the body's ability to use sugar, or glucose. But it also causes destructive changes in the blood vessels throughout the body, including the brain. Also, if blood glucose levels are high at the time of a stroke, then brain damage is usually more severe and extensive than when blood glucose is well-controlled. Treating diabetes can delay the onset of complications that increase the risk of stroke.

Do You Know Your Stroke Risk?

Some of the most important risk factors for stroke can be determined during a physical exam at your doctor's office. If you are over 55 years old, the tables below can help you estimate your risk of stroke and show the benefit of risk-factor control.

The worksheet was developed from NINDS-supported work in the well-known Framingham Study. Working with your doctor, you can develop a strategy to lower your risk to average or even below average for your age.

Many risk factors for stroke can be managed, some very successfully. Although risk is never zero at any age, by starting early and controlling your risk factors you can lower your risk of death or disability from stroke. With good control, the risk of stroke in most age groups can be kept below that for accidental injury or death.

Americans have shown that stroke is preventable and treatable. In recent years, a better understanding of the causes of stroke has helped Americans make lifestyle changes that have cut the stroke death rate nearly in half.

Scientists at the NINDS predict that, with continued attention to reducing the risks of stroke and by using currently available therapies and developing new ones, Americans should be able to prevent 80 percent of all strokes.

Stroke Risk Scorecard

To reduce your risk for stroke:

1. Know your blood pressure. If high, work with your doctor to lower it.

2. Find out from your doctor if you have atrial fibrillation.

3. If you smoke, stop.

4. If you drink alcohol, do so in moderation.

5. Find out if you have high cholesterol. If so, work with your doctor to control it.

6. If you are diabetic, follow your doctor's recommendations carefully to control your diabetes.

7. Include exercise in the activities you enjoy in your daily routine.

8. Enjoy a lower sodium (salt), lower fat diet.

9. Ask your doctor how you can lower your risk of stroke.

10. Know the symptoms of stroke.

If you have any stroke symptoms, seek immediate medical attention. Symptoms include:

- sudden numbness or weakness of face, arm or leg—especially on one side of the body;

- sudden confusion, trouble speaking, or understanding;

- sudden trouble seeing in one or both eyes;

Table 8.1. Score Your Stroke Risk for the Next 10 Years—Men

Points	0	+1	+2	+3	+4	+5	+6	+7	+8	+9	+10
Age	55–56	57–59	60–62	63–65	66–68	69–72	73–75	76–78	79–81	83–84	85
SBD-untrd	97–105	106–115	116–125	126–135	136–145	146–155	156–165	166–175	176–185	186–195	196–205
or											
SBP-trtd	97–105	106–112	113–117	118–123	124–129	130–135	136–142	143–150	151–161	162–176	177–205
Diabetes	No		Yes								
Cigarettes	No			Yes							
CVD	No				Yes						
AF	No				Yes						
LVH	No					Yes					

Key: SBP = systolic blood pressure (score one line only, untreated or treated); Diabetes = history of diabetes; Cigarettes = smokes cigarettes; CVD (cardiovascular disease) = history of heart disease; AF = history of atrial fibrillation; LVH = diagnosis of left ventricular hypertrophy

Table 8.2. Your 10-Year Stroke Probability—Men

Your Points	10-Year Probability	Your Points	10-Year Probability
1	3%	16	22%
2	3%	17	26%
3	4%	18	29%
4	4%	19	33%
5	5%	20	37%
6	5%	21	42%
7	6%	22	47%
8	7%	23	52%
9	8%	24	57%
10	10%	25	63%
11	11%	26	68%
12	13%	27	74%
13	15%	28	79%
14	17%	29	84%
15	20%	30	88%

Table 8.3. Your Stroke Risk Compared to Your Peers—Men

Compare with Your Age Group	Average 10-Year Probability of Stroke
55–59	5.9%
60–64	7.8%
65–69	11.0%
70–74	13.7%
75–79	18.0%
80–84	22.3%

Table 8.4. Score Your Stroke Risk for the Next 10 Years—Women

Points	0	+1	+2	+3	+4	+5	+6	+7	+8	+9	+10
Age	55–56	57–59	60–62	63–64	65–67	68–70	71–73	74–76	77–78	79–81	82–84
SBP-untrd		95–106	107–118	119–130	131–143	144–155	156–167	168–180	181–192	193–204	205–216
or											
SBP-trtd		95–106	107–113	114–119	120–125	126–131	132–139	140–148	149–160	161–204	205–216
Diabetes	No			Yes							
Cigarettes	No			Yes							
CVD	No		Yes								
AF	No						Yes				
LVH	No				Yes						

Key: SBP = systolic blood pressure (score one line only, untreated or treated); Diabetes = history of diabetes; Cigarettes = smokes cigarettes; CVD (cardiovascular disease) = history of heart disease; AF = history of atrial fibrillation; LVH = diagnosis of left ventricular hypertrophy

Table 8.5. Your 10-Year Stroke Probability—Women

Your Points	10-Year Probability	Your Points	10-Year Probability
1	1%	15	16%
2	1%	16	19%
3	2%	17	23%
4	2%	18	27%
5	2%	19	32%
6	3%	20	37%
7	4%	21	43%
8	4%	22	50%
9	5%	23	57%
10	6%	24	64%
11	8%	25	71%
12	9%	26	78%
13	11%	27	84%
14	13%		

Table 8.6. Your Stroke Risk Compared to Your Peers—Women

Compare with Your Age Group	Average 10-Year Probability of Stroke
55–59	3.0%
60–64	4.7%
65–69	7.2%
70–74	10.9%
75–79	15.5%
80–84	23.9%

Source: D'Agostino, R.B.; Wolf, P.A.; Belanger, A.J.; & Kannel, W.B. "Stroke Risk Profile: The Framingham Study." *Stroke,* Vol. 25, No. 1, pp. 40–43, January 1994.

- sudden trouble walking, dizziness, loss of balance, or coordination; and/or

- sudden severe headache with no known cause.

If you have experienced any of these symptoms, you may have had a TIA [transient ischemic attack] or a stroke—call 911 immediately!

Table 8.7. Scoring Your Stroke Risk

Risk Factor	High Risk	Caution	Low Risk
Blood Pressure	>140/90 or I don't know	120–139/80–89	<120/80
Cholesterol	>240 or I don't know	200–239	<200
Diabetes	Yes	Borderline	No
Smoking	I still smoke	I'm trying to quit	I am a nonsmoker
Atrial Fibrillation	I have an irregular heartbeat	I don't know	My heartbeat is not irregular
Diet	I am overweight	I am slightly overweight	My weight is healthy
Exercise	I am a couch potato	I exercise sometimes	I exercise regularly
I have stroke in my family	Yes	Not sure	No

Score (each box=1). Each box that applies to you equals 1 point. Total your score at the bottom of each column. If your "High Risk" score is 3 or more, please ask your doctor about stroke prevention right away. If your "Caution" score is 4–6, you're off to a good start. Keep working on it! If your "Low Risk" score is 6–8, congratulations! You're doing very well at controlling your risk for stroke.

Chapter 9

Racial and Ethnic Disparities in Stroke

The disparities in stroke death rates between blacks and whites in the United States have been well documented, with blacks consistently having dramatically higher stroke death rates than whites. The national health agenda outlined in Healthy People 2000 called for a 49% reduction in age-adjusted stroke death rates from 1987 through 2000 for blacks and a 34% reduction for the total population. Neither of these objectives have been met. During 1990–1998, stroke death rates decreased only 11% for blacks and 9% for the total population. Although the amount of the reduction was slightly greater for blacks than whites, the substantial gap between age-adjusted stroke death rates (for those ages 35 years and older) for blacks (156/100,000) and whites (113/100,000) still existed in 1998.

Disparities in stroke death rates among other racial and ethnic groups in the United States have not been examined as extensively, but a 2001 study indicated substantial gaps among the largest racial and ethnic groups in the United States. The largest disparities occurred among adults ages 35–64 years. To address these problems, the Department of Health and Human Services launched the Initiative to Eliminate Racial and Ethnic Disparities in Health in 1998. This initiative seeks to eliminate disparities in six targeted health status

Excerpted from Casper ML, Barnett E, Williams GI Jr., Halverson JA, Braham VE, Greenlund KJ. *Atlas of Stroke Mortality: Racial, Ethnic, and Geographic Disparities in the United States.* Atlanta, GA: Department of Health and Human Services, Centers for Disease Control and Prevention; January 2003; updated May 12, 2006.

81

areas, including heart disease and stroke. In addition, one of the two overarching goals of the updated Healthy People 2010 is to "eliminate health disparities among segments of the population including differences that occur by gender, race or ethnicity, education or income, disability, geographic location, or sexual orientation."

In this text, we provide information regarding racial and ethnic disparities in the distribution of types of stroke (i.e., hemorrhagic and ischemic) and the age distribution of stroke deaths. We use the terms "black" and "African American," as well as the terms "Latina/Latino" and "Hispanic," interchangeably throughout this publication.

Specific Categories of Stroke Deaths

There are two main types of stroke: ischemic and hemorrhagic. Ischemic strokes are caused by a blockage of the arterial blood supply to the brain. According to research studies in which detailed tests were performed to determine the type of stroke, 70%–80% of all stroke deaths are ischemic. Hemorrhagic strokes are less prevalent but more lethal. Hemorrhagic strokes occur when blood vessels rupture and cause bleeding either in the brain or the space between the brain and the skull.

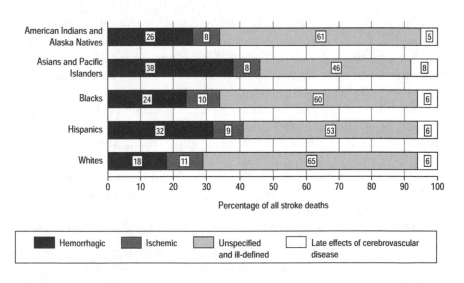

Figure 9.1. Categories of Stroke Deaths Among People Ages Greater Than or Equal to 35 Years, by Racial and Ethnic Group, 1991–1998

The percentage of definite hemorrhagic strokes varied substantially among racial and ethnic groups (Figure 9.1). Asians and Pacific Islanders had the largest percentage (38%), followed by Hispanics (32%), American Indians and Alaska Natives (26%), blacks (24%), and whites (18%). The range of percentages for definite ischemic stroke was much narrower—from 8% for American Indians and Alaska Natives and Asians and Pacific Islanders to 11% for whites. Unspecified and ill-defined stroke deaths accounted for a large percentage of stroke deaths among all racial and ethnic groups. This was due in part to the low rate of CT [computed tomography] scans performed on people who died of a stroke and the difficulty in accurately diagnosing the exact type of stroke in the absence of a CT scan.

Age Distribution of Stroke Deaths

Stroke death rates increase dramatically with age, but there are substantial racial and ethnic disparities in the age distribution of stroke deaths (Figure 9.2). Among whites, only 25% of stroke deaths occurred before age 75; among the other racial and ethnic groups, the percentage of deaths before age 75 ranged from 45% for Asians and Pacific Islanders to 49% for blacks. For each of the younger adult age

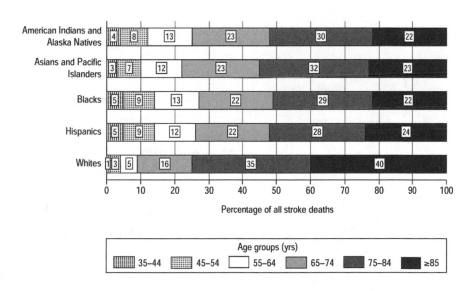

Figure 9.2. *Age Distribution of Stroke Deaths Among People Ages Greater Than or Equal to 35 Years, by Racial and Ethnic Group, 1991–1998*

groups, whites consistently experienced a relatively smaller proportion of total stroke deaths.

Trends in Stroke Death Rates During 1991–1998

Although stroke death rates declined substantially in the 1970s and 1980s, the rate of decline slowed in the 1990s. Trend data presented in this publication indicate that stroke death rates for all racial and ethnic groups declined little in the 1990s for people ages 35 years and older (Figure 9.3). On average, stroke death rates during 1991–1998 fell only 0.8% per year for all racial and ethnic groups combined. (The average annual percentage change in death rate was calculated by subtracting the 1991 rate from the 1998 rate, dividing by the 1991 rate, and then dividing by 7.) The largest declines were experienced by

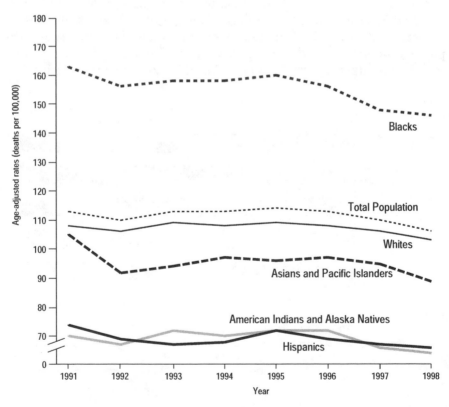

Figure 9.3. *Trends in Stroke Death Rates Among People Ages Greater than or Equal to 35 Years, by Racial and Ethnic Group, 1991–1998*

Asians and Pacific Islanders (2.0% per year), followed by Hispanics and blacks (1.4% per year for both groups). American Indians and Alaska Natives experienced a decline of only 1.1% per year, and whites experienced a decline of 0.8% per year.

In addition, disparities in the level of stroke death rates among the five racial and ethnic groups were observed during 1991–1998 (Figure 9.3). African Americans experienced dramatically higher death rates than the other groups. Rates for whites were the next highest, followed by those for Asians and Pacific Islanders. Hispanics and American Indians and Alaska Natives had the lowest rates, and their rates were similar. Throughout this period, the differences between the lowest rates (Hispanics, American Indians and Alaska Natives) and the highest rates (blacks) were more than twofold.

In 1998, stroke death rates for blacks were 2.1 times higher than the rates for Hispanics and American Indians and Alaska Natives, 1.6 times higher than the rates for Asians and Pacific Islanders, and 1.4 times higher than the rates for whites. However, death rates for American Indians and Alaska Natives, Asians and Pacific Islanders, and Hispanics may be underestimated because of misreporting of race and ethnicity on death certificates. Furthermore, the relatively low stroke death rates for Asians and Pacific Islanders mainly reflect the mortality experience of Asians because Pacific Islanders make up only 5% of this population. Mortality studies conducted in the 1980s and 1990s reported that stroke death rates among Native Hawaiians were higher than those among Chinese, Filipino, and Japanese people living in Hawaii.

Chapter 10

Family History and Gender Influence Risk of Stroke

Chapter Contents

Section 10.1

Family History and Stroke Risk

"Genetics and family history" is from the Centers for Disease
Control and Prevention (CDC, www.cdc.gov), National Office of Public
Health Genomics, December 2007.

Stroke is the third leading cause of death and a major cause of disability in the United States. A stroke occurs when the blood supply to part of the brain is blocked, or when a blood vessel in the brain bursts, causing damage to a part of the brain.

Some health conditions and behavioral and lifestyle factors can put individuals at a higher risk for stroke. The most important risk factors are high blood pressure, heart disease, diabetes, and cigarette smoking.

Individuals can help prevent a stroke by making behavioral and lifestyle changes that lower their risk.

Genetics and Family History

Genes play a role in the development of risk factors that can lead to a stroke, such as high blood pressure, heart disease, diabetes, and vascular conditions. An increased risk for stroke within a family may also be due to common factors, such as a sedentary lifestyle or poor eating habits. Thus, family health history is an important tool for identifying people at increased risk for stroke because it reflects both an individual's genes and shared environmental risk factors.

In a 2003 study in Utah, 86% of all early strokes occurred in just 11% of families. This shows that a relatively small subset of families in the population with history of stroke account for the majority of cases. These families may benefit the most from screening and lifestyle interventions.

Stroke also occurs as a complication of several genetic disorders, the most common of these being sickle cell disease. Other genetic disorders such as CADASIL (cerebral autosomal dominant arteriopathy with subcortical infarcts and leukoencephalopathy) have stroke as the primary feature, but these disorders are quite rare. Research in inherited

88

diseases that include stroke is providing insights into how genes contribute to stroke risk with the goal of developing new approaches for prediction, prevention, and treatment of the disease.

Section 10.2

Why Your Sex Matters: Gender Differences Associated with Stroke

"Why Your Sex Matters: Stroke and Gender Differences,"
February 7, 2006. Reprinted with permission from the University of
Connecticut Health Center (www.uchc.edu).

Women tend to think stroke is a men's disease. But the truth is, each year more women than men die from stroke. Annually, of the 700,000 Americans who have a stroke, 39 percent who die are men, 62 percent are women, according to the National Stroke Association.

"Both stroke incidence and mortality have increased in women over the past three decades, which has not been true for men," says Louise McCullough, M.D., Ph.D., director of stroke research at the University of Connecticut Health Center. "Heart disease and stroke take more women's lives than the next five leading causes of death combined—cancer, chronic respiratory diseases, diabetes, Alzheimer's, and unintentional injuries."

Stroke related to gender has historically been an understudied topic, according to McCullough. She is trying to change that. She is a board certified vascular neurologist and a basic science researcher who has found what happens in the lab may not hold true when tested in humans. Even though estrogen appears to offer a protective effect against stroke when administered to lab animals, clinical trials in humans found hormone replacement therapy could actually increase stroke risk, she explained.

McCullough is also looking closely at the way women are treated for stroke compared to men. Studies have found that women are less likely to receive prescriptions for blood pressure medications or advised to take aspirin, both of which have been shown to reduce stroke risk. In contrast, women are more likely than men to receive anti-anxiety medication.

Researchers conducting lab work, using tissue cultures or animal models, found certain drugs that protect male brains from stroke do nothing to protect female brains. In fact, some medications could do more harm than good. "Clinical trials need to be carefully considered before testing them on humans," said McCullough. "And in the future, gender-based designer drugs may be the answer."

It's important to note that 80 percent of strokes are preventable and there are lifestyle changes you can make to lower your risk. Some risk factors are the same for men and women: high blood pressure, high cholesterol, smoking, diabetes, being overweight, and not exercising. Other risks are unique to women: taking birth control pills, using hormone replacement therapy, having a thick waist and high triglyceride level, and being a migraine headache sufferer.

Common stroke symptoms are seen in both men and women: weakness or numbness in the face, arms or legs, especially on one side of the body; visual changes in one or both eyes; severe headache; dizziness or loss of balance; and trouble speaking or understanding. And women may experience some unique warning signs such as sudden hiccups, nausea, chest pain, and shortness of breath.

Knowing these symptoms is crucial in order to receive treatment as quickly as possible. If the stroke is caused by a blood clot, the most common type, a medication called tPA (tissue plasminogen activator) dissolves clots, and should be given within three hours after symptoms begin.

"Too many women ignore the symptoms," says Dr. McCullough. "So many women have told me they thought their symptoms would disappear if they took a nap or just rested awhile. And then by the time they get to the emergency room, it's too late."

A stroke is a form of cardiovascular disease that affects the arteries traveling towards and inside the brain. A stroke results when one of these vessels becomes blocked or bursts and the brain is deprived of blood and oxygen. Stroke is the third leading cause of death in America and the number one cause of adult disability.

The University of Connecticut Health Center includes the schools of medicine and dental medicine, John Dempsey Hospital, the UConn Medical Group and University Dentists. Founded in 1961, the Health Center pursues a mission of providing outstanding health care education in an environment of exemplary patient care, research, and public service. To learn more about the UConn Health Center, visit our website at www.uchc.edu.

Section 10.3

More Women Than Men Having Mid-Life Stroke

More women than men appear to be having a stroke in middle age, according to a study published June 20, 2007, in the online edition of *Neurology*, the medical journal of the American Academy of Neurology. Researchers say heart disease and increased waist size may be contributing to this apparent mid-life stroke surge among women.

For the study, researchers analyzed data from 17,000 people over the age of 18 who participated in the National Health and Nutrition Examination Survey. Of the participants, 606 people experienced a stroke.

The study found women in the 45 to 54 age range were more than twice as likely as men in the same age group to have had a stroke. There were no sex differences in stroke rates found in the 35 to 44 and the 55 to 64 age groups.

"While our analysis shows increased waist size and coronary artery disease are predictors of stroke among women aged 45 to 54, it is not immediately clear why there is a sex disparity in stroke rates among this age group," said study author Amytis Towfighi, M.D., with the Stroke Center and Department of Neurology at the University of California at Los Angeles, and member of the American Academy of Neurology. "While further study is needed, this mid-life stroke surge among women suggests prompt and close attention may need to be paid to the cardiovascular health of women in their mid-30s to mid-50s with a goal of mitigating this burden."

In addition, Towfighi says several vascular risk factors including systolic blood pressure and total cholesterol levels increased at higher rates among women compared to men in each older age group.

"For instance, with each decade, men's blood pressure increased by an average of four to five points, whereas women's blood pressure increased by eight to 10 points. Similarly, men had significantly higher total cholesterol levels than women at age 35 to 44, but men's total cholesterol remained stable while women's total cholesterol increased by 10 to 12 points with each decade, so that by age 55 to 64, women had significantly higher total cholesterol than men," said Towfighi.

Towfighi says the study also found a greater than expected stroke surge among men who were nearing the end of middle age. Men aged 55 to 64 were three times more likely than men aged 45 to 54 to have had a stroke. Towfighi says the reasons behind this increase warrant further investigation.

Chapter 11

Children and Stroke

Children and newborn babies can develop a stroke. A stroke is the interruption of blood to the brain. The brain cells in the immediate area die and those in the surrounding areas are affected by the reduced blood flow. Once brain cells die, their functions die with them. However, the brains of young children seem to be sufficiently immature (and therefore flexible enough) to recover from stroke better than adults. Stroke is relatively rare amongst children, with only 2.5 children out of 100,000 affected every year. Most cases occur in the under two years of age group. A major underlying cause of stroke in children seems to be congenital heart disorders. However, in approximately one third of cases, the exact cause cannot be found.

Types of Stroke

An ischaemic stroke means that an embolism (either a clot of blood or a piece of debris) blocks a blood vessel in the brain, interrupting blood flow. A haemorrhagic stroke refers to a ruptured blood vessel bleeding into the brain. In newborns, bleeding into the space surrounding the brain can occur, and this is called a subarachnoid haemorrhage.

General Symptoms of Stroke

Children often experience different symptoms of stroke to adults, such as seizures, headache and fever. However, many of the symptoms of stroke in children are similar to those experienced by adults. Depending on the areas of the brain affected by stroke, the symptoms can include:

- Brief attacks of weakness
- Clumsiness
- Numbness or pins and needles of the face, arm or leg on one side of the body
- Slurring speech or difficulty finding words
- If blood vessels in the eye are affected, brief loss of vision in one or both eyes.

Causes of Stroke in Children

In around one third of cases, the cause of stroke remains unknown. The most common known causes of stroke in children include:

- Heart disorders, such as congenital structural defects
- Blood disorders, such as sickle cell disease or blood clotting problems
- Genetic disorders
- Infections in the skull
- Abnormalities of the blood vessels of the head
- Injury or trauma to the head.

Treatment Options

Treatment of stroke is similar in both children and adults, and can include:

- Hospitalisation
- Maintaining optimum pressure inside the skull, by drainage if necessary
- Treating any underlying or associated illnesses

- Investigating and treating the cause to prevent further attacks
- Rehabilitation.

Long-Term Effects

Generally, the brain of a young child is more resilient than an adult brain and tends to recover from stroke more easily. In some cases, particularly if the stroke was flagged with a seizure, the outlook for the child is poor. The long term effect of severe stroke for a young child may include:

- Epilepsy
- Movement disorders
- Learning disabilities
- Mental retardation.

Seek Urgent Medical Attention

Stroke is a medical emergency. If your child experiences symptoms such as seizures, loss of speech or paralysis, seek urgent medical attention.

Where to Get Help

- Your doctor
- In an emergency, always call 000 for an ambulance. [Editorial Note: In the United States, dial 911.]

Things to Remember

- Stroke is rare amongst children, with only 2.5 cases per 100,000 occurring every year.
- The most common cause is congenital heart disease.
- Symptoms of stroke in children include seizures, fever, speech impairment, and paralysis.

Chapter 12

Younger Stroke Survivors Have Reduced Access to Care and Medications

Summary: Stroke survivors under the age 65 are more likely to have problems having access to physicians to care for them and affording the medicines they need than do those who are over the age of 65 and more likely to be eligible for Medicare.

Why it's important: More than 5 million people in the United States have survived stroke. To avoid subsequent strokes, recover from the one they have had, and live life as healthily as possible, they need care including changes in the way they live their lives and drugs that can reduce the likelihood of a second stroke. Access to physicians skilled in treating them along with specific medications is a critical part of this recovery. Young individuals are more likely to live longer after stroke. Accessing the care that is needed is a critical part of their recovery and their ability to get on with their lives. Not only is it important to them, but it is also important to the nation as disability will raise the national health care bill.

What's already known: As many as 5.4 million U.S. residents have survived a stroke. However, they face an increased risk of having another stroke. Studies have shown that the annual risk for another stroke is between 5 percent and 15 percent. Stroke survivors

---

"Younger Stroke Survivors Have Reduced Access to Physician Care and Medications: National Health Interview Survey From Years 1998 to 2002," Reprinted with permission from www.americanheart.org. © 2006 American Heart Association.

also face an increased risk of other diseases involving the heart and blood vessels, including heart attack. The care of physicians trained and skilled in avoiding second strokes and heart disease is critical in assuring further good health. However, studies have shown that many stroke survivors do not receive treatments that would reduce their risk of a second stroke, including prescription of diet and drugs to reduce the level of fat and cholesterol in the blood. It is fair to question whether patients have access to the care they need. Such questions should start with patients under the age of 65 because they are more likely to lack health insurance. Most of those 65 and older qualify for Medicare health insurance.

How this study was done: This study analyzed answers from the National Health Interview Survey, an ongoing household survey of people in the United States. The interviews in this survey are conducted in person by personnel from the National Center for Health Statistics. This study used an analysis of responses from the adult surveys conducted from 1998 to 2002. In this survey, the researchers, led by Deborah A. Levine, M.D., M.P.H., of the Birmingham (Ala.) Veterans Affairs Medical Center and the University of Birmingham at Alabama, singled out responses from people who said they had had a stroke and were 45 and older.

These people had been asked if they had had a stroke, if they had seen a general or specialist physician in the preceding year, and if they could not afford the prescriptions they needed during that period of time.

What was found: Of the 3,681 stroke survivors in the survey, 2,509 were 65 or older and 1,172 were 45 to 64. Those in the younger group were more likely to be black, male, and lack health insurance. Fourteen percent of younger stroke survivors said they had not visited a general physician in the past year compared to 10 percent of older ones. Eight percent of the younger stroke survivors had not visited either a general or specialist physician in the preceding 12 months compared to 5 percent of the older ones, and 15 percent of younger stroke survivors said they could not afford medicines they needed compared to 6 percent of the older ones.

The authors wrote: "Lack of health insurance was associated with reduced access to care on all three outcome measures. . . . The percentage of stroke survivors reporting no general doctor visits, no general doctor or medical specialist visit, and the inability to afford medications decreased with increasing age category."

"Clinicians may assume that stroke survivors have health insurance owing to misunderstandings about qualifications for insurance based on disability," they wrote. "Our data show that these assumptions may well be unwarranted for younger stroke survivors. Moreover, most of the uninsured stroke survivors in this study were not born outside the United States; only 16 percent and 43 percent of uninsured younger and older stroke survivors, respectively, were foreign born. . . . Given the increasing number of uninsured nonelderly Americans and the high costs associated with recurrent stroke (which are increased compared with first stroke) and other cardiovascular events, the potential costs of reduced access to health care among younger stroke survivors are substantial. Expanding health insurance by providing affordable Medicare insurance or, more radically, immediate Medicare insurance to uninsured patients with stroke would be expected to improve access to care and increase the use of basic clinical services like physician visits. Affordable prescription coverage would be necessary to increase access to medications."

The bottom line: Younger people who survive stroke are less likely to be able to afford the care and medicine that could be expected to prevent recurrent stroke and enhance their ability to recover from it. Maintaining health insurance coverage is an important factor in maintaining good health for everyone. Studies such as this one provide good indicators for people considering national health policy.

Journal: *Archives of Neurology*

Journal citation: Arch Neurol. 2007; 64: (doi:10.1001/archneur.64.1 .noc60002).

Chapter 13

Atherosclerosis and Hypercholesterolemia

Chapter Contents

Section 13.1

Understanding Atherosclerosis and Its Causes

Excerpted from "Atherosclerosis," by the National Heart,
Lung, and Blood Institute (NHLBI, www.nhlbi.nih.gov), part
of the National Institutes of Health, July 2006.

What Is Atherosclerosis?

Atherosclerosis is a disease in which plaque builds up on the insides of your arteries. Arteries are blood vessels that carry oxygen-rich blood to your heart and other parts of your body.

Plaque is made up of fat, cholesterol, calcium, and other substances found in the blood. Over time, plaque hardens and narrows your arteries. The flow of oxygen-rich blood to your organs and other parts of your body is reduced. This can lead to serious problems, including heart attack, stroke, or even death.

Overview

Atherosclerosis can affect any artery in the body, including arteries in the heart, brain, arms, legs, and pelvis. As a result, different diseases may develop based on which arteries are affected.

- **Coronary artery disease (CAD).** This is when plaque builds up in the coronary arteries. These arteries supply oxygen-rich blood to your heart. When blood flow to your heart is reduced or blocked, it can lead to chest pain and heart attack. CAD also is called heart disease, and it's the leading cause of death in the United States.

- **Carotid artery disease.** This happens when plaque builds up in the carotid arteries. These arteries supply oxygen-rich blood to your brain. When blood flow to your brain is reduced or blocked, it can lead to stroke.

- **Peripheral arterial disease (PAD).** This occurs when plaque builds up in the major arteries that supply oxygen-rich blood to

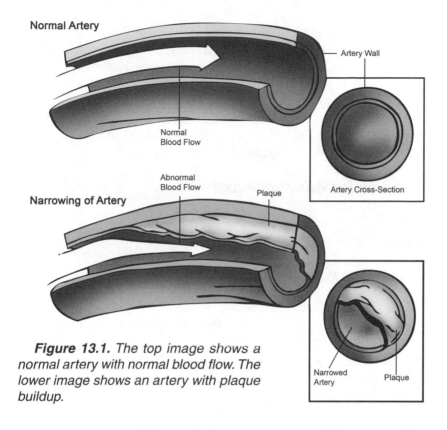

Normal Artery

Artery Wall

Normal
Blood Flow

Artery Cross-Section

Abnormal
Blood Flow

Plaque

Narrowing of Artery

Narrowed
Artery

Plaque

Figure 13.1. *The top image shows a normal artery with normal blood flow. The lower image shows an artery with plaque buildup.*

the legs, arms, and pelvis. When blood flow to these parts of your body is reduced or blocked, it can lead to numbness, pain, and sometimes dangerous infections.

Some people with atherosclerosis have no signs or symptoms. They may not be diagnosed until after a heart attack or stroke.

The main treatment for atherosclerosis is lifestyle changes. You also may need medicines and medical procedures. These, along with ongoing medical care, can help you live a healthier life.

The cause of atherosclerosis isn't known. However, certain conditions may raise your chances of developing it. These conditions are known as risk factors. You can control some risk factors, such as lack of physical activity, smoking, and unhealthy eating. Others you can't control, such as age and family history of heart disease.

Outlook

Better treatments have reduced the number of deaths from atherosclerosis-related diseases. These treatments also have improved the quality of life for people with these diseases. Still, the number of people diagnosed with atherosclerosis remains high.

You may be able to prevent or delay atherosclerosis and the diseases it can cause, mainly by maintaining a healthy lifestyle. This, along with ongoing medical care, can help you avoid the problems of atherosclerosis and live a long, healthy life.

Other Names for Atherosclerosis

- Arteriosclerosis
- Hardening of the arteries

What Causes Atherosclerosis?

The exact cause of atherosclerosis isn't known. However, studies show that atherosclerosis is a slow, complex disease that may start in childhood. It develops faster as you age.

Atherosclerosis may start when certain factors damage the inner layers of the arteries. These factors include:

- smoking;
- high amounts of certain fats and cholesterol in the blood;
- high blood pressure; and
- high amounts of sugar in the blood due to insulin resistance or diabetes.

When damage occurs, your body starts a healing process. Fatty tissues release compounds that promote this process. This healing causes plaque to build up where the arteries are damaged.

Over time, the plaque may crack. Blood cells called platelets clump together to form blood clots where the cracks are. This narrows the arteries more and worsens angina (chest pain) or causes a heart attack.

Researchers continue to look at why atherosclerosis develops. They hope to find answers to such questions as:

- Why and how do the arteries become damaged?

- How does plaque develop and change over time?

- Why does plaque break open and lead to clots?

Who Is at Risk for Atherosclerosis?

Coronary artery disease (atherosclerosis of the coronary arteries) is the leading cause of death in the United States.

The exact cause of atherosclerosis isn't known. However, certain traits, conditions, or habits may raise your chance of developing it. These conditions are known as risk factors. Your chances of developing atherosclerosis increase with the number of risk factors you have.

You can control most risk factors and help prevent or delay atherosclerosis. Other risk factors can't be controlled.

Major Risk Factors

- **Unhealthy blood cholesterol levels.** This includes high LDL cholesterol (sometimes called bad cholesterol) and low HDL cholesterol (sometimes called good cholesterol).

- **High blood pressure.** Blood pressure is considered high if it stays at or above 140/90 mmHg over a period of time.

- **Smoking.** This can damage and tighten blood vessels, raise cholesterol levels, and raise blood pressure. Smoking also doesn't allow enough oxygen to reach the body's tissues.

- **Insulin resistance.** This condition occurs when the body can't use its own insulin properly. Insulin is a hormone that helps move blood sugar into cells where it's used.

- **Diabetes.** This is a disease in which the body's blood sugar level is high because the body doesn't make enough insulin or doesn't use its insulin properly.

- **Overweight or obesity.** Overweight is having extra body weight from muscle, bone, fat, and/or water. Obesity is having a high amount of extra body fat.

- **Lack of physical activity.** Lack of activity can worsen other risk factors for atherosclerosis.

- **Age.** As you get older, your risk for atherosclerosis increases. Genetic or lifestyle factors cause plaque to build in your arteries as you age. By the time you're middle-aged or older, enough plaque has built up to cause signs or symptoms.

- In men, the risk increases after age 45.
- In women, the risk increases after age 55.
- **Family history of early heart disease.** Your risk for athero-sclerosis increases if your father or a brother was diagnosed with heart disease before 55 years of age, or if your mother or a sister was diagnosed with heart disease before 65 years of age.

Although age and a family history of early heart disease are risk factors, it doesn't mean that you will develop atherosclerosis if you have one or both.

Making lifestyle changes and/or taking medicines to treat other risk factors can often lessen genetic influences and prevent athero-sclerosis from developing, even in older adults.

Emerging Risk Factors

Scientists continue to study other possible risk factors for athero-sclerosis.

High levels of a protein called C-reactive protein (CRP) in the blood may raise the risk for atherosclerosis and heart attack. High levels of CRP are proof of inflammation in the body. Inflammation is the body's response to injury or infection. Damage to the arteries' inner walls seems to trigger inflammation and help plaque grow.

People with low CRP levels may get atherosclerosis at a slower rate than people with high CRP levels. Research is under way to find out whether reducing inflammation and lowering CRP levels also can reduce the risk of atherosclerosis.

High levels of fats called triglycerides in the blood also may raise the risk of atherosclerosis, particularly in women.

Other Factors That Affect Atherosclerosis

Other risk factors also may raise your risk for developing athero-sclerosis. These include:

- **Sleep apnea.** Sleep apnea is a disorder in which your breath-ing stops or gets very shallow while you're sleeping. Untreated sleep apnea can raise your chances of having high blood pres-sure, diabetes, and even a heart attack or stroke.
- **Stress.** Research shows that the most commonly reported "trig-ger" for a heart attack is an emotionally upsetting event—partic-ularly one involving anger.

- **Alcohol.** Heavy drinking can damage the heart muscle and worsen other risk factors for atherosclerosis. Men should have no more than two drinks containing alcohol a day. Women should have no more than one drink containing alcohol a day.

What Are the Signs and Symptoms of Atherosclerosis?

Atherosclerosis usually doesn't cause signs and symptoms until it severely narrows or totally blocks an artery. Many people don't know they have the disease until they have a medical emergency, such as a heart attack or stroke.

Some people may have other signs and symptoms of the disease. These depend on which arteries are severely narrowed or blocked.

The coronary arteries supply oxygen-rich blood to your heart. When plaque narrows or blocks these arteries (a condition called coronary artery disease, or CAD), a common symptom is angina.

Angina is chest pain or discomfort that occurs when your heart muscle doesn't get enough oxygen-rich blood. Angina may feel like pressure or a squeezing pain in your chest. You also may feel it in your shoulders, arms, neck, jaw, or back.

This pain tends to get worse with activity and goes away when you rest. Emotional stress also can trigger the pain.

Other symptoms of CAD are shortness of breath and arrhythmias (irregular heartbeats).

The carotid arteries supply oxygen-rich blood to your brain. When plaque narrows or blocks these arteries (a condition called carotid artery disease), you may have symptoms of a stroke. These symptoms include sudden numbness, weakness, and dizziness.

Plaque also can build up in the major arteries that supply oxygen-rich blood to the legs, arms, and pelvis (a condition called peripheral arterial disease). When these arteries are narrowed or blocked, it can lead to numbness, pain, and sometimes dangerous infections.

How Is Atherosclerosis Diagnosed?

Your doctor will diagnose atherosclerosis based on:

- your medical and family histories;
- your risk factors; and
- the results of a physical exam and diagnostic tests.

Specialists Involved

If you have atherosclerosis, a doctor, internist, or general practitioner may handle your care. Your doctor may send you to other health care specialists if you need expert care. These specialists may include:

- A cardiologist (a doctor who specializes in treating people with heart problems). You may see a cardiologist if you have coronary artery disease (CAD).

- A vascular specialist (a doctor who specializes in treating people with blood vessel problems). You may see a vascular specialist if you have peripheral arterial disease (PAD).

- A neurologist (a doctor who specializes in treating people with disorders of the nervous system). You may see a neurologist if you've had a stroke due to carotid artery disease.

Physical Exam

During the physical exam, your doctor may listen to your arteries for an abnormal whooshing sound called a bruit. Your doctor can hear a bruit when placing a stethoscope over an affected artery. A bruit may indicate poor blood flow due to plaque.

Your doctor also may check to see whether any of your pulses (for example, in the leg or foot) are weak or absent. A weak or absent pulse can be a sign of a blocked artery.

Diagnostic Tests and Procedures

Your doctor may order one or more tests to diagnose atherosclerosis. These tests also can help your doctor learn the extent of your disease and plan the best treatment.

Blood tests. Blood tests check the levels of certain fats, cholesterol, sugar, and proteins in your blood. Abnormal levels may show that you have risk factors for atherosclerosis.

EKG (Electrocardiogram). An EKG is a simple test that detects and records the electrical activity of your heart. An EKG shows how fast your heart is beating and whether it has a regular rhythm. It also shows the strength and timing of electrical signals as they pass through each part of your heart.

Certain electrical patterns that the EKG detects can suggest whether CAD is likely. An EKG also can show signs of a previous or current heart attack.

Chest x-ray. A chest x-ray takes a picture of the organs and structures inside the chest, including your heart, lungs, and blood vessels. A chest x-ray can reveal signs of heart failure.

Ankle/brachial index. This test compares the blood pressure in your ankle with the blood pressure in your arm to see how well your blood is flowing. This test can help diagnose PAD.

Echocardiography. This test uses sound waves to create a moving picture of your heart. Echocardiography provides information about the size and shape of your heart and how well your heart chambers and valves are working.

The test also can identify areas of poor blood flow to the heart, areas of heart muscle that aren't contracting normally, and previous injury to the heart muscle caused by poor blood flow.

Computed tomography scan. A computed tomography, or CT, scan creates computer-generated images of the heart, brain, or other areas of the body. The test can often show hardening and narrowing of large arteries.

Stress testing. During stress testing, you exercise to make your heart work hard and beat fast while heart tests are performed. If you can't exercise, you're given medicine to speed up your heart rate.

When your heart is beating fast and working hard, it needs more blood and oxygen. Arteries narrowed by plaque can't supply enough oxygen-rich blood to meet your heart's needs. A stress test can show possible signs of CAD, such as:

- abnormal changes in your heart rate or blood pressure;

- symptoms such as shortness of breath or chest pain; and

- abnormal changes in your heart rhythm or your heart's electrical activity.

During the stress test, if you can't exercise for as long as what's considered normal for someone your age, it may be a sign that not enough blood is flowing to your heart. But other factors besides CAD can prevent you from exercising long enough (for example, lung diseases, anemia, or poor general fitness).

Some stress tests use a radioactive dye, sound waves, positron emission tomography (PET), or cardiac magnetic resonance imaging (MRI) to take pictures of your heart when it's working hard and when it's at rest.

These imaging stress tests can show how well blood is flowing in the different parts of your heart. They also can show how well your heart pumps blood when it beats.

Angiography. Angiography is a test that uses dye and special x-rays to show the insides of your arteries. This test can show whether plaque is blocking your arteries and how severe the plaque is.

A thin, flexible tube called a catheter is put into a blood vessel in your arm, groin (upper thigh), or neck. A dye that can be seen on x-ray is then injected into the arteries. By looking at the x-ray picture, your doctor can see the flow of blood through your arteries.

How Is Atherosclerosis Treated?

Treatments for atherosclerosis may include lifestyle changes, medicines, and medical procedures or surgery.

Goals of Treatment

The goals of treatment are to:

- relieve symptoms;
- reduce risk factors in an effort to slow, stop, or reverse the buildup of plaque;
- lower the risk of blood clots forming;
- widen or bypass clogged arteries; and
- prevent diseases related to atherosclerosis.

Lifestyle Changes

Making lifestyle changes can often help prevent or treat atherosclerosis. For some people, these changes may be the only treatment needed.

- Follow a healthy eating plan to prevent or reduce high blood pressure and high blood cholesterol and to maintain a healthy weight.

- Increase your physical activity. Check with your doctor first to find out how much and what kinds of activity are safe for you.

- Lose weight, if you're overweight or obese.

- Quit smoking, if you smoke. Avoid exposure to secondhand smoke.

- Reduce stress.

Follow a Healthy Eating Plan

Therapeutic Lifestyle Changes (TLC). Your doctor may recommend TLC if you have high cholesterol. TLC is a three-part program that includes a healthy diet, physical activity, and weight management.

With the TLC diet, less than 7 percent of your daily calories should come from saturated fat. This kind of fat is mainly found in meat and poultry, including dairy products. No more than 25 to 35 percent of your daily calories should come from all fats, including saturated, trans, monounsaturated, and polyunsaturated fats.

You also should have less than 200 mg a day of cholesterol. The amounts of cholesterol and the different kinds of fat in prepared foods can be found on the Nutrition Facts label.

Foods high in soluble fiber also are part of a healthy eating plan. They help block the digestive tract from absorbing cholesterol. These foods include:

- whole grain cereals such as oatmeal and oat bran;

- fruits such as apples, bananas, oranges, pears, and prunes; and

- legumes such as kidney beans, lentils, chickpeas, black-eyed peas, and lima beans.

A diet high in fruits and vegetables can increase important cholesterol-lowering compounds in your diet. These compounds, called plant stanols or sterols, work like soluble fiber.

Fish are an important part of a heart healthy diet. They're a good source of omega-3 fatty acids, which may help protect the heart from blood clots and inflammation and reduce the risk for heart attack. Try to have about two fish meals every week. Fish high in omega-3 fats are salmon, tuna (canned or fresh), and mackerel.

You also should try to limit the amount of sodium (salt) that you eat. This means choosing low-sodium and low-salt foods and "no added salt" foods and seasonings at the table or when cooking. The Nutrition Facts label on food packaging shows the amount of sodium in the item.

Try to limit drinks with alcohol. Too much alcohol will raise your blood pressure and triglyceride level. (Triglycerides are a type of fat found in the blood.) Alcohol also adds extra calories, which will cause weight gain. Men should have no more than two drinks containing alcohol a day. Women should have no more than one drink containing alcohol a day.

Dietary Approaches to Stop Hypertension (DASH) eating plan. Your doctor may recommend the DASH eating plan if you have high blood pressure. The DASH eating plan focuses on fruits, vegetables, whole grains, and other foods that are heart healthy and lower in salt/sodium.

This eating plan is low in fat and cholesterol. It also focuses on fat-free or low-fat milk and dairy products, fish, poultry, and nuts. The DASH eating plan is reduced in red meats (including lean red meat), sweets, added sugars, and sugar-containing beverages. It's rich in nutrients, protein, and fiber.

The DASH eating plan is a good heart healthy eating plan, even for those who don't have high blood pressure.

Increase Physical Activity

Regular physical activity can lower many atherosclerosis risk factors, including LDL ("bad") cholesterol, high blood pressure, and excess weight. Physical activity also can lower your risk for diabetes and raise your levels of HDL cholesterol (the "good" cholesterol that helps prevent atherosclerosis).

Check with your doctor about how much and what kinds of physical activity are safe for you. Unless your doctor tells you otherwise, try to get at least 30 minutes of moderate-intensity activity on most or all days of the week. You can do the activity all at once or break it up into shorter periods of at least 10 minutes each.

Moderate-intensity activities include brisk walking, dancing, bowling, bicycling, gardening, and housecleaning.

More intense activities, such as jogging, swimming, and various sports, also may be appropriate for shorter periods.

Maintain a Healthy Weight

Maintaining a healthy weight can decrease your risk factors for atherosclerosis. A general goal to aim for is a body mass index (BMI) of less than 25.

BMI measures your weight in relation to your height and gives an estimate of your total body fat. You can calculate your BMI using the NHLBI's online calculator [http://www.nhlbisupport.com/bmi], or your health care provider can calculate your BMI.

A BMI between 25 and 29 is considered overweight. A BMI of 30 or more is considered obese. A BMI of less than 25 is the goal for preventing and treating atherosclerosis. Your doctor or other health care provider can help you determine an appropriate goal for you.

Quit Smoking

If you smoke or use tobacco, quit. Smoking can damage and tighten blood vessels and raise your risk for atherosclerosis.

Reduce Stress

Research shows that the most commonly reported "trigger" for a heart attack is an emotionally upsetting event—particularly one involving anger. Also, some of the ways people cope with stress, such as drinking, smoking, or overeating, aren't heart healthy.

Physical activity can help relieve stress and reduce other atherosclerosis risk factors. Many people also find that meditation or relaxation therapy helps them reduce stress.

Medicines

To help slow or reverse atherosclerosis, your doctor may prescribe medicines to help lower your cholesterol or blood pressure or prevent blood clots from forming.

For successful treatment, take all medicines as your doctor prescribes.

Medical Procedures and Surgery

If you have severe atherosclerosis, your doctor may recommend one of several procedures or surgeries.

Angioplasty is a procedure to open blocked or narrowed coronary (heart) arteries. Angioplasty can improve blood flow to the heart, relieve chest pain, and possibly prevent a heart attack. Sometimes a small mesh tube called a stent is placed in the artery to keep it open after the procedure.

Coronary artery bypass grafting (CABG) is a type of surgery. In CABG, arteries or veins from other areas in your body are used to bypass (that is, go around) your narrowed coronary arteries. CABG can improve blood flow to your heart, relieve chest pain, and possibly prevent a heart attack.

Bypass grafting also can be used for leg arteries. In this surgery, a healthy blood vessel is used to bypass a narrowed or blocked blood vessel in one of your legs. The healthy blood vessel redirects blood around the artery, improving blood flow to the leg.

Carotid artery surgery removes plaque buildup from the carotid arteries in the neck. This opens the arteries and improves blood flow to the brain. Carotid artery surgery can help prevent a stroke.

How Can Atherosclerosis Be Prevented or Delayed?

Taking action to control your risk factors can help prevent or delay atherosclerosis and its related diseases. Your chance of developing atherosclerosis goes up with the number of risk factors you have.

Making lifestyle changes and taking prescribed medicines are important steps.

Know your family history of health problems related to atherosclerosis. If you or someone in your family has this disease, be sure to tell your doctor. Also, let your doctor know if you smoke.

Living with Atherosclerosis

Improved treatments have reduced deaths from atherosclerosis-related diseases. These treatments also have improved the quality of life for people with these diseases.

You may be able to prevent or delay atherosclerosis and the problems it can cause, mainly by maintaining a healthy lifestyle. This, along with ongoing medical care, can help you avoid the problems of atherosclerosis and live a long, healthy life.

Research continues to look for ways to improve the health of people who have atherosclerosis or may get it. The goals of research are to:

- find more effective medicines;
- identify people at greatest risk earlier; and
- find out how well alternative treatments work.

Ongoing Health Care Needs

If you have atherosclerosis, work closely with your doctor and other health care providers to avoid serious problems, like heart attack and stroke.

Talk to your doctor about how often you should schedule office visits or blood tests. Be sure to let your doctor know if you develop new symptoms or if your symptoms worsen.

Support Groups

Community resources are available to help you learn more about atherosclerosis. Contact your local public health departments, hospitals, and local chapters of national health organizations to learn more about available resources in your area.

Talk about your lifestyle changes with your spouse, family, or friends—whoever can provide support or needs to understand why you're changing your habits. They may be able to help you make lifestyle changes, like helping you plan healthier meals.

Because atherosclerosis tends to run in families, your lifestyle changes may help many of your family members, too.

Section 13.2

Inflammation, C-Reactive Protein, and Stroke Risk

Could a new blood test give physicians the upper hand in predicting stroke or heart attack in patients who show no other risk factors?

Researchers at the Center for Cardiovascular Disease Prevention at Baylor College of Medicine and The Methodist DeBakey Heart Center see the test as an indicator that may help identify risk in patients for whom other factors are less clear.

The test identifies levels of C-reactive protein in the blood. C-reactive protein is an indicator of inflammation. High levels of C-reactive protein have been linked to increased risk of heart attack, stroke, and type 2 (non-insulin dependent) diabetes.

Researchers have found the new high sensitivity test to be helpful in identifying potential problems in those who fall neither into a "low risk" or "high risk" category using the traditional risk factors. The C-reactive protein test is only one of several new markers Baylor scientists are researching in the lab.

"C-reactive protein is not a substitute for the factors we've been telling people to keep an eye on," said Christie Ballantyne, M.D., director of the center and a professor in Baylor's department of medicine. "The major risk factors are still age, hypertension, diabetes, high density lipoprotein (the so-called good) cholesterol, and cigarettes. We still look at those five factors and we determine the intensity of therapy based on them."

However, he said, there are millions of people who fall in the "gray zone" because their traditional risk factors put them in an equivocal area that is neither high nor low. This could be a test to help that patient and doctor determine they need a more aggressive treatment.

"If you have low cholesterol and have no risk factors, this is probably not a test that you need," he said. "If you have all the risk factors or already have heart disease or diabetes, again, this is probably not a test you need. However if you have even a borderline cholesterol or low high density lipoprotein with some risk factors this may be a useful test"

In January 2003, the American Heart Association and the federal Centers for Disease Control and Prevention in Atlanta, Georgia, issued guidelines for the use of C-reactive protein testing by physicians in practice. The group suggests that screening should be reserved for people with moderate cardiovascular risk, with 10-year coronary heart disease risk in the range of 10% to 20%, and that it should not replace assessment for major risk factors. Screening should consist of two C-reactive protein measurements, fasting or non-fasting, approximately two weeks apart. Values higher than 10 milligrams/liter may suggest active infection or inflammation.

Ballantyne notes, however, that the test isn't flawless. "The problem is that C-reactive protein levels rise in the presence of any acute illness," he said. "A cold can send your levels up."

In the coming years, Ballantyne and his research team are hoping to develop a complete panel of new markers, including C-reactive protein, that are associated with inflammation or atherosclerosis. These markers will be used to identify those heading toward a problem early.

"I really think in the next four or five years we'll have this complete panel of markers ready to use," he said.

Health Reference Series *Medical Advisor's Notes and Updates*

Since the original publication of this article, a number of additional studies have confirmed that persistently elevated levels of C-reactive protein predict increased stroke risk, as well as risk for other forms of cardiovascular disease. As stated above, it appears to be most useful among patients at intermediate risk for strokes, rather than those in very low- or high-risk groups.

Section 13.3

Hardening of the Neck Arteries Can Increase Stroke Risk

"Stroke secondary to carotid stenosis"
© 2008 A.D.A.M., Inc. Reprinted with permission.

Definition

Stroke secondary to carotid stenosis is a group of brain disorders involving loss of brain function.

Causes

Stroke secondary to carotid stenosis occurs when blood flow to the brain is blocked. This is usually related to hardening of the arteries (atherosclerosis), particularly those arteries in the neck. Carotid stenosis means hardening of the neck arteries.

Atherosclerosis occurs when a sticky substance called plaque builds up in the inner lining of the arteries. The plaque may block or narrow an artery. A blood clot may occur at the site of the plaque. If a piece of plaque breaks off and travels to an artery in the brain, it can cause a blockage or even a stroke. The risks for stroke secondary to carotid stenosis are the same as atherosclerosis.

Stroke secondary to carotid stenosis is most common in older people. Often times, patients with stroke secondary to carotid stenosis have atherosclerotic heart disease or diabetes.

Radiation therapy to the area may also cause carotid stenosis.

Symptoms

- Weakness or total inability to move a body part
- Numbness, loss of sensation
- Tingling or other abnormal sensations
- Decreased or lost vision (may be partial or temporary)
- Language difficulties (aphasia)
- Inability to recognize or identify sensory stimuli (agnosia)
- Loss of memory
- Loss of coordination
- Swallowing difficulties
- Personality changes
- Mood and emotion changes
- Urinary incontinence (lack of control over bladder)
- Lack of control over the bowels
- Consciousness changes:
  - Sleepiness
  - Stupor, lethargy
  - Coma, unconsciousness

Exams and Tests

An exam may show:

- Blood clots in the retina
- Reflex problems
- Muscle weakness
- Decreased sensation

- A bruit (an abnormal sound heard with the stethoscope) over the carotid arteries of the neck

  The following tests may be done:

- Serum lipids blood test (may show high levels of triglycerides and cholesterol)
- Carotid or cerebral angiography
- Carotid duplex or Doppler ultrasound
- MRI of the head
- MRA (magnetic resonance angiography) of the brain vessels and neck vessels

Treatment

Medicine may be prescribed for:

- High blood pressure
- Cholesterol problem

Surgery to remove the plaque from the carotid (neck) arteries may be needed, especially if more than 70% of the carotid artery is blocked. The procedure is called carotid endarterectomy.

Outlook (Prognosis)

Stroke is a leading cause of death in the United States. About 25% of people who have a stroke die from the stroke itself or complications. About half have long-term problems.

However, 25% of people who have a stroke recover most or all of their function.

When to Contact a Medical Professional

Go to the emergency room or call the local emergency number (such as 911) if symptoms occur.

Prevention

High blood pressure, diabetes, heart disease, and other risk factors should be treated.

119

If you smoke, you should stop.

Treatment of TIA (transient ischemic attack, "warning strokes") may prevent future strokes.

Aspirin therapy (81 mg a day or 100 mg every other day) is now recommended for stroke prevention in women under 65 as long as the benefits outweigh the risks. It should be considered for women over age 65 only if their blood pressure is controlled and the benefit is greater than the risk of gastrointestinal bleeding and brain hemorrhage.

Chapter 14

Atrial Fibrillation

What Is Atrial Fibrillation?

Atrial fibrillation, or AF, is the most common arrhythmia. An arrhythmia is a problem with the speed or rhythm of the heartbeat. A disorder in the heart's electrical system causes AF and other types of arrhythmia.

AF occurs when rapid, disorganized electrical signals in the heart's two upper chambers, called the atria, cause them to contract very fast and irregularly (this is called fibrillation). As a result, blood pools in the atria and isn't pumped completely into the heart's two lower chambers, called the ventricles. When this happens, the heart's upper and lower chambers don't work together as they should.

Often, people who have AF may not even feel symptoms. However, even when not noticed, AF can lead to an increased risk of stroke. In many patients, particularly when the rhythm is extremely rapid, AF can cause chest pain, heart attack, or heart failure. AF may occur rarely or every now and then, or it may become a persistent or permanent heart rhythm lasting for years.

Understanding the Heart's Electrical System

The heart has an internal electrical system that controls the speed and rhythm of the heartbeat. With each heartbeat, an electrical signal

Excerpted from "Atrial Fibrillation," by the National Heart, Lung, and Blood Institute (NHLBI, www.nhlbi.nih.gov), part of the National Institutes of Health, June 2007.

spreads from the top of the heart to the bottom. As it travels, the signal causes the heart to contract and pump blood. The process repeats with each new heartbeat.

Each electrical signal begins in a group of cells called the sinus node, or sinoatrial (SA) node. The SA node is located in the right atrium, which is the upper right chamber of the heart. In a healthy adult heart at rest, the SA node fires off an electrical signal to begin a new heartbeat 60 to 100 times a minute. (This rate may be slower in very fit athletes.)

From the SA node, the electrical signal travels through special pathways to the right and left atria. This causes the atria to contract and pump blood into the heart's two lower chambers, the ventricles. The electrical signal then moves down to a group of cells called the atrioventricular (AV) node, located between the atria and the ventricles. Here, the signal slows down just a little, allowing the ventricles time to finish filling with blood.

The electrical signal then leaves the AV node and travels along a pathway called the bundle of His. This pathway divides into a right bundle branch and a left bundle branch. The signal goes down these branches to the ventricles, causing them to contract and pump blood out to the lungs and the rest of the body. The ventricles then relax, and the heartbeat process starts all over again in the SA node.

Understanding the Electrical Problem in Atrial Fibrillation

In AF, the heart's electrical signal begins in a different part of the atria or the nearby pulmonary veins and is conducted abnormally. The signal doesn't travel through normal pathways, but may spread throughout the atria in a rapid, disorganized way. This can cause the atria to beat more than 300 times a minute in a chaotic fashion. The atria's rapid, irregular, and uncoordinated beating is called fibrillation.

The abnormal signal from the SA node floods the AV node with electrical impulses. As a result, the ventricles also begin to beat very fast. However, the AV node can't conduct the signals to the ventricles as fast as they arrive, so even though the ventricles may be beating faster than normal, they aren't beating as fast as the atria. The atria and ventricles no longer beat in a coordinated fashion, creating a fast and irregular heart rhythm. In AF, the ventricles may beat up to 100–175 times a minute, in contrast to the normal rate of 60–100 beats a minute.

When this happens, blood isn't pumped into the ventricles as well as it should be, and the amount of blood pumped out of the ventricles is based on the randomness of the atrial beats. In AF, instead of the body receiving a constant, regular amount of blood from the ventricles, it receives rapid, small amounts and occasional random, larger amounts, depending on how much blood has flowed from the atria to the ventricles with each beat.

Most of the symptoms of AF are related to how fast the heart is beating. If medicines or age slow the heart rate, the effect of the irregular beats is minimized.

AF may be brief, with symptoms that come and go and end on their own, or it may be persistent and require treatment. Or, AF can be permanent, in which case medicines or other interventions can't restore a normal rhythm.

Outlook

People who have AF can live normal, active lives. For some people, treatment can cure AF and return their heartbeat to a normal rhythm. For people who have permanent AF, treatment can successfully control symptoms and prevent complications. Treatment consists primarily of different kinds of medicines or nonsurgical procedures.

How the Heart Works

The heart is a muscle about the size of your fist. The heart works like a pump and beats about 100,000 times a day.

The heart has two sides, separated by an inner wall called the septum. The right side of the heart pumps blood to the lungs to pick up oxygen. Then, oxygen-rich blood returns from the lungs to the left side of the heart, and the left side pumps it to the body.

The heart has four chambers and four valves and is connected to various blood vessels. Veins are the blood vessels that carry blood from the body to the heart. Arteries are the blood vessels that carry blood away from the heart to the body.

Heart Chambers

The heart has four chambers or "rooms."

- The atria are the two upper chambers that collect blood as it comes into the heart.
- The ventricles are the two lower chambers that pump blood out of the heart to the lungs or other parts of the body.

Heart Valves

Four valves control the flow of blood from the atria to the ventricles and from the ventricles into the two large arteries connected to the heart.

- The tricuspid valve is in the right side of the heart, between the right atrium and the right ventricle.

- The pulmonary valve is in the right side of the heart, between the right ventricle and the entrance to the pulmonary artery, which carries blood to the lungs.

- The mitral valve is in the left side of the heart, between the left atrium and the left ventricle.

- The aortic valve is in the left side of the heart, between the left ventricle and the entrance to the aorta, the artery that carries blood to the body.

Valves are like doors that open and close. They open to allow blood to flow through to the next chamber or to one of the arteries, and then they shut to keep blood from flowing backward.

When the heart's valves open and close, they make a "lub-DUB" sound that a doctor can hear using a stethoscope.

- The first sound—the "lub"—is made by the mitral and tricuspid valves closing at the beginning of systole. Systole is when the ventricles contract, or squeeze, and pump blood out of the heart.

- The second sound—the "DUB"—is made by the aortic and pulmonary valves closing at beginning of diastole. Diastole is when the ventricles relax and fill with blood pumped into them by the atria.

Arteries

The arteries are major blood vessels connected to your heart.

- The pulmonary artery carries blood pumped from the right side of the heart to the lungs to pick up a fresh supply of oxygen.

- The aorta is the main artery that carries oxygen-rich blood pumped from the left side of the heart out to the body.

- The coronary arteries are the other important arteries attached to the heart. They carry oxygen-rich blood from the aorta to the heart muscle, which must have its own blood supply to function.

Veins

The veins are also major blood vessels connected to your heart.

- The pulmonary veins carry oxygen-rich blood from the lungs to the left side of the heart so it can be pumped out to the body. The part of the pulmonary veins that connects to the left atrium has recently been found to often be the source of the abnormal electrical signals that can begin AF.

- The vena cava is a large vein that carries oxygen-poor blood from the body back to the heart.

Types of Atrial Fibrillation

Paroxysmal Atrial Fibrillation

In paroxysmal atrial fibrillation (AF), the abnormal electrical signals and rapid heart rate begin suddenly and then stop on their own. Symptoms can be mild or severe and last for seconds, minutes, hours, or days.

Persistent Atrial Fibrillation

Persistent AF is a condition in which the abnormal heart rhythm continues until it's stopped with treatment.

Permanent Atrial Fibrillation

Permanent AF is a condition in which the normal heart rhythm can't be restored with the usual treatments. Both paroxysmal and persistent atrial fibrillation may become more frequent and eventually result in permanent AF.

Other Names for Atrial Fibrillation

- A fib
- Auricular fibrillation

What Causes Atrial Fibrillation?

Atrial fibrillation (AF) occurs when the electrical signals traveling through the heart are conducted abnormally and become disorganized and very rapid.

This is the result of damage to the heart's electrical system. This damage is most often the result of other conditions, such as coronary artery disease or high blood pressure, that affect the health of the heart. Sometimes, the cause of AF is unknown.

Who Is at Risk for Atrial Fibrillation?

Populations Affected

More than 2 million people in the United States have atrial fibrillation (AF), and it affects both men and women. AF generally occurs in older people, mostly because they're more likely to have heart disease or conditions that increase the risk of AF. AF is uncommon among young people.

Major Risk Factors

AF is more common in people with heart diseases or conditions, including:

- coronary artery disease;
- heart failure;
- rheumatic heart disease;
- structural defects, such as mitral valve disorders;
- pericarditis (inflammation of the tissues surrounding the heart);
- congenital heart defects; and
- sick sinus syndrome (a condition in which the heart's electrical signals don't fire properly and the heart rate slows down; sometimes the heart will switch back and forth between a too-slow rate and a too-fast rate).

AF also is more common in people who are having a heart attack or who have just had surgery.

Other conditions that increase AF risk include hyperthyroidism, obesity, high blood pressure (hypertension), diabetes, and lung diseases.

Recent evidence suggests that patients who receive high-dose steroid therapy are at increased risk of AF. This therapy, which is commonly used for asthma and certain inflammatory conditions, may act as a trigger in people who already have other risk factors for AF.

What Are the Signs and Symptoms of Atrial Fibrillation?

Signs and Symptoms

Atrial fibrillation (AF) usually causes the ventricles to contract faster than normal. When this happens, the ventricles don't have enough time to fill completely with blood to pump to the lungs and body. This inefficient pumping can cause signs and symptoms, such as:

- palpitations (a strong feeling of a fast heartbeat or a "thumping" in the chest);
- shortness of breath;
- weakness or difficulty exercising;
- chest pain;
- dizziness or fainting;
- fatigue (tiredness); and
- confusion.

Complications

AF has two major complications—stroke and heart failure. Heart attack is another, rarer complication.

Stroke

During AF, the atria don't pump all of their blood to the ventricles. Some blood pools in the atria. When this happens, a blood clot (also called a thrombus) can form. If the clot breaks off and travels to the brain, it can cause a stroke. (A clot that forms in one part of the body and travels in the bloodstream to another part of the body is called an embolus.)

Blood-thinning medicines to reduce the risk of stroke are a very important part of treatment for patients who have AF.

Heart Failure

Heart failure occurs when the heart can't pump enough blood to meet the body's needs. Because the ventricles are beating very fast and aren't able to properly fill with blood to pump out to the body, AF can lead to heart failure.

Fatigue and shortness of breath are common symptoms of heart failure. A buildup of fluid in the lungs causes these symptoms. Fluid also can build up in the feet, ankles, and legs, causing weight gain.

Lifestyle changes, medicines, and sometimes special care (rarely, a mechanical heart pump or heart transplant) are the main treatments for heart failure.

How Is Atrial Fibrillation Diagnosed?

Sometimes people have atrial fibrillation (AF), but don't have symptoms. For these people, AF is often found during a physical exam or EKG (electrocardiogram) test done for another purpose. Other times, AF is diagnosed after a person goes to the doctor because of symptoms.

To understand why a person has AF and the best way to treat it, the doctor will want to discover any immediate or underlying causes. Doctors use several methods to diagnose AF, including family and medical history, a physical exam, and several diagnostic tests and procedures.

Specialists Involved

A primary care doctor often is involved in the initial diagnosis and treatment of AF. These doctors can include family practitioners and internists.

Doctors who specialize in the diagnosis and treatment of heart disease also may be involved, such as cardiologists (doctors who take care of adults with heart problems) and electrophysiologists (cardiologists who specialize in arrhythmias).

Family and Medical History

The doctor will ask questions about:

- **Symptoms.** What symptoms are you having? Have you had palpitations (a feeling of a strong or fast heartbeat)? Are you dizzy or short of breath? Are your feet or ankles swollen (a possible sign of heart failure)? Do you have any chest pain?

- **Medical history.** This includes other health problems, such as a history of heart disease, high blood pressure, lung disease, diabetes, or thyroid problems.

- **Family medical history.** Does anyone in your family have a history of AF? Has anyone in your family ever had heart disease or high blood pressure? Has anyone had thyroid problems? Are there other illnesses or health problems in your family?

- **Health habits.** These include smoking and alcohol or caffeine use.

Physical Exam

The doctor will do a complete cardiac exam, listening to the rate and rhythm of your heartbeat and taking your pulse and blood pressure reading. The doctor will likely check to see whether you have any sign of problems with your heart muscle or valves. He or she will listen to your lungs to check for signs of heart failure.

The doctor also will check for swelling in the legs or feet and look for an enlarged thyroid gland or other signs of hyperthyroidism.

Diagnostic Tests and Procedures

EKG. An EKG is a simple test that detects and records the electrical activity of your heart. It is the most useful test for diagnosing AF. It shows how fast the heart is beating and its rhythm (steady or irregular). It also records the timing of the electrical signals as they pass through each part of the heart.

A standard EKG test only records the heartbeat for a few seconds. It won't detect an AF episode that doesn't happen during the test. To diagnose paroxysmal AF, the doctor may ask you to wear a portable EKG monitor that can record your heartbeat for longer periods. The two most common types of portable EKGs are Holter and event monitors.

Holter Monitor. Also called an ambulatory EKG, this device records the electrical signals of the heart for a full 24- or 48-hour period. You wear small patches called electrodes on your chest that are connected by wires to a small, portable recorder. The recorder can be clipped to a belt, kept in a pocket, or hung around your neck.

During the time you're wearing a Holter monitor, you do your usual daily activities and keep a notebook, noting any symptoms you have and the time they occurred. You then return both the recorder and the notebook to the doctor to read the results. The doctor can see how your heart was beating at the time you had symptoms.

Event Monitor. Event monitors are useful to diagnose AF that occurs only once in a while. The device is worn continuously, but only records the heart's electrical activity when you push a button. You push the button on the device when you feel symptoms. Event monitors can be worn for 1 to 2 months, or as long as it takes to get a recording of the heart when symptoms are occurring.

Other Tests Used to Diagnose Atrial Fibrillation

Echocardiogram. This test uses sound waves to create a moving picture of your heart. An echocardiogram provides information about the size and shape of your heart and how well your heart chambers and valves are functioning. The test also can identify areas of poor blood flow to the heart, areas of heart muscle that aren't contracting normally, and previous injury to the heart muscle caused by poor blood flow.

This test is sometimes called a transthoracic echocardiogram. It's noninvasive and is done by placing an echo "probe" on your chest wall. The procedure is the same technique used for obtaining sonograms in pregnant women.

Transesophageal Echocardiogram. A transesophageal echocardiogram, or TEE, takes pictures of the heart through your esophagus (the tube leading from your mouth to your stomach). The atria are deep in the chest and often can't be seen very well on a regular echocardiogram. A doctor can see the atria much better with a TEE. In this test, the transducer is attached to the end of a flexible tube that's guided down your throat and into your esophagus. TEE is usually done while the patient is under some sedation. TEE is used to detect clots that may be developing in the atria because of AF.

Blood Tests. These tests check the level of thyroid hormone and the balance of your body's electrolytes. Electrolytes are minerals in your blood and body fluids that are essential for normal health and functioning of your body's cells and organs.

How Is Atrial Fibrillation Treated?

Treatment for atrial fibrillation (AF) depends on how severe or frequent the symptoms are and whether you already have heart disease. General treatment options include medicines, medical procedures, and lifestyle changes.

Treatment of AF is designed to:

- prevent blood clots from forming, and thereby reduce the risk for stroke.

- control how many times a minute the ventricles contract. This is called rate control. Rate control is important because it allows the ventricles enough time to completely fill with blood. With this approach, the irregular heart rhythm continues, but the person feels better and has fewer symptoms.

- restore the heart to a normal rhythm. This is called rhythm control. Rhythm control allows the atria and ventricles to work together again to efficiently pump blood to the body.

- treat any underlying disorder that's causing or raising the risk of AF—for example, hyperthyroidism.

Who Needs Treatment for Atrial Fibrillation?

People with no symptoms and no related heart problems may not need treatment. AF may even go back to a permanent normal heart rhythm on its own. In some people who have AF for the first time, doctors may choose to use an electrical procedure or medicine to re-store the heart rhythm to normal.

Repeated episodes of AF tend to cause changes to the electrical system of the heart, leading to persistent or permanent AF. Most people with persistent or permanent AF need treatment to control their heart rate and prevent complications.

Specific Types of Treatment

Blood Clot Prevention. The risk of a blood clot traveling from the heart to the brain and causing a stroke is increased in people who have AF. Preventing the formation of blood clots is probably the most im-portant part of treating AF. Doctors prescribe blood-thinning medicines to prevent blood clots. These medicines include warfarin (Coumadin®), heparin, and aspirin.

Warfarin is the most effective medicine in people with risk factors for stroke. People taking warfarin must have regular blood tests to check how well the medicine is working.

Rate Control. Doctors also prescribe medicines to slow down the rate at which the ventricles are beating. These medicines help bring the heart rate to a normal level.

Rate control is the recommended strategy for most patients with AF, even though the heart rhythm continues to be abnormal and the heart doesn't work as efficiently as it could. Most people feel better and can function well if their heart rate is well controlled.

Medicines used to control the heart rate include beta blockers (for example, metoprolol and atenolol), calcium channel blockers (diltiazem and verapamil), and digitalis (digoxin). Several other medicines also are available.

Rhythm Control. Doctors use medicines or procedures to restore and maintain the heart's rhythm. This treatment approach is recommended for people who aren't functioning well with rate control treatment or who have only recently started having AF.

The longer you have AF, the less likely it is that an abnormal heart rhythm can be restored to a normal heart rhythm. This is especially true for people who have had AF for 6 months or more.

Restoring a normal rhythm also becomes less likely if the atria become enlarged or if any underlying heart disease becomes more severe. In these situations, the chance that AF will recur is high, even if you're taking a medicine to help convert AF to a normal rhythm.

Medicines. Medicines used to control a person's heart rhythm include amiodarone, sotalol, flecainide, propafenone, dofetilide, ibutilide, and occasionally older medicines such as quinidine, procainamide, and disopyramide.

Medicines must be carefully tailored to the person taking them because they can cause a different kind of irregular, slow, or rapid heartbeat (arrhythmia) or can be harmful in people who have underlying diseases of the heart or other organs. This is particularly true for those patients who have an unusual heart rhythm problem called Wolff-Parkinson-White syndrome.

To convert AF to a normal heart rhythm, people can be given AF medicines regularly by injection at a doctor's office, clinic, or hospital. Or, to try to control AF or prevent recurrences, people may take pills on an ongoing basis. If the doctor knows how a person will react to a medicine, a specific dose may be prescribed according to the "pill in the pocket" technique. This means that a patient takes a specific dose of a medicine as needed only if he or she has an episode of AF, but not on a regular, daily basis.

Procedures. Doctors use several procedures to restore a normal heart rhythm, including:

- Electrical cardioversion, which is a jolt of electricity delivered to the heart to "convert" the rhythm from AF back to a normal heart rhythm. This shock can break the pattern of abnormal electrical signals and restore a normal rhythm. Electrical cardioversion isn't the same as the emergency heart shocking procedure often seen on TV programs. It's planned in advance and done under carefully controlled conditions with the person heavily sedated. Before doing electrical cardioversion, the doctor may recommend a transesophageal echocardiogram (TEE) to rule out the presence of blood clots in the atria. If clots are present, the patient may need to receive blood-thinning medicines to help eliminate the clots before the electrical cardioversion.

- Radiofrequency ablation, which is used to restore a normal heart rhythm when medicines or electrical cardioversion don't work. In this procedure, a wire is inserted through a vein in the leg or arm and threaded to the heart. Radiowave energy is sent through the wire to destroy abnormal tissue that's believed to be disrupting the normal flow of electrical signals. This procedure is usually done in the hospital and is performed by an electrophysiologist.

- Maze procedure, in which a surgeon makes small cuts or burns in the atria to reduce the chances of chaotic electrical activity happening in the atria. This procedure requires open-heart surgery, so it's usually performed when a person requires heart surgery for other reasons, such as for valve disease, which can increase the risk of AF.

Approaches to Treating Underlying Causes and Reducing Risk Factors. The doctor also may suggest other approaches designed to treat the underlying condition that may be causing AF or to reduce risk factors for AF. These approaches include prescribing medicines to treat an overactive thyroid, reduce blood pressure and overweight, or treat other underlying causes of AF.

The doctor also may recommended lifestyle changes, such as reducing stress, quitting smoking, reducing salt intake (to help lower blood pressure), and eating healthily. Limiting or avoiding stress as well as alcohol, caffeine, or other stimulants that may increase your heart rate also may help to reduce the risk of AF.

How Can Atrial Fibrillation Be Prevented?

You may be able to prevent atrial fibrillation (AF) by leading a healthy lifestyle and taking steps to lower your risk for heart disease. These steps include:

- not smoking;

- following a heart healthy diet that is low in saturated fat, trans fat, and cholesterol and that includes a variety of grains, fruits, and vegetables daily;

- getting regular physical activity; and

- maintaining a healthy weight.

If you have heart disease or risk factors, you should work with your doctor to control your condition and lower your risk of complications, such as AF. In addition to following the healthy lifestyle steps above, which also can help control heart disease, your doctor may advise you to take one or more of the following steps:

- Follow the DASH [Dietary Approaches to Stop Hypertension] eating plan to help lower your blood pressure.

- Keep your cholesterol (total cholesterol, high-density lipoprotein [HDL], and low-density lipoprotein [LDL]) and triglycerides at healthy levels with dietary changes and/or medicines.

- Limit or avoid alcohol.

- Control blood glucose (blood sugar) levels if you have diabetes.

- Get regular checkups.

- Take medicines as directed.

Living with Atrial Fibrillation

People who have atrial fibrillation (AF)—even permanent AF—can live normal, active lives.

If you have AF, you should:

- Keep all your medical appointments.

- Bring all the medicines you're taking to every doctor and emergency room visit. This will help your doctor know exactly what medicines you're taking.

- Follow your doctor's instructions for taking medicines. Be careful about taking over-the-counter medicines, nutritional supplements, or cold and allergy medicines, because some contain stimulants that can trigger rapid heart rhythms.

- Some over-the-counter medicines can have harmful interactions with heart rhythm medicines.

- Tell your doctor if you're having side effects from your medicines, if your symptoms are getting worse, or if you have new symptoms.

- If you're taking blood-thinning medicines, you will need to be monitored carefully, including getting regular blood tests to check how the medicines are working. Talk with your doctor about your monitoring program.

- Talk with your doctor about diet, physical activity, weight control, and alcohol use.

Chapter 15

Congenital Conditions That Increase Stroke Risk

Chapter Contents

Section 15.1

Arteriovenous Malformations

"Arteriovenous Malformations and Other Vascular Lesions of the Central Nervous System Fact Sheet" is from the National Institute of Neurological Disorders and Stroke (NINDS, www.ninds.nih.gov), February 9, 2007.

What are arteriovenous malformations?

Arteriovenous malformations (AVMs) are defects of the circulatory system that are generally believed to arise during embryonic or fetal development or soon after birth. They are comprised of snarled tangles of arteries and veins. Arteries carry oxygen-rich blood away from the heart to the body's cells; veins return oxygen-depleted blood to the lungs and heart. The presence of an AVM disrupts this vital cyclical process. Although AVMs can develop in many different sites, those located in the brain or spinal cord—the two parts of the central nervous system—can have especially widespread effects on the body.

AVMs of the brain or spinal cord (neurological AVMs) are believed to affect approximately 300,000 Americans. They occur in males and females of all racial or ethnic backgrounds at roughly equal rates.

What are the symptoms?

Most people with neurological AVMs experience few, if any, significant symptoms, and the malformations tend to be discovered only incidentally, usually either at autopsy or during treatment for an unrelated disorder. But for about 12 percent of the affected population (about 36,000 of the estimated 300,000 Americans with AVMs), these abnormalities cause symptoms that vary greatly in severity. For a small fraction of the individuals within this group, such symptoms are severe enough to become debilitating or even life-threatening. Each year about 1 percent of those with AVMs will die as a direct result of the AVM.

Seizures and headaches are the most generalized symptoms of AVMs, but no particular type of seizure or headache pattern has been identified. Seizures can be partial or total, involving a loss of control over movement, convulsions, or a change in a person's level of consciousness. Headaches can vary greatly in frequency, duration, and intensity, sometimes becoming as severe as migraines. Sometimes a headache consistently affecting one side of the head may be closely linked to the site of an AVM. More frequently, however, the location of the pain is not specific to the lesion and may encompass most of the head.

AVMs also can cause a wide range of more specific neurological symptoms that vary from person to person, depending primarily upon the location of the AVM. Such symptoms may include muscle weakness or paralysis in one part of the body; a loss of coordination (ataxia) that can lead to such problems as gait disturbances; apraxia, or difficulties carrying out tasks that require planning; dizziness; visual disturbances such as a loss of part of the visual field; an inability to control eye movement; papilledema (swelling of a part of the optic nerve known as the optic disk); various problems using or understanding language (aphasia); abnormal sensations such as numbness, tingling, or spontaneous pain (paresthesia or dysesthesia); memory deficits; and mental confusion, hallucinations, or dementia. Researchers have recently uncovered evidence that AVMs may also cause subtle learning or behavioral disorders in some people during their childhood or adolescence, long before more obvious symptoms become evident.

One of the more distinctive signs indicating the presence of an AVM is an auditory phenomenon called a bruit, coined from the French word meaning noise. (A sign is a physical effect observable by a physician, but not by a patient.) Doctors use this term to describe the rhythmic, whooshing sound caused by excessively rapid blood flow through the arteries and veins of an AVM. The sound is similar to that made by a torrent of water rushing through a narrow pipe. A bruit can sometimes become a symptom—that is, an effect experienced by a patient—when it is especially severe. When audible to patients, the bruit may compromise hearing, disturb sleep, or cause significant psychological distress.

Symptoms caused by AVMs can appear at any age, but because these abnormalities tend to result from a slow buildup of neurological damage over time they are most often noticed when people are in their twenties, thirties, or forties. If AVMs do not become symptomatic by the time people reach their late forties or early fifties, they tend to remain stable and rarely produce symptoms. In women, pregnancy sometimes causes a sudden onset or worsening of symptoms, due to accompanying cardiovascular changes, especially increases in blood volume and blood pressure.

In contrast to the vast majority of neurological AVMs, one especially severe type causes symptoms to appear at, or very soon after, birth. Called a vein of Galen defect after the major blood vessel involved, this lesion is located deep inside the brain. It is frequently associated with hydrocephalus (an accumulation of fluid within certain spaces in the brain, often with visible enlargement of the head), swollen veins visible on the scalp, seizures, failure to thrive, and congestive heart failure. Children born with this condition who survive past infancy often remain developmentally impaired.

How do AVMs damage the brain and spinal cord?

AVMs become symptomatic only when the damage they cause to the brain or spinal cord reaches a critical level. This is one of the reasons why a relatively small fraction of people with these lesions experiences significant health problems related to the condition. AVMs damage the brain or spinal cord through three basic mechanisms: by reducing the amount of oxygen reaching neurological tissues; by causing bleeding (hemorrhage) into surrounding tissues; and by compressing or displacing parts of the brain or spinal cord.

AVMs compromise oxygen delivery to the brain or spinal cord by altering normal patterns of blood flow. Arteries and veins are normally interconnected by a series of progressively smaller blood vessels that control and slow the rate of blood flow. Oxygen delivery to surrounding tissues takes place through the thin, porous walls of the smallest of these interconnecting vessels, known as capillaries, where the blood flows most slowly. The arteries and veins that make up AVMs, however, lack this intervening capillary network. Instead, arteries dump blood directly into veins through a passageway called a fistula. The flow rate is uncontrolled and extremely rapid—too rapid to allow oxygen to be dispersed to surrounding tissues. When starved of normal amounts of oxygen, the cells that make up these tissues begin to deteriorate, sometimes dying off completely.

This abnormally rapid rate of blood flow frequently causes blood pressure inside the vessels located in the central portion of an AVM directly adjacent to the fistula—an area doctors refer to as the nidus, from the Latin word for nest—to rise to dangerously high levels. The arteries feeding blood into the AVM often become swollen and distorted; the veins that drain blood away from it often become abnormally constricted (a condition called stenosis). Moreover, the walls of the involved arteries and veins are often abnormally thin and weak. Aneurysms—balloon-like bulges in blood vessel walls that are susceptible to rupture—may develop in association with approximately half of all neurological AVMs due to this structural weakness.

Bleeding can result from this combination of high internal pressure and vessel wall weakness. Such hemorrhages are often microscopic in size, causing limited damage and few significant symptoms. Even many nonsymptomatic AVMs show evidence of past bleeding. But massive hemorrhages can occur if the physical stresses caused by extremely high blood pressure, rapid blood flow rates, and vessel wall weakness are great enough. If a large enough volume of blood escapes from a ruptured AVM into the surrounding brain, the result can be a catastrophic stroke. AVMs account for approximately 2 percent of all hemorrhagic strokes that occur each year.

Even in the absence of bleeding or significant oxygen depletion, large AVMs can damage the brain or spinal cord simply by their presence. They can range in size from a fraction of an inch to more than 2.5 inches in diameter, depending on the number and size of the blood vessels making up the lesion. The larger the lesion, the greater the amount of pressure it exerts on surrounding brain or spinal cord structures. The largest lesions may compress several inches of the spinal cord or distort the shape of an entire hemisphere of the brain. Such massive AVMs can constrict the flow of cerebrospinal fluid—a clear liquid that normally nourishes and protects the brain and spinal cord—by distorting or closing the passageways and open chambers (ventricles) inside the brain that allow this fluid to circulate freely. As cerebrospinal fluid accumulates, hydrocephalus results. This fluid buildup further increases the amount of pressure on fragile neurological structures, adding to the damage caused by the AVM itself.

Where do neurological AVMs tend to form?

AVMs can form virtually anywhere in the brain or spinal cord—wherever arteries and veins exist. Some are formed from blood vessels located in the dura mater or in the pia mater, the outermost and innermost, respectively, of the three membranes surrounding the brain and spinal cord. (The third membrane, called the arachnoid, lacks blood vessels.) AVMs affecting the spinal cord are of two types, AVMs of the dura mater, which affect the function of the spinal cord by transmitting excess pressure to the venous system of the spinal cord, and AVMs of the spinal cord itself, which affect the function of the spinal cord by hemorrhage, by reducing blood flow to the spinal cord, or by causing excess venous pressure. Spinal AVMs frequently cause attacks of sudden, severe back pain, often concentrated at the roots of nerve fibers where they exit the vertebrae; the pain is similar to that caused by a slipped disk. These lesions also can cause sensory disturbances, muscle weakness, or paralysis in the parts of the body served by the spinal cord or the damaged nerve fibers. Spinal cord injury by the AVM by either of the mechanisms described above can lead to degeneration of the nerve fibers within the spinal cord below the level of the lesion, causing widespread paralysis in parts of the body controlled by those nerve fibers.

Dural and pial AVMs can appear anywhere on the surface of the brain. Those located on the surface of the cerebral hemispheres—the uppermost portions of the brain—exert pressure on the cerebral cortex, the brain's "gray matter." Depending on their location, these AVMs may damage portions of the cerebral cortex involved with thinking, speaking, understanding language, hearing, taste, touch, or initiating and controlling voluntary movements. AVMs located on the frontal lobe close to the optic nerve or on the occipital lobe, the rear portion of the cerebrum where images are processed, may cause a variety of visual disturbances.

AVMs also can form from blood vessels located deep inside the interior of the cerebrum. These AVMs may compromise the functions of three vital structures: the thalamus, which transmits nerve signals between the spinal cord and upper regions of the brain; the basal ganglia surrounding the thalamus, which coordinate complex movements; and the hippocampus, which plays a major role in memory.

AVMs can affect other parts of the brain besides the cerebrum. The hindbrain is formed from two major structures: the cerebellum, which is nestled under the rear portion of the cerebrum, and the brainstem, which serves as the bridge linking the upper portions of the brain with the spinal cord. These structures control finely coordinated movements, maintain balance, and regulate some functions of internal organs, including those of the heart and lungs. AVM damage to these parts of the hindbrain can result in dizziness, giddiness, vomiting, a loss of the ability to coordinate complex movements such as walking, or uncontrollable muscle tremors.

What are the health consequences of AVMs?

The greatest potential danger posed by AVMs is hemorrhage. Researchers believe that each year between 2 and 4 percent of all AVMs hemorrhage. Most episodes of bleeding remain undetected at the time they occur because they are not severe enough to cause significant neurological damage. But massive, even fatal, bleeding episodes do occur. The present state of knowledge does not permit doctors to predict whether or not any particular person with an AVM will suffer an extensive hemorrhage. The lesions can remain stable or can suddenly begin to grow. In a few cases, they have been observed to regress spontaneously. Whenever an AVM is detected, the individual should be carefully and consistently monitored for any signs of instability that may indicate an increased risk of hemorrhage.

A few physical characteristics appear to indicate a greater-than-usual likelihood of clinically significant hemorrhage. Smaller AVMs have a greater likelihood of bleeding than do larger ones. Impaired drainage by unusually narrow or deeply situated veins also increases the chances of hemorrhage. Pregnancy also appears to increase the likelihood of clinically significant hemorrhage, mainly because of increases in blood pressure and blood volume. Finally, AVMs that have hemorrhaged once are about nine times more likely to bleed again during the first year after the initial hemorrhage than are lesions that have never bled.

The damaging effects of a hemorrhage are related to lesion location. Bleeding from AVMs located deep inside the interior tissues, or parenchyma, of the brain typically causes more severe neurological damage than does hemorrhage by lesions that have formed in the dural or pial membranes or on the surface of the brain or spinal cord. (Deeply located bleeding is usually referred to as an intracerebral or parenchymal hemorrhage; bleeding within the membranes or on the surface of the brain is known as subdural or subarachnoid hemorrhage.) Thus, location is an important factor to consider when weighing the relative risks of surgical versus non-surgical treatment of AVMs.

What other types of vascular lesions affect the central nervous system?

Besides AVMs, three other main types of vascular lesion can arise in the brain or spinal cord: cavernous malformations, capillary telangiectases, and venous malformations. These lesions may form virtually anywhere within the central nervous system, but unlike AVMs, they are not caused by high-velocity blood flow from arteries into veins. In contrast, cavernous malformations, telangiectases, and venous malformations are all low-flow lesions. Instead of a combination of arteries and veins, each one involves only one type of blood vessel. These lesions are less unstable than AVMs and do not pose the same relatively high risk of significant hemorrhage.

In general, low-flow lesions tend to cause fewer troubling neurological symptoms and require less aggressive treatment than do AVMs.

- **Cavernous malformations.** These lesions are formed from groups of tightly packed, abnormally thin-walled, small blood vessels that displace normal neurological tissue in the brain or spinal cord. The vessels are filled with slow-moving or stagnant blood that is usually clotted or in a state of decomposition. Like AVMs, cavernous malformations can range in size from a few fractions of an inch to several inches in diameter, depending on the number of blood vessels involved. Some people develop multiple lesions. Although cavernous malformations usually do not hemorrhage as severely as AVMs do, they sometimes leak blood into surrounding neurological tissues because the walls of the involved blood vessels are extremely fragile. Although they are often not as symptomatic as AVMs, cavernous malformations can cause seizures in some people. After AVMs, cavernous malformations are the type of vascular lesion most likely to require treatment.

- **Capillary telangiectases.** These lesions consist of groups of abnormally swollen capillaries and usually measure less than an inch in diameter. Capillaries are the smallest of all blood vessels, with diameters smaller than that of a human hair; they have the capacity to transport only small quantities of blood, and blood flows through these vessels very slowly. Because of these factors, telangiectases rarely cause extensive damage to surrounding brain or spinal cord tissues. Any isolated hemorrhages that occur are microscopic in size. Thus, the lesions are usually benign. However, in some inherited disorders in which people develop large numbers of these lesions, telangiectases can contribute to the development of nonspecific neurological symptoms such as headaches or seizures.

- **Venous malformations.** These lesions consist of abnormally enlarged veins. The structural defect usually does not interfere with the function of the blood vessels, which is to drain oxygen-depleted blood away from the body's tissues and return it to the lungs and heart. Venous malformations rarely hemorrhage. As with telangiectases, most venous malformations do not produce symptoms, remain undetected, and follow a benign course.

What causes vascular lesions?

Although the cause of these vascular anomalies of the central nervous system is not yet well understood, scientists believe that they most often result from mistakes that occur during embryonic or fetal development. These mistakes may be linked to genetic mutations in some cases. A few types of vascular malformations are known to be hereditary and thus are known to have a genetic basis. Some evidence also suggests that at least some of these lesions are acquired later in life as a result of injury to the central nervous system.

During fetal development, new blood vessels continuously form and then disappear as the human body changes and grows. These changes in the body's vascular map continue after birth and are controlled by angiogenic factors, chemicals produced by the body that stimulate new blood vessel formation and growth. Researchers have recently identified changes in the chemical structures of various angiogenic factors in some people who have AVMs or other vascular abnormalities of the central nervous system. However, it is not yet clear how these chemical changes actually cause changes in blood vessel structure.

By studying patterns of familial occurrence, researchers have established that one type of cavernous malformation involving multiple lesion formation is caused by a genetic mutation in chromosome 7. This genetic mutation appears in many ethnic groups, but it is especially frequent in a large population of Hispanic Americans living in the Southwest; these individuals share a common ancestor in whom the genetic change occurred. Some other types of vascular defects of the central nervous system are part of larger medical syndromes known to be hereditary. They include hereditary hemorrhagic telangiectasia (also known as Osler-Weber-Rendu disease), Sturge-Weber syndrome, Klippel-Trenaunay syndrome, Parkes-Weber syndrome, and Wyburn-Mason syndrome.

How are AVMs and other vascular lesions detected?

Physicians now use an array of traditional and new imaging technologies to uncover the presence of AVMs. Angiography provides the most accurate pictures of blood vessel structure in AVMs. The technique requires injecting a special water-soluble dye, called a contrast agent, into an artery. The dye highlights the structure of blood vessels so that it can be recorded on conventional X-rays. Although angiography can record fine details of vascular lesions, the procedure is somewhat invasive and carries a slight risk of causing a stroke. Its safety, however, has recently been improved through the development of more precise techniques for delivering dye to the site of an AVM. Superselective angiography involves inserting a thin, flexible tube called a catheter into an artery; a physician guides the tip of the catheter to the site of the lesion and then releases a small amount of contrast agent directly into the lesion.

Two of the most frequently employed noninvasive imaging technologies used to detect AVMs are computed axial tomography (CT) and magnetic resonance imaging (MRI) scans. CT scans use X-rays to create a series of cross-sectional images of the head, brain, or spinal cord and are especially useful in revealing the presence of hemorrhage. MRI imaging, however, offers superior diagnostic information by using magnetic fields to detect subtle changes in neurological tissues. A recently developed application of MRI technology—magnetic resonance angiography (MRA)—can record the pattern and velocity of blood flow through vascular lesions as well as the flow of cerebrospinal fluid throughout the brain and spinal cord. CT, MRI, and MRA can provide three-dimensional representations of AVMs by taking images from multiple angles.

How can AVMs and other vascular lesions be treated?

Medication can often alleviate general symptoms such as headache, back pain, and seizures caused by AVMs and other vascular lesions. However, the definitive treatment for AVMs is either surgery or focused irradiation therapy. Venous malformations and capillary telangiectases rarely require surgery; moreover, their structures are diffuse and usually not suitable for surgical correction and they usually do not require treatment anyway. Cavernous malformations are usually well defined enough for surgical removal, but surgery on these lesions is less common than for AVMs because they do not pose the same risk of hemorrhage.

The decision to perform surgery on any individual with an AVM requires a careful consideration of possible benefits versus risks. The natural history of an individual AVM is difficult to predict; however, left untreated, they have the potential of causing significant hemorrhage, which may result in serious neurological deficits or death. On the other hand, surgery on any part of the central nervous system carries its own risks as well; AVM surgery is associated with an estimated 8 percent risk of serious complications or death. There is no easy formula that can allow physicians and their patients to reach a decision on the best course of therapy—all therapeutic decisions must be made on a case-by-case basis.

Today, three surgical options exist for the treatment of AVMs: conventional surgery, endovascular embolization, and radiosurgery. The choice of treatment depends largely on the size and location of an AVM.

Conventional surgery involves entering the brain or spinal cord and removing the central portion of the AVM, including the fistula, while causing as little damage as possible to surrounding neurological structures. This surgery is most appropriate when an AVM is located in a superficial portion of the brain or spinal cord and is relatively small in size. AVMs located deep inside the brain generally cannot be approached through conventional surgical techniques because there is too great a possibility that functionally important brain tissue will be damaged or destroyed.

Endovascular embolization and radiosurgery are less invasive than conventional surgery and offer safer treatment options for some AVMs located deep inside the brain. In endovascular embolization the surgeon guides a catheter though the arterial network until the tip reaches the site of the AVM. The surgeon then introduces a substance that will plug the fistula, correcting the abnormal pattern of blood flow. This process is known as embolization because it causes an embolus (a blood clot) to travel through blood vessels, eventually becoming lodged in a vessel and obstructing blood flow. The materials used to create an artificial blood clot in the center of an AVM include fast-drying biologically inert glues, fibered titanium coils, and tiny balloons. Since embolization usually does not permanently obliterate the AVM, it is usually used as an adjunct to surgery or to radiosurgery to reduce the blood flow through the AVM and make the surgery safer.

Radiosurgery is an even less invasive therapeutic approach. It involves aiming a beam of highly focused radiation directly on the AVM. The high dose of radiation damages the walls of the blood vessels making up the lesion. Over the course of the next several months, the irradiated vessels gradually degenerate and eventually close, leading to the resolution of the AVM.

Embolization frequently proves incomplete or temporary, although in recent years new embolization materials have led to improved results. Radiosurgery often has incomplete results as well, particularly when an AVM is large, and it poses the additional risk of radiation damage to surrounding normal tissues. Moreover, even when successful, complete closure of an AVM takes place over the course of many months following radiosurgery. During that period, the risk of hemorrhage is still present. However, both techniques now offer the possibility of treating deeply situated AVMs that had previously been

147

inaccessible. And in many patients, staged embolization followed by conventional surgical removal or by radiosurgery is now performed, resulting in further reductions in mortality and complication rates.

Because so many variables are involved in treating AVMs, doctors must assess the danger posed to individual patients largely on a case-by-case basis. The consequences of hemorrhage are potentially disastrous, leading many clinicians to recommend surgical intervention whenever the physical characteristics of an AVM appear to indicate a greater-than-usual likelihood of significant bleeding and resultant neurological damage.

What research is being done?

Within the federal government, the National Institute of Neurological Disorders and Stroke (NINDS), a division of the National Institutes of Health (NIH), has primary responsibility for sponsoring research on neurological disorders. As part of its mission, the NINDS conducts research on AVMs and other vascular lesions of the central nervous system and supports studies through grants to major medical institutions across the country.

In partnership with the medical school of Columbia University, the NINDS has established a long-term Arteriovenous Study Group to learn more about the natural course of AVMs in patients and to improve the surgical treatment of these lesions.

Another group of NINDS-sponsored researchers is currently studying large populations of patients with AVMs to formulate criteria that will allow doctors to predict more accurately the risk of hemorrhage in individual patients. Of particular importance is the role that high blood pressure within the lesion plays in the onset of hemorrhage. Other scientists are examining the genetic basis of familial cavernous malformations and other hereditary syndromes that cause neurological vascular lesions, including ataxia telangiectasia.

Other scientists are seeking to refine the techniques now available to treat AVMs. Radiosurgery is a special area of interest because this technology is still in its infancy. An ongoing study is closely examining the precise effects that radiation exposure has on vascular tissue in order to improve the predictability and consistency of treatment results.

Finally, several ongoing studies are devoted to developing new noninvasive neuroimaging technologies to increase the effectiveness and safety of AVM surgery. Some scientists are pioneering the use of MRI to measure amounts of oxygen present in the brain tissue of patients with vascular lesions in order to predict the brain's response to surgical therapies. Others are developing a new micro-imager that may be inserted into catheters to increase the accuracy of angiography. In addition, new types of noninvasive imaging devices are being developed that detect functional brain activity through changes in tissue light emission or reflectance. This technology may prove more sensitive than MRI and other imaging devices currently available, giving surgeons a new tool for improving the efficacy and safety of AVM surgery.

Section 15.2

Sickle Cell Anemia

Excerpted from "Facts About Sickle Cell Disease," by the Centers for Disease Control and Prevention (CDC), National Center on Birth Defects and Developmental Disabilities (NCBDDD, www.cdc.gov/ncbddd), January 2007.

Sickle cell disease (SCD) is a group of inherited red blood cell disorders. Healthy red blood cells are round, and they move through small blood vessels to carry oxygen to all parts of the body. In sickle cell disease, the red blood cells become hard and sticky and look like a C-shaped farm tool called a "sickle." The sickle cells die early, which causes a constant shortage of red blood cells. Also, when they travel through small blood vessels, they get stuck and clog the blood flow. This can cause pain and other serious problems.

What causes sickle cell disease?

Sickle cell disease is a genetic condition that is present at birth. It is inherited when a child receives two sickle cell genes—one from each parent.

How is it diagnosed?

Sickle cell disease is diagnosed with a simple blood test. It is most often found at birth during routine newborn screening tests at the hospital. In addition, sickle cell disease can be diagnosed before birth.

Because children with sickle cell disease are at an increased risk of infection and other health problems, early diagnosis and treatment are important.

What are the symptoms and complications and how are they treated?

People with sickle cell disease start to have symptoms during the first year of life, usually around 5 months of age. Symptoms and complications of sickle cell disease are different for each person and can range from mild to severe. They include:

- hand-foot syndrome;
- pain episode or crisis;
- anemia;
- infection;
- acute chest syndrome;
- splenic sequestration;
- vision loss;
- leg ulcers;
- stroke; and
- other complications.

How does sickle cell disease increase the risk of stroke?

A stroke can happen if sickle cells get stuck in a blood vessel and clog blood flow to the brain. About 10% of children with sickle cell disease will have a stroke. Stroke can cause lifelong disabilities and learning problems.

Prevention: Doctors can sometimes identify children who are at risk for stroke using a special type of exam called transcranial Doppler ultrasound. In some cases, a doctor might recommend frequent blood transfusions to help prevent a stroke. People who have frequent blood transfusions must be watched closely because there are serious side effects. For example, too much iron can build up in the body, causing life-threatening damage to the organs.

Is there a cure?

The only cure for SCD is bone marrow/stem cell transplant.

Bone marrow is a soft, fatty tissue inside the center of the bones where blood cells are made. A bone marrow/stem cell transplant is a procedure that takes healthy cells that form blood from one person—the donor—and puts them into someone whose bone marrow is not working properly.

Bone marrow/stem cell transplants are very risky, and can have serious side effects, including death. For the transplant to work, the bone marrow must be a close match. Usually, the best donor is a brother or sister. Bone marrow/stem cell transplants are used only in cases of severe sickle cell disease for children who have minimal organ damage from the disease.

Chapter 16

Diabetes and Stroke

Diabetes is increasing in people of all ages and in the United Kingdom there are over two million people with diabetes. This text describes the main symptoms of diabetes, explains who is at increased risk of developing diabetes, and why being diabetic increases your risk of stroke. It also describes how you can make changes in your lifestyle to reduce the risk of stroke.

What Is Diabetes?

Diabetes is a condition which occurs when the level of glucose (sugar) in the blood is too high because the body is not processing it properly. Glucose comes from the digestion of starchy and sugary foods and also from the liver, which produces glucose.

The hormone insulin is produced by the pancreas (a gland behind the stomach). Insulin enables glucose to be broken down and used as fuel. It controls the levels of glucose in the blood.

There are two types of diabetes:

- **Type 1** usually—but not always—begins in childhood or adolescence. It develops when the cells in the pancreas that produce insulin have been destroyed and the body cannot produce any insulin. This results in higher than normal levels of glucose building up in the bloodstream—this is called hyperglycemia.

- **Type 2** is much more common—85–95 percent of people with diabetes have this type. It develops gradually—usually occurring in adulthood. Type 2 diabetes occurs when the body is unable to respond effectively to any insulin produced (this is known as insulin resistance) or when the body cannot produce enough insulin.

Diabetes during Pregnancy

Some pregnant women develop high levels of glucose in their blood and their body is unable to produce enough insulin to process it. This is known as gestational diabetes. This usually stops after giving birth, however it may increase the risk of developing Type 2 diabetes later in life.

The Link with Stroke

Insulin is the key to diabetes. People with Type 1 diabetes do not produce insulin, whilst those with Type 2 either do not produce enough or the insulin produced does not work effectively. However, diabetes is not simply a problem of glucose. In the long term, uncontrolled high levels of glucose in the bloodstream can lead to other health problems.

Diabetes is progressive and if it goes untreated or uncontrolled it increases the risk of developing serious problems with the nerves, eyes, kidneys, and blood vessels. Men may also experience impotence.

Having diabetes also increases the risk of vascular disease—disease of the blood vessels due to hardening and narrowing of the artery walls. This can lead to stroke, heart disease, or complications with the legs and feet.

Disease of the blood vessel walls is called atherosclerosis. The inside walls of the arteries become thickened and hardened as fatty deposits including surplus cholesterol build up. The blood vessels become narrowed and the flow of blood is restricted. This damage may also lead to the formation of blood clots. If a clot blocks the flow of blood to the brain, this causes an ischemic stroke; if a clot obstructs the flow of blood to the heart, then this causes a heart attack.

If you have diabetes, you are most at risk of having an ischemic stroke. This is the most common type of stroke and is caused by a blood clot blocking the blood supply to the brain. Research shows that the risk of ischemic stroke is multiplied two to three times in people with diabetes. However, the risk of having a hemorrhagic stroke (caused by bleeding in and around the brain) is probably similar to that of people who do not have diabetes.

Recognizing the Symptoms of Diabetes

The main symptoms of diabetes are:

- increased thirst;
- increased urination—especially at night;
- extreme tiredness;
- weight loss;
- genital itching or regular episodes of thrush; and
- blurred vision.

In the United Kingdom it is estimated that there are up to one million people living with undiagnosed diabetes. If you have Type 2 diabetes, you may not notice these symptoms at all, or at least not when they first develop. Ask your doctor to test you for Type 2 diabetes every few years, particularly if you have any of the following risk factors.

Risk Factors

You are at an increased risk of developing diabetes if any of the following apply:

- **Age**—if you are Caucasian and over 40 or if you are over 25 and are of African, African-Caribbean, or Asian descent.

- **A family history of diabetes**—particularly if a close relative such as a parent or sibling has the condition.

- **Your ethnicity**—in the United Kingdom, Type 2 diabetes is up to six times more common in people of South Asian descent and up to three times more common in people of African or African-Caribbean descent, compared to the Caucasian population.

- **Obesity**—Type 2 diabetes which is much more common, is closely linked to obesity. The organization Diabetes UK states that over 80 percent of people diagnosed with Type 2 diabetes are overweight. Being overweight reduces the body's ability to respond to insulin and extra fat around the waist can reduce the liver's sensitivity to insulin—this is associated with Type 2 diabetes. The 'apple shape' created by extra fat around the waist is called central obesity and applies to women whose waist measurement is 31.5 inches (80 cm) or over. Caucasian, African, and African-Caribbean men with a waist measurement of 37 inches (94 cm) or over and Asian men with a waist measurement of 35 inches (89 cm) or over.

- You have had **diabetes during pregnancy**.

Treatment

If you are diagnosed with diabetes, you will work with a diabetes care team—a group of health professionals (including your GP [general practitioner, or doctor]) appropriate for your needs. This team will normally include a diabetes specialist nurse and a dietitian. Other specialists you may see include an eye specialist—ophthalmologist or optometrist, a pharmacist, a chiropodist or podiatrist, a psychologist, and a consultant.

Some mild forms of diabetes may be controlled through healthy eating and regular exercise, and you may not need to take medication. The diabetes care team will advise and support you in making any necessary changes. They will also guide you in knowing your own levels of blood pressure, blood glucose, and cholesterol as well as monitoring the condition of your feet and eyes and making appropriate appointments with specialists.

For those who need medication to help control their blood glucose levels, there are different types of medication available and your diabetes care team will work with you to find the most suitable one for you.

There are many different drugs available with different 'trade' names. The following section describes the different groups of drugs—your medication will have its own, different trade name.

Diabetes Tablets

There are different groups of tablets available:

- **Sulfonylureas**—work on the pancreas into producing more insulin and ensure that the body uses insulin efficiently.

- **Biguanide**—work on the liver to stop the production of new glucose and help insulin to carry glucose efficiently into muscle and fat cells, combating insulin resistance.

- **Prandial glucose regulator**—taken with meals, they stimulate the pancreas into making more insulin.

- **Thiazolidinediones or glitazones**—combat insulin resistance and help the body to respond to its own insulin more efficiently.

- **Alpha glucosidase inhibitors**—slow down the absorption of starchy foods from the intestine, this slows the increase in blood glucose after eating.

- **DPP-4 inhibitors**—a new type of medication, Januvia belongs to this group and is available for people with Type 2 diabetes. It increases levels of incretins—hormones that promote the production of insulin when it is needed by the body and reduce the levels of glucose made by the liver when it is not needed.

Insulin Injections

People with Type 1 diabetes (and some people with Type 2) require insulin injections every day to manage their blood sugar levels.

As an alternative to using traditional syringes, insulin pens are available where a cartridge of insulin is inserted into the pen and the user 'dials' the dose before injecting.

Incretin Mimetics

Byetta is the first type of this class of drug; it is taken by injection but it is not insulin. It is for adults with Type 2 diabetes and it promotes the production of insulin when it is needed, reduces the liver's production of glucose when this is not needed, slows the rate of food digestion in the stomach—slowing the release of glucose into the blood, and reduces appetite.

As with all medication, some people may experience side effects to certain drugs. The diabetes care team will work with you to find the most appropriate medication for you.

Reducing Your Risk

If you have diabetes, you will need to keep a tight control over your blood glucose levels. Check your blood or urine for glucose regularly to ensure it stays at a healthy level. Persistently high levels of blood glucose are a sign that your diabetes is not properly controlled and you may need to adjust your diet and/or medication or insulin.

It's also important to attend regular checkups with your doctor or at a diabetes clinic to ensure your blood glucose and blood pressure stay at healthy levels. Most people will need to attend a diabetes clinic at least once a year.

You should also aim to keep your blood pressure as low as possible. Doctors now recommend that people with diabetes should have a lower level of blood pressure than those without diabetes. Ideally, your blood pressure should be 130/80 or lower. Blood pressure can be controlled through lifestyle, but you may also need drug treatment with antihypertensive (blood pressure lowering) medication.

Reducing your cholesterol levels may also help reduce your risk of stroke, as well as other conditions such as heart disease. For some people, lowering their cholesterol can be achieved through eating a diet low in saturated fat. However, for others this may not be adequate and they may also require medication to lower their cholesterol levels.

Helping Yourself

Take regular exercise. As well as helping to reduce blood pressure, regular physical activity can help to control blood glucose levels, reduce cholesterol levels, and maintain overall fitness.

The Department of Health recommends that adults take at least 30 minutes of moderate exercise five days a week and children take at least one hour, five days a week. (Moderate exercise includes brisk walking, badminton, golf, tennis, and cycling). For older people these recommendations depend on ability.

Eat a healthy, balanced diet. Eating little and often prevents fluctuations in blood glucose levels. A healthy diet is one that is low in salt, fat, and sugar and is based around foods that convert slowly to energy, such as complex carbohydrates (whole-meal bread, brown rice, and whole-wheat cereals), beans, lentils, vegetables, and fruit.

Control your weight. Excess weight can raise blood pressure and increase the strain on your heart, so it's important to try to shed any excess pounds. Weight loss also improves the body's ability to respond to insulin and helps to control glucose levels.

Don't smoke. Smoking damages blood vessels that may already be damaged as a result of diabetes. Smoking is also linked to higher blood pressure.

For More Information

Diabetes UK
Macleod House
10 Parkway
London NW1 7AA
Diabetes Careline: 0845 120 2960
Email: info@diabetes.org.uk
Website: www.diabetes.org.uk

This national charity has regional offices and contacts across England, Northern Ireland, Scotland, and Wales.

Chapter 17

Fibromuscular Dysplasia Increases Stroke Risk

Definition

Stroke secondary to fibromuscular dysplasia (FMD) is an interruption of blood flow to the brain due to problems with the structure of the arteries that supply the brain with blood.

Causes

A stroke is an interruption of the blood supply to any part of the brain. Stroke secondary to fibromuscular dysplasia (FMD) primarily affects women, especially those older than 50.

FMD is an inherited disorder involving the ongoing destruction of arterial blood vessels. There are areas of increased muscle and fibrous (scar-like) tissue in the wall of the affected arteries, which alternate with enlarged (dilated) areas of destroyed tissue. This irregularity in the arteries increases the risk for stroke.

The disease may affect the neck arteries (carotids) that supply blood to the brain, or the arteries within the brain (cerebral) and cause stroke. It may also affect the following arteries:

- Kidneys (renal)
- Intestinal tract (mesenteric)
- Heart (coronary)

"Stroke secondary to FMD" © 2008 A.D.A.M., Inc. Reprinted with permission.

- Groin (iliac)

Secondary symptoms include high blood pressure, leg pain, heart attack, kidney failure, and other disorders.

Risks include a personal or family history of FMD.

Symptoms

- Weakness or total inability to move a body part
- Numbness, tingling, or other abnormal sensations
- Decreased or lost vision, partial or temporary
- Language difficulties (aphasia)
- Inability to recognize or identify visual cues (agnosia)
- Loss of memory
- Vertigo (abnormal sensation of movement)
- Loss of coordination
- Swallowing difficulties
- Personality changes
- Mood and emotion changes
- Urinary incontinence (lack of control over bladder)
- Lack of control over the bowels
- Consciousness changes:
  - Sleepiness
  - Stupor, lethargy
  - Coma, loss of consciousness

Exams and Tests

The exact location and extent of the stroke, and changes in the arteries indicating FMD may be seen on:

- Head CT [computed tomography] scan
- Ultrasound of the arteries involved
- Head MRI [magnetic resonance imaging]/MRA [magnetic resonance angiography]

An arteriography or angiography of the head may show blood vessel changes such as narrowing of the arteries.

An artery biopsy confirms the diagnosis of FMD (this is not performed on brain blood vessels).

Treatment

Stroke is a serious condition. The sooner treatment is received, the better the person will do, and the lower the chance of permanent disability or death.

Treatment depends on the severity of the stroke and its effects. Careful monitoring can reveal problems with the arteries before injury occurs. In some circumstances, surgery to repair any blockages can prevent complications.

Evaluation and treatment of hypertension (high blood pressure) associated with kidney disorders may be appropriate in some people with stroke secondary to FMD.

Outlook (Prognosis)

The outcome from any stroke depends on the initial severity, and ability to treat it quickly. Although FMD is associated with an increased risk of stroke and other complications, many patients can do well with good treatment and close attention to any secondary complications. As with other types of stroke, strokes from FMD can result in death or severe disability. Complete or significant recovery from a stroke is also possible.

Possible Complications

- Problems due to loss of mobility (joint contractures, pressure sores)

- Permanent loss of movement or sensation of a part of the body

- Bone fractures

- Muscle spasticity

- Permanent loss of brain functions

- Reduced communication or social interaction

- Reduced ability to function or care for self

- Decreased life span

- Side effects of medications
- Aspiration
- Malnutrition

When to Contact a Medical Professional

Stroke is a medical emergency. Immediately go to the emergency room or call the local emergency number (911 in the United States) if signs of a stroke occur.

Prevention

Awareness of personal or family history of FMD can allow earlier diagnosis of the cause of stroke.

Aspirin therapy (81 mg a day or 100 mg every other day) is now recommended for stroke prevention in women under 65 as long as the benefits outweigh the risks.

It should be considered for women over age 65 only if their blood pressure is controlled and the benefit is greater than the risk of gastrointestinal bleeding and brain hemorrhage.

Chapter 18

High Blood Pressure and Stroke

High blood pressure, or hypertension, usually has no symptoms and, if not treated and kept under control, is one of the major risk factors for stroke. Both lifestyle changes and medication can help to control your blood pressure. This text explains what high blood pressure is.

What Is Blood Pressure?

Blood pressure is a measure of the force with which the blood presses on the walls of the arteries as it is pumped around the body. This pumping action is driven by your heart which beats, on average, around 70 to 80 times a minute and pumps the blood to the arteries and out to various parts of the body.

How Blood Pressure Is Measured

Measuring blood pressure is quick, simple, and painless, and can be carried out at your doctor's surgery or at some pharmacies. An inflatable cuff will be placed around one arm and a stethoscope will be used to listen to the blood flow. Readings are measured against a column of mercury or by using an automatic digital machine. An Ambulatory Blood Pressure Monitoring (ABPM) machine, attached to a belt, is sometimes used to record blood pressure over a 24-hour period.

"High blood pressure after stroke," © 2006 The Stroke Association (www .stroke.org.uk). Reprinted with permission.

Blood pressure is measured with two readings, firstly when the heart beats (systolic pressure) and secondly when the heart relaxes between beats (diastolic pressure). Blood pressure is always higher when the heart beats than when it is relaxing. The readings are expressed as a fraction and the systolic reading is always written before the diastolic figure. Both pressures are measured in millimeters of mercury, written as mmHg.

Normal Blood Pressure

The optimal blood pressure is less than 120/80 mmHg. If, on multiple readings, the systolic blood pressure is between 120 and 139, or the diastolic blood pressure is between 80 and 89, this is called prehypertension and high blood pressure is likely to develop at some point.

High Blood Pressure, or Hypertension

Your blood pressure varies throughout the day. It can go down if you are asleep or sitting quietly, and can go up if you are rushing about or stressed. Hypertension, or high blood pressure, develops when the pressure of the blood running through the vessels is consistently too high. A person is usually considered to have high blood pressure if they have a measurement that is consistently above 140/90 mmHg. Drug treatment should be considered in this case.

Before giving a diagnosis of hypertension, your doctor may take a few readings over a period of days or weeks to make sure that a higher reading was not due to something simple like rushing to your appointment (sometimes referred to as "white coat hypertension"). If your blood pressure is high, your doctor will discuss with you ways to reduce it, especially if you are at particular risk, for instance, if you have diabetes or circulatory problems, or if you smoke or are overweight.

What Are the Symptoms of High Blood Pressure?

High blood pressure is very often a silent condition that shows no symptoms. Unfortunately, it can also be dangerous. There is no clear way of knowing you have high blood pressure, apart from having it measured. The damage that is caused by raised blood pressure occurs over time. People with high blood pressure usually only get symptoms when the strain on their arteries leads to blockages or bleeds. Studies have shown that around four fifths of men and two thirds of women with high blood pressure are not being treated.

Why High Blood Pressure Is Dangerous

If high blood pressure is not treated and kept under control, it puts you at much greater risk of a stroke. High blood pressure is the single most important risk factor for stroke. It causes about 50 percent of ischemic strokes and also increases the risk of strokes due to bleeding in the brain (hemorrhage).

High blood pressure puts a strain on blood vessels all over the body, including vital arteries to the brain, and the heart has to work much harder to keep the blood circulation going.

This strain can cause vessels to become clogged up or to weaken, and this in turn can lead to narrow blood vessels and blood clots. When a clot forms a blockage in an artery leading to the brain, or in a blood vessel inside the brain, it can result in a stroke or transient ischemic attack (TIA or mini-stroke). More rarely, this extra strain may cause a cerebral hemorrhage where a blood vessel bursts inside the brain and blood spills into surrounding tissues. This is also a type of stroke. The symptoms of stroke include numbness or weakness down one side of the body, blurred vision, and slurred speech.

A person with high blood pressure is also more at risk of having a heart attack or developing other forms of heart disease in the future. Because of the increased strain on your heart and blood vessels, untreated hypertension puts you at risk of angina which can cause chest pain and breathlessness and may lead to a heart attack. High blood pressure can also cause kidney damage and retinopathy (sight problems).

Risk Factors for High Blood Pressure

High blood pressure develops for a variety of reasons. Factors such as being overweight, drinking too much alcohol, getting little exercise, and eating an unhealthy diet all contribute to high blood pressure.

It is also more common in middle-aged and elderly people as blood pressure tends to rise as you get older. It is estimated that nearly 40 percent of middle-aged people and more than two thirds of those aged 75 and over have high blood pressure.

In some people, high blood pressure may be caused by another underlying condition, such as certain kidney disorders. Also, some people are more at risk than others. For instance, blood pressure problems can run in families, and certain ethnic groups, such as African-Caribbean people, are particularly at risk.

How Often Should Blood Pressure Be Checked?

All adults should have their blood pressure checked regularly. For those whose pressure has previously been normal, that means at least once every five years, preferably more often. Women taking the contraceptive pill or who are pregnant or on hormone replacement therapy (HRT), and some people taking specific medicines, also need blood pressure checks more often.

If you've had a high or borderline reading in the past, but do not currently need medicines, your blood pressure should be measured at least once a year. And if you are already taking medicines to control your blood pressure, you will need a check at least twice a year. You can help protect yourself by ensuring your blood pressure is checked regularly at intervals suggested by your doctor.

Treatment of High Blood Pressure

Doctors treat high blood pressure to reduce the risk of strokes, heart attacks, and other circulatory problems. Medical advice, for all but the mildest forms of hypertension, is likely to include the daily use of drugs to bring blood pressure down.

Both lifestyle changes and medication can bring blood pressure down to a normal level. If your blood pressure is below 140/90, you will normally not need any treatment with medicines. If you have higher levels, your doctor will aim to reduce the systolic or upper figure of your blood pressure to below 140 and the diastolic or lower figure to below 85. If you have diabetes or have already had a stroke or heart attack, the aim will be to reduce your blood pressure even further to below 130/80 mmHg. This is not always possible, but even small reductions in blood pressure can significantly reduce your risk of heart disease or stroke.

Chapter 19

Medication Use and Stroke Risk

Chapter Contents

Section 19.1

Do Statins Have a Role in Acute Stroke Prevention?

"Do Statins Have a Role in Acute Stroke Prevention?"
by Colby Stong, *Neurology Reviews,* August 2006. © Quadrant
HealthCom Inc. Reprinted with permission.

Increasing evidence indicates that hypercholesterolemia, as well as increased low-density lipoprotein (LDL) cholesterol levels and decreased high-density lipoprotein (HDL) cholesterol levels, may be a risk factor for carotid atheroma and ischemic stroke, according to Ralph L. Sacco, M.D. Mounting data also suggest that taking statins, especially by patients in certain high-risk categories, may help reduce that risk.

"I do believe, and I think the data suggest, that cholesterol is a stroke risk factor," said Dr. Sacco, at the 58th Annual Meeting of the American Academy of Neurology. "It may not be the strongest, but it is prevalent and may be important when we think about the number of strokes attributed to elevated cholesterol. It may be differential by stroke subtype. Statins clearly reduce stroke risk among high-risk patients—for example, those with coronary artery disease, diabetes, and hypertension—and have a role in secondary stroke prevention."

Dr. Sacco is a Professor of Neurology and Epidemiology at the Neurological Institute of Columbia University College of Physicians and Surgeons in New York City and Chair of the Stroke Advisory Committee of the American Stroke Association.

Advances in primary and secondary stroke prevention could have a significant impact in the overall treatment of stroke, according to Dr. Sacco. The prevalence of hypercholesterolemia makes it a prime target in that effort, as about 43% of men and 36% of women in the United States have an elevated LDL cholesterol level, defined as greater than 130, noted Dr. Sacco. "So even if it is a mild risk factor, its prevalence implies that it would have a big effect in terms of number of strokes attributed to this risk factor," he said.

Stroke and Cholesterol

The relationship between stroke and cholesterol levels has been a somewhat controversial issue in the past, as epidemiologic studies did not establish a strong association. But this may be due, in part, to the heterogeneity of stroke, Dr. Sacco theorized. "This heterogeneity of stroke may actually impair our ability to look at the specificity of certain risk factors like cholesterol in overall ischemic stroke," he said.

In addition, whereas older trials did not involve statins, more recent randomized clinical trials with 3-hydroxy-3-methylglutaryl co-enzyme A reductase inhibitors have shown that effective lowering of cholesterol levels substantially reduces the risk of cardiac disease and stroke, said Dr. Sacco. "The good news is that there are multiple studies regarding statins that are randomized, and therefore the evidence is great," he said.

The latest endorsement for the use of statins in stroke prevention was provided by the Stroke Prevention by Aggressive Reduction in Cholesterol Levels (SPARCL) trial, results of which were reported at the 15th European Stroke Conference. Investigators found that atorvastatin, 80 mg/day, significantly reduced the risk of recurrent stroke in patients without coronary heart disease who had normal cholesterol levels. The 10-year international study included more than 4,700 patients with a stroke or transient ischemic attack within the previous six months. The atorvastatin regimen reduced stroke risk by 16%, major coronary events by 35%, coronary heart disease events by 42%, and revascularization procedures by 45%.

"This landmark study now expands the evidence of the benefits of statins to all ischemic stroke patients, and specifically for the prevention of recurrent stroke as an outcome," Dr. Sacco commented to *Neurology Reviews*.

Who Benefits?

A number of studies have shown a correlation between various risk groups and the degree of benefit derived from taking statins. For example, the Treating to New Targets Study showed that strokes were significantly reduced among patients with coronary heart disease and diabetes who took an 80-mg/day regimen of atorvastatin. The Anglo-Scandinavian Cardiac Outcomes Trial—Lipid Lowering Arm showed that strokes were reduced in patients with hypertension but without coronary heart disease. The Collaborative Atorvastatin Diabetes Study found a reduced risk of first cardiovascular disease event, including stroke, in patients with type 2 diabetes mellitus who did not have a high LDL cholesterol level.

Other statin trials involving medium- to lower-risk patients have not been as clear in terms of stroke outcome. The Prospective Study of Pravastatin in the Elderly at Risk trial found a reduced risk of coronary artery disease, though stroke risk was unaffected. "The effect of statins for primary stroke prevention may be less than that, say, for higher-risk individuals," said Dr. Sacco.

Multiple Benefits of Statins

Pierre Amarenco, M.D., conducted a meta-analysis of clinical trials in which statin therapy had been used in the prevention and treatment of stroke and found that the greater the LDL cholesterol reduction, the greater the stroke risk reduction. "However, others have questioned whether some of the effect of statins may go beyond that of LDL, particularly when you [consider that] LDL is not as strong a risk factor for overall ischemic stroke," said Dr. Sacco.

In addition to aiding cholesterol reduction, statins may also lead to improved endothelial function, reduced inflammation, stabilization and reduction in atherosclerotic plaques, and attenuated thrombogenic responses, suggested Dr. Sacco. "Some of these cholesterol-independent effects are important and have brought us more basic science evidence to go from the bedside back to the bench and maybe even back to the bedside with some translational work," he said.

Retrospective data have also revealed favorable outcomes among those who took statins at the time of a stroke. Elkind et al, in the Northern Manhattan Study, observed a lower 90-day mortality among patients taking statins at the time of stroke. Parra and colleagues found that in patients with acute aneurysmal subarachnoid hemorrhage, those who used statins demonstrated significant improvement in 14-day functional outcomes. "So there is beginning evidence in humans, retrospectively albeit for now, that suggests that statins may have an effect that would go beyond what we would expect by just LDL lowering," said Dr. Sacco.

Furthermore, preclinical studies have demonstrated neuroprotective effects of higher doses of statins after acute stroke. Drs. Elkind and Sacco, as part of the NINDS [National Institute of Neurological Disorders and Stroke]-funded Specialized Program on Translational Research in Acute Stroke, are conducting the Neuroprotection with Statin Therapy for Acute Recovery Trial, under way to determine if lovastatin can be administered safely in increasing doses from 1 to

10 mg/kg daily for three days, beginning 24 hours after acute ischemic stroke. "The next step will be [to show] whether there is any efficacy or hint of efficacy before we move to phase II and III trials," noted Dr. Sacco. "Animal model data are beginning to suggest that there may be some other approaches for statins in the future, but it is still quite early to do anything yet clinically.

"I think in the future, based on the results of this translational work, statins could have a role as an acute stroke therapy," Dr. Sacco continued. "The availability of more effective preventive treatments for stroke will greatly improve our ability to modify the risk of ischemic stroke and substantially reduce the number of persons killed or disabled by stroke each year."

Suggested Reading

1. Amarenco P. Effect of statins in stroke prevention. *Curr Opin Lipidol*. 2005;16:614–618.

2. Colhoun HM, Betteridge DJ, Durrington PN, et al. Primary prevention of cardiovascular disease with atorvastatin in type 2 diabetes in the Collaborative Atorvastatin Diabetes Study (CARDS): multicentre randomised placebo-controlled trial. *Lancet*. 2004;364:685–696.

3. Elkind MS, Flint AC, Sciacca RR, Sacco RL. Lipid-lowering agent use at ischemic stroke onset is associated with decreased mortality. *Neurology*. 2005;65:253–258.

4. Parra A, Kreiter KT, Williams S, et al. Effect of prior statin use on functional outcome and delayed vasospasm after acute aneurysmal subarachnoid hemorrhage: a matched controlled cohort study. *Neurosurgery*. 2005;56:476–484.

5. Sever PS, Dahlof B, Poulter NR, et al. Prevention of coronary and stroke events with atorvastatin in hypertensive patients who have average or lower-than-average cholesterol concentrations, in the Anglo-Scandinavian Cardiac Outcomes Trial—Lipid Lowering Arm (ASCOT-LLA): a multicentre randomised controlled trial. *Lancet*. 2003;361:1149–1158.

6. Shepherd J, Barter P, Carmena R, et al. Effect of lowering LDL cholesterol substantially below currently recommended levels in patients with coronary heart disease and diabetes: the Treating to New Targets (TNT) study. *Diabetes Care*. 2006;29:1220–1226.

7. Shepherd J, Blauw GJ, Murphy MB, et al. Pravastatin in elderly individuals at risk of vascular disease (PROSPER): a randomised controlled trial. *Lancet.* 2002;360:1623–1630.

Section 19.2

Patients Who Abandon Statins after Stroke Increase Risk of Death

Patients who stop taking cholesterol-lowering drugs within a year of surviving a stroke had a two-fold increased risk of death, researchers reported in *Stroke: Journal of the American Heart Association*.

Statins can benefit patients who have suffered an ischemic stroke (caused by a clot). However, stroke survivors often stop taking these drugs—an issue previously not studied in a clinical setting, said Furio Colivicchi, M.D., lead study author.

"To the best of our knowledge, this is the first evidence linking discontinuation of statin therapy to increased death rates in stroke survivors who have no other clinical evidence of heart disease," he and colleagues wrote.

Statins effectively lower blood levels of low-density lipoprotein cholesterol (LDL), known as "bad" cholesterol. The drugs have major side effects.

The observational study ran for four-and-a-half years at San Filippo Neri Hospital in Rome, in collaboration with the Institute for Clinical Research Santa Lucia Foundation of Rome. Researchers identified 631 consecutive stroke survivors (322 men and 309 women, average age 70 years). None had any other major illness, including heart disease. All patients were discharged from the hospital with orders to take a drug regimen including statin therapy.

Trained nurses interviewed the patients and researchers examined their primary care physicians' records for 12 months after their stroke.

Researchers recorded the date and possible reasons for any cardio-vascular drug discontinuation.

By the end of the study, 38.9 percent of the patients—246 patients—had stopped taking statins. The average time to discontinuation was 48.6 days.

Seventy-one patients (28.8 percent) cited mild side effects, the most common of which was indigestion. In the other 175 cases (71.2 percent), neither the patient nor the primary care physician could give specific medical reasons for discontinuation. Similar figures have been reported in studies in other Western countries, including the United States.

"Because medication costs are covered by the Italian National Health Service, except for a small co-pay, cost cannot be related to these patients discontinuing their prescribed therapy," said senior author Carlo Caltagirone, M.D., Scientific Director of Santa Lucia Foundation. "In these studies the specific reasons for discontinuation are usually unknown, and they are difficult to analyze. However, contributing factors are probably related to patients' and their healthcare providers' behavior and beliefs, and probably also to features of the healthcare system itself."

Compared to the entire study group, patients who stopped taking the statins were older (71.4 vs. 69.5, on average) and more often female.

Patients were less likely to stop taking the statins if they had diabetes or a previous stroke.

During the study, 116 patients died. Eighty percent of these deaths were attributed to cardiovascular causes.

Statistical analysis determined that discontinuing statin therapy was independently and significantly associated with increased risk of death from any cause. Patients who had stopped taking statins within a year of stroke were more than twice as likely to die (2.78 hazard ratio) than others in the study group.

Other independent predictors of death were discontinuing antiplatelet drugs (80 percent increased risk); stroke severity at the time of hospital admission (11 percent increased risk per unit on the NIH [National Institutes of Health] Stroke Scale); and age (8 percent increased risk).

"Patients who stop taking the statins have a significantly increased chance of death in the first year after their stroke—and the earlier they stop, the higher the risk they face," Colivicchi said. "In fact, the risk factors for the association between statin discontinuation and death gradually decreased with time. Effective clinical strategies are needed to bring out a significant increase in patients who maintain their drug therapies."

Researchers said future studies should also evaluate whether interventions designed to improve patients' self-care behaviors and lifestyles might also improve the percentage of patients who continue their medication.

Other co-authors are Andrea Bassi, M.D., and Massino Santini, M.D.

Statements and conclusions of study authors that are published in the American Heart Association scientific journals are solely those of the study authors and do not necessarily reflect association policy or position. The American Heart Association makes no representation or warranty as to their accuracy or reliability.

Section 19.3

Contraceptives and Stroke Risk

Excerpted from "Stroke," by the National Women's Health Information Center (NWHIC, www.4women.gov), part of the Office on Women's Health, May 2006.

Does taking birth control pills increase my risk for stroke?

Taking birth control pills is generally safe for young, healthy women. But birth control pills can raise the risk of stroke for some women, especially women over 35; women with high blood pressure, diabetes, or high cholesterol; and women who smoke. Talk with your doctor if you have questions about the pill.

If you are taking birth control pills, and you have any of the symptoms listed below, call 911:

- eye problems such as blurred or double vision;
- pain in the upper body or arm;
- bad headaches;
- problems breathing;
- spitting up blood;
- swelling or pain in the leg;

176

- yellowing of the skin or eyes;

- breast lumps; or

- unusual (not normal) heavy bleeding from your vagina.

Does using the birth control patch increase my risk for stroke?

The patch is generally safe for young, healthy women. The patch can raise the risk of stroke for some women, especially women over 35; women with high blood pressure, diabetes, or high cholesterol; and women who smoke.

Recent studies show that women who use the patch may be exposed to more estrogen (the female hormone in birth control pills and the patch that keeps users from becoming pregnant) than women who use the birth control pill. Research is underway to see if the risk for blood clots (which can lead to heart attack or stroke) is higher in patch users. Talk with your doctor if you have questions about the patch.

If you are using the birth control patch, and you have any of the symptoms listed below, call 911:

- eye problems such as blurred or double vision;

- pain in the upper body or arm;

- bad headaches;

- problems breathing;

- spitting up blood;

- swelling or pain in the leg;

- yellowing of the skin or eyes;

- breast lumps; or

- unusual (not normal) heavy bleeding from your vagina.

Section 19.4

Menopausal Hormone Therapy: Does It Increase Stroke Risk?

Excerpted from "Facts about Menopausal Hormone Therapy," by the
National Heart, Lung, and Blood Institute (NHLBI, www.nhlbi.nih.gov),
part of the National Institutes of Health, June 2005.

Menopausal hormone therapy once seemed the answer for many of the conditions women face as they age. It was thought that hormone therapy could ward off heart disease, osteoporosis, and cancer, while improving women's quality of life.

But beginning in July 2002, findings emerged from clinical trials that showed this was not so. In fact, long-term use of hormone therapy poses serious risks and may increase the risk of heart attack and stroke. This text discusses those findings.

Menopause and Hormone Therapy

As you age, significant internal changes take place that affect your production of the two female hormones, estrogen and progesterone. The hormones, which are important in regulating the menstrual cycle and having a successful pregnancy, are produced by the ovaries, two small oval-shaped organs found on either side of the uterus.

During the years just before menopause, known as perimenopause, your ovaries begin to shrink. Levels of estrogen and progesterone fluctuate as your ovaries try to keep up hormone production. You can have irregular menstrual cycles, along with unpredictable episodes of heavy bleeding during a period. Perimenopause usually lasts several years.

Eventually, your periods stop. Menopause marks the time of your last menstrual period. It is not considered the last until you have been period-free for 1 year without being ill, pregnant, breastfeeding, or using certain medicines, all of which also can cause menstrual cycles to cease. There should be no bleeding, even spotting, during that year. Natural menopause usually happens sometime between the ages of 45 and 54.

You also can undergo menopause as the result of surgery. A surgical procedure, called a hysterectomy, removes the uterus. This surgery puts an end to your menstrual cycle but does not affect menopause, which still occurs naturally.

You go through menopause immediately if both of your ovaries are also removed at surgery. Whether you go through menopause naturally or surgically, symptoms can result as your body adjusts to the drop in estrogen levels. These symptoms vary greatly—one woman may go through menopause with few symptoms, while another has difficulty. Symptoms may last for several months or years, or persist.

The most common symptoms are hot flashes or flushes, night sweats, and sleep disturbances. (A hot flash is a feeling of heat in your face and over the surface of your body, which may cause the skin to appear flushed or red as blood vessels expand. It can be followed by sweating and shivering. Hot flashes that occur during sleep are called night sweats.) But the drop in estrogen also can contribute to changes in the vaginal and urinary tracts, which can cause painful intercourse and urinary infections.

To relieve the symptoms of menopause, doctors may prescribe hormone therapy. This can involve the use of either estrogen alone or with another hormone called progesterone, or progestin in its synthetic form. The two hormones normally help to regulate a woman's menstrual cycle.

Progestin is added to estrogen to prevent the overgrowth (or hyperplasia) of cells in the lining of the uterus. This overgrowth can lead to uterine cancer. If you haven't had a hysterectomy, you'll receive estrogen plus progesterone or a progestin; if you have had a hysterectomy, you'll receive only estrogen. Hormones may be taken daily (continuous use) or on only certain days of the month (cyclic use).

They also can be taken in several ways, including orally, through a patch on the skin, as a cream or gel, or with an IUD (intrauterine device) or vaginal ring. How the therapy is taken can depend on its purpose. For instance, a vaginal estrogen ring or cream can ease vaginal dryness, urinary leakage, or vaginal or urinary infections, but does not relieve hot flashes.

Hormone therapy may cause side effects, such as bleeding, bloating, breast tenderness or enlargement, headaches, mood changes, and nausea. Further, side effects vary by how the hormone is taken. For instance, a patch may cause irritation at the site where it's applied.

There also are nonhormonal approaches to easing the symptoms of menopause.

Postmenopausal Use

Menopause may cause other changes that produce no symptoms yet affect your health. For instance, after menopause, women's rate of bone loss increases. The increased rate can lead to osteoporosis, which may in turn increase the risk of bone fractures. The risk of heart disease increases with age, but is not clearly tied to the menopause.

Through the years, studies were finding evidence that estrogen might help with some of these postmenopausal health risks—especially heart disease and osteoporosis. With more than 40 million American women over age 50, the promise seemed great. Although many women think it is a "man's disease," heart disease is the leading killer of American women. Women typically develop it about 10 years later than men.

Furthermore, women are more prone to osteoporosis than men. Menopause is a time of increased bone loss. Bone is living tissue. Old bone is continuously being broken down and new bone formed in its place. With menopause, bone loss is greater and, if not enough new bone is made, the result can be weakened bones and osteoporosis, which increases the risk of breaks. One of every two women over age 50 will have an osteoporosis-related fracture during her life.

Many scientists believed these increased health risks were linked to the postmenopausal drop in estrogen produced by the ovaries and that replacing estrogen would help protect against the diseases.

Early Findings

Early studies seemed to support hormone therapy's ability to protect women against the diseases that tend to occur after menopause. For instance, research showed that the treatment does prevent osteoporosis. However, other findings lacked evidence or were unclear. No large clinical trials had proved that hormone therapy prevents heart disease or fractures. Answers also were needed about other possible effects of long-term use of hormones, especially on such conditions as breast and colorectal cancers.

Further, prior research on menopausal hormone therapy's effect on heart disease had involved mainly observational studies, which can indicate possible relationships between behaviors or treatments and disease, but cannot establish a cause-and-effect tie.

There were some clinical trials, considered the "gold standard" in establishing a cause-and-effect connection between a behavior or treatment and a disease, but most looked at the therapy's effects on the risk factors or predictors of various diseases.

Two important clinical trials were the "Postmenopausal Estrogen/ Progestin Interventions Trial" (PEPI) and the "Heart and Estrogen- Progestin Replacement Study" (HERS).

PEPI looked at the effect of therapies on key heart disease risk factors and bone mass. It found generally positive results, including a reduction by both types of therapy of "bad" LDL cholesterol and an increase of "good" HDL cholesterol. (LDL, or low density lipoprotein, carries cholesterol to tissues, while HDL, or high density lipoprotein, carries it away, aiding in its removal from the body.)

HERS tested whether estrogen plus progestin would prevent a second heart attack or other coronary event. It found no reduction in risk from such hormone therapy over 4 years. In fact, the therapy increased women's risk for a heart attack during the first year of hormone use. The risk declined thereafter. HERS also found that the therapy caused an increase in blood clots in the legs and lungs. The "HERS Follow-Up Study," which tracked the participants for about 3 more years, found no lasting decrease in heart disease from estrogen- plus progestin therapy.

The Women's Health Initiative

In 1991, the National Heart, Lung, and Blood Institute (NHLBI) and other units of the National Institutes of Health (NIH) launched the Women's Health Initiative (WHI), one of the largest studies of its kind ever undertaken in the United States.

It consists of a set of clinical trials, an observational study, and a community prevention study, which altogether involve more than 161,000 healthy postmenopausal women.

The observational study is looking for predictors and biological markers for disease and is being conducted at more than 40 centers across the United States. The community prevention study, which has ended, sought to find ways to get women to adopt healthful behaviors and was done with the Federal Government's Centers for Disease Control and Prevention.

WHI's three clinical trials, conducted at the same U.S. centers, are designed to test the effects of menopausal hormone therapy, diet modification, and calcium and vitamin D supplements on heart disease, osteoporotic fractures, and breast and colorectal cancer risk.

The hormone trials also were checking whether the therapies' possible benefits outweighed possible risks from breast cancer, endometrial (or uterine) cancer, and blood clots. The hormone therapy trials have ended.

181

The menopausal hormone therapy clinical trial had two parts. The first involved 16,608 postmenopausal women with a uterus who took either estrogen plus-progestin therapy or a placebo. (The added progestin protects women against uterine cancer.) The second involved 10,739 women who had had a hysterectomy and took estrogen alone or a placebo. (A placebo is a substance that looks like the real drug but has no biologic effect.)

The estrogen-plus-progestin trial used 0.625 milligrams of conjugated equine estrogens taken daily plus 2.5 milligrams of medroxyprogesterone acetate (Prempro™) taken daily. The estrogen-alone trial used 0.625 milligrams of conjugated equine estrogens (Premarin™) taken daily.

Prempro and Premarin were chosen for two key reasons: They contain the most commonly prescribed forms of estrogen-alone and combined therapies in the United States, and, in several observational studies, these drugs appeared to benefit women's health.

Women in the trials were aged 50 to 79—their average age at enrollment was about 64 for both trials. They enrolled in the studies between 1993 and 1998. Their health was carefully monitored by an independent panel, called the Data and Safety Monitoring Board (DSMB).

Both hormone studies were to have continued until 2005, but were stopped early. The estrogen plus-progestin study was halted in July 2002, and the estrogen-alone study at the end of February 2004. Women in both trials are now in a follow-up phase, due to last until 2007. During the follow-up, their health will be closely monitored.

Effects on Disease and Death

Briefly, the combination therapy study was stopped because of an increased risk of breast cancer and because, overall, risks from use of the hormones outnumbered the benefits. "Outnumbered" means that more women had adverse effects from the therapy than benefited from it. For breast cancer, the risk was greatest among women who had used estrogen plus progestin before entering the study, indicating that the therapy may have a cumulative effect. The combination therapy also increased the risk for heart attack, stroke, and blood clots. For heart attack, the risk was particularly high in the first year of hormone use and continued for several years thereafter. Unlike HERS, which involved women with heart disease, there was an overall increased risk from the hormone therapy over the 5.6 years of the trial. The risk for blood clots was greatest during the first 2 years of hormone use—four times higher than that of placebo users. By the end of the study, the risk for blood clots had decreased to two times greater—or 18 more women with blood clots each year for every 10,000 women.

Estrogen plus progestin also reduced the risk for hip and other fractures, and colorectal cancer. The reduction in colorectal cancer risk appeared after 3 years of hormone use and became more marked thereafter. However, the number of cases of colorectal cancer was relatively small, and more research is needed to confirm the finding.

The estrogen-alone study was stopped after almost 7 years because the hormone therapy increased the risk of stroke and did not reduce the risk of coronary heart disease. It also increased the risk for venous thrombosis (blood clots deep in a vein, usually in the leg). There also was a trend towards increased risk for pulmonary embolism (blood clots in the lungs), but it was not statistically significant. The therapy had no significant effect on the risk of heart disease or colorectal cancer. Its effect on breast cancer was uncertain. Although the risk for breast cancer for those on estrogen alone appeared to be lower, this finding was not statistically significant. Estrogen alone reduced the risk for hip and other fractures. The reduction began early in the study and persisted throughout the follow-up period.

Neither estrogen plus progestin nor estrogen alone affected the risk of death.

Chapter 20

Migraines and Stroke

Around 15 per cent of women and five per cent of men experience migraine. Stroke and migraine share certain symptoms, which may lead someone with a migraine to fear they are having a stroke. A migraine is a type of headache, caused by spasms of the arteries leading into the head. A stroke is the interruption of blood to the brain, which kills the cells in the immediate area and affects those in the surrounding areas. The most common type of stroke is the ischaemic stroke, which is caused by an embolism (clot or debris) blocking a blood vessel in the brain. A migraine doesn't cause brain damage, either in the short or long term. A stroke results in brain damage that varies from mild to disabling. In severe cases, a stroke can cause coma or death. Despite the similarities in symptoms, it is possible to tell the difference between migraine and stroke.

Migraine Aura

Around one in five migraine sufferers experience what are known as "focal neurological symptoms" (migraine aura). Migraine aura often causes visual disturbances, such as flashing lights, zigzagging lines, or partial loss of vision. Other symptoms may include numbness, tingling, speech difficulties, and muscle weakness on one side of the body. These disturbing symptoms usually disappear within an hour. Unlike stroke, where similar symptoms are caused by an interruption of blood flow to the brain, migraine aura is thought to be caused by over-activity of the brain cells. The gradual onset of migraine aura is due to the slow spreading of hyperactive nerve activity across the brain surface.

Symptoms of Stroke

Stroke and migraine aura can have similar symptoms. Depending on the area of brain affected, the symptoms of stroke may include:

- Problems with vision, such as vision loss
- Numbness and tingling of the face, sometimes on one side only
- Speech disturbances
- Muscle weakness, sometimes on one side of the body.

Transient Ischaemic Attack

Problems can occur if what's known as a transient ischaemic attack is mistaken for a migraine. A transient ischaemic attack (TIA) is a minor stroke and a powerful warning that a severe stroke may follow. The symptoms of a TIA are identical to those of a full stroke, but disappear within 24 hours. TIAs can appear hours, days, weeks, or months before a full stroke. Just like full strokes, TIAs need emergency treatment. It seems that TIAs are caused by tiny blockages to blood vessels. These blockages cause temporary symptoms before they dissolve. Migraine aura and TIAs share similar symptoms, such as speech disturbances, weakness, and problems with vision. Since the symptoms of TIAs go away within hours, the person may mistakenly believe they suffered nothing more than a migraine.

Differences between TIA and Migraine Symptoms

It is extremely dangerous for people to diagnose themselves and they should always seek medical advice. The broad differences between a migraine and a TIA include:

- **Visual disturbances**—in TIA, the only disturbance is vision loss, whereas visual disturbance in migraine includes flashing lights and zigzagging lines as well.

- **Speed of attack**—in TIA, the symptoms occur suddenly. In migraine, symptoms spread slowly over a few minutes.

- **Age of onset**—migraine tends to first occur when an individual is young, whereas stroke is more common in older people.

Slightly Increased Risk of Stroke

People who suffer from migraine may have a slightly greater risk of stroke. One study found that the risk of stroke for women in their 20s is 1.4 cases per 100,000. For young women with migraine, the risk rises to 4.2 cases per 100,000. The link between migraine and stroke risk is unknown. However, stroke is generally caused by a number of factors working in combination. Other factors which can increase the risk of stroke include the use of oral contraceptives and cigarette smoking. A young woman who experiences frequent migraine can reduce her minimal risk of stroke by quitting cigarettes and using other forms of birth control.

Treatment Options

Recurring migraine should be medically investigated to confirm the diagnosis and to ensure appropriate and effective treatment. In some people, what seems to be a migraine aura may turn out to be stroke or a transient ischaemic attack (TIA). A person with a suspected stroke or TIA should seek medical advice immediately. If in doubt, see your doctor or call an ambulance.

Where to Get Help

- Your doctor
- In an emergency, call 000 for an ambulance. [Editorial Note: In the United States, dial 911.]

Things to Remember

- Migraine and stroke may present similar symptoms, including visual disturbances, speech problems, and weakness down one side.

- People who suffer from migraine may have a slightly greater risk of experiencing stroke in the future.

- You can reduce your risk of stroke by making healthy lifestyle choices, such as quitting cigarettes.

Chapter 21

Obesity and Physical Inactivity

Chapter Contents

Section 21.1

The Health Risks of Overweight and Obesity

Excerpted from "What Are the Health Risks of Overweight and Obesity?" by the National Heart, Lung, and Blood Institute (NHLBI, www.nhlbi.nih .gov), part of the National Institutes of Health, September 2007.

Being overweight or obese isn't a cosmetic problem. It greatly raises the risk in adults for many diseases and conditions.

Overweight and Obesity-Related Health Problems in Adults

Heart Disease. This condition occurs when a fatty material called plaque builds up on the inside walls of the coronary arteries (the arteries that supply blood and oxygen to your heart). Plaque narrows the coronary arteries, which reduces blood flow to your heart. Your chances for having heart disease and a heart attack get higher as your body mass index (BMI) increases. Obesity also can lead to congestive heart failure, a serious condition in which the heart can't pump enough blood to meet your body's needs.

High Blood Pressure (Hypertension). This condition occurs when the force of the blood pushing against the walls of the arteries is too high. Your chances for having high blood pressure are greater if you're overweight or obese.

Stroke: Being overweight or obese can lead to a buildup of fatty deposits in your arteries that form a blood clot. If the clot is close to your brain, it can block the flow of blood and oxygen and cause a stroke. The risk of having a stroke rises as BMI increases.

Type 2 Diabetes. This is a disease in which blood sugar (glucose) levels are too high. Normally, the body makes insulin to move the blood sugar into cells where it's used. In type 2 diabetes, the cells don't respond enough to the insulin that's made. Diabetes is a leading cause of early death, heart disease, stroke, kidney disease, and blindness. More than 80 percent of people with type 2 diabetes are overweight.

Abnormal Blood Fats. If you're overweight or obese, you have a greater chance of having abnormal levels of blood fats. These include high amounts of triglycerides and low-density lipoprotein (LDL) cholesterol (a fat-like substance often called "bad" cholesterol), and low high-density lipoprotein (HDL) cholesterol (often called "good" cholesterol). Abnormal levels of these blood fats are a risk for heart disease.

Metabolic Syndrome. This is the name for a group of risk factors linked to overweight and obesity that raise your chance for heart disease and other health problems such as diabetes and stroke. A person can develop any one of these risk factors by itself, but they tend to occur together. Metabolic syndrome occurs when a person has at least three of these heart disease risk factors:

- A large waistline. This is also called abdominal obesity or "having an apple shape." Having extra fat in the waist area is a greater risk factor for heart disease than having extra fat in other parts of the body, such as on the hips.
- Abnormal blood fat levels, including high triglycerides and low HDL cholesterol.
- Higher than normal blood pressure.
- Higher than normal fasting blood sugar levels.

Cancer. Being overweight or obese raises the risk for colon, breast, endometrial, and gallbladder cancers.

Osteoarthritis. This is a common joint problem of the knees, hips, and lower back. It occurs when the tissue that protects the joints wears away. Extra weight can put more pressure and wear on joints, causing pain.

Sleep Apnea. This condition causes a person to stop breathing for short periods during sleep. A person with sleep apnea may have more fat stored around the neck. This can make the breathing airway smaller so that it's hard to breathe.

Reproductive Problems. Obesity can cause menstrual irregularity and infertility in women.

Gallstones. These are hard pieces of stone-like material that form in the gallbladder. They're mostly made of cholesterol and can cause abdominal or back pain. People who are overweight or obese have a greater chance of having gallstones. Also, being overweight may result in an enlarged gallbladder that may not work properly.

Section 21.2

Obese Women Have Thicker Carotid Walls, Higher Stroke Risk

Obesity in middle-aged women is independently associated with premature thickening of the carotid arteries, a sign of impending heart disease, researchers report in [the November 14, 2002] rapid access issue of *Stroke: Journal of the American Heart Association.*

Carotid arteries are in the neck and supply blood to the brain. Thickening of the carotid artery wall is an early sign of atherosclerotic disease and a risk factor for stroke.

The association between obesity—regardless of other risk factors, such as high blood pressure—and atherosclerotic disease has been controversial, says the study's author Paolo Rubba, M.D., professor of internal medicine and director of the clinical unit for vascular medicine Federico II University, Naples, Italy.

"There is an established link between obesity and damage to the heart, but whether obesity also has an independent effect on the carotid arteries is less well known," he says.

Researchers investigated whether overall obesity and obesity specific to the abdominal area were associated with thickening of the carotid arteries. They analyzed data from the Progetto ATENA study, an ongoing study of chronic disease in more than 5,000 middle-aged women from Southern Italy. In this region, increased caloric intake, increased animal fat intake, and sedentary habits have led to a high prevalence of overweight and obesity, the researchers say.

Researchers took a subsample of 310 study participants (average age 55) who had ultrasound testing to examine the intima-media thickness (IMT), which is the lining and middle muscle layers of the carotid artery. They also examined the intima-media area (IM). The researchers compared body mass index (BMI) and waist-to-hip ratio—which both indicate obesity—to the health of the carotid arteries.

They found a significant association between the estimates of obesity and the level of wall thickness, which was still significant after accounting for other risk factors, such as age, blood pressure, and cholesterol.

Women with BMI of 30 kilograms per meter squared (kg/m2) or greater had higher blood pressure, triglycerides, glucose, and insulin and lower high-density lipoprotein (HDL, the "good" cholesterol.)

A gradual increase in IMT was found with increasing weight. Lean women (23.0 BMI) had an average IMT of 0.94 millimeters (mm), overweight women (27.2 BMI) had an average of 0.98 mm and obese women (33.8 BMI) had an average of 1.02 mm.

IM was 20 mm for lean women, 21 for overweight women and 23 for obese women.

Women with high waist-to-hip ratios also had higher triglycerides, glucose and insulin and decreased HDL. The wall thickness measurements were higher for women with higher waist-to-hip ratios.

Hence, BMI and waist-to-hip ratio were significant predictors of carotid wall thickness, independent of other risk factors. Researchers conclude that general and abdominal obesity are associated with carotid artery wall thickening in middle-aged women.

"Controlling blood pressure is not enough to prevent the cardiovascular damage from being overweight," Rubba says. "Doctors should face the difficult challenge of encouraging patients to lose weight to prevent premature atherosclerosis and stroke. With the information in this study, women also should be aware of further health implications if they don't reduce their weight."

The study suggests that ultrasound screening in obese women may help identify those at high risk and those who may require aggressive therapy to prevent early atherosclerosis, he says. By seeing the early warning signs, women and their doctors might be better motivated to aggressively treat obesity and the benefits of their efforts might be evident in follow-up evaluations years later.

Future studies should focus on whether atherosclerosis in obese women progresses faster than in women who are not obese, Rubba says.

Co-authors are Mario De Michele, M.D.; Salvatore Panico, M.D.; Arcangelo Iannuzzi, M.D.; Egidio Celentano, M.D.; Anna V. Ciardullo, M.D.; Rocco Galasso, M.D.; Lucia Sacchetti, Ph.D.; Federica Zarrilli, Ph.D.; and M. Gene Bond, Ph.D.

Section 21.3

Physical Inactivity

"Physical Inactivity" is from the Centers for Disease Control and Prevention (CDC, www.cdc.gov), July 23, 2003. This document was reviewed by David A. Cooke, M.D., March 3, 2008.

What's the problem?

Increasingly, researchers are learning that regular exercise and good nutrition are critical to sustained good health. In fact, estimates are that some 300,000 deaths each year in the United States likely are the results of physical inactivity and poor eating habits. These deaths range across a number of diseases, from heart disease and stroke to colon cancer and diabetes.

Good exercise and nutrition habits, especially if formed in childhood (although it is never too late to change one's habits), can help prevent high blood pressure and elevated cholesterol, which contribute to heart disease and stroke.

They can reduce obesity, which is closely associated with these diseases, as well as with diabetes and certain types of cancer. They also help in building strong bones, which are needed to prevent osteoporosis later in life. Other benefits include anxiety and stress reduction, improved self-esteem, and general feelings of well being.

Physical activity levels tend to decrease as a person ages. Of youths aged 12 and 13, 69% are regularly physically active, but, the number drops to 38% for young people between 18 and 21. A physically inactive child is more likely to become a physically inactive adult, which can lead to chronic disease and premature death.

Between 1991 and 1997, the percentage of students who attended a daily physical education class dropped from 42% to 27%. The lack of organized physical activity in our nation's schools sends a false message to young people that being active isn't important.

Daily opportunities to burn calories have diminished. We now see fewer sidewalks and a greater emphasis on driving rather than walking or bicycling. Also, our society is more automated and we have labor-saving devices at work and home.

These problems, along with popular sedentary activities such as watching TV and using computers, have all contributed to the decline of physical activity.

Who's at risk?

Young people and adults are at risk for health problems when they are inactive. Physical activity declines dramatically during adolescence. Nearly half of young people between 12 and 21 do not regularly engage in vigorous physical activity; participation in all types of physical activity declines strikingly as people age. Only about a third of adults meet current public health recommendations for regular moderate physical activity (five times a week for at least 30 minutes), and about a quarter report no leisure-time physical activity at all.

Can it be prevented?

Yes. Physical activity and a healthy diet can enhance health and prevent disease. Both children and adults need to find ways to increase the amount of weight-bearing (e.g., running, walking) and aerobic (e.g., biking, swimming) exercise. They also need to give greater attention to diets low in fat, high in fiber, calcium, and fruits and vegetables to promote better health.

Chapter 22

Peripheral Arterial Disease Increases Stroke Risk

What Is Peripheral Arterial Disease?

Peripheral arterial disease (PAD) occurs when a fatty material called plaque builds up on the inside walls of the arteries that carry blood from the heart to the head, internal organs, and limbs. PAD is also known as atherosclerotic peripheral arterial disease.

The buildup of plaque on the artery walls is called atherosclerosis, or hardening of the arteries. Atherosclerosis causes the arteries to narrow or become blocked, which can reduce or block blood flow. PAD most commonly affects blood flow to the legs.

Blocked blood flow can cause pain and numbness. It also can increase a person's chance of getting an infection, and it can make it difficult for the person's body to fight the infection. If severe enough, blocked blood flow can cause tissue death (gangrene). PAD is the leading cause of leg amputation.

Important General Information

Atherosclerosis can affect arteries anywhere in the body, including the arteries that carry blood to the heart and brain. When atherosclerosis affects the arteries of the heart, it is called coronary artery

From "Peripheral Arterial Disease," by the National Heart, Lung, and Blood Institute (NHLBI, www.nhlbi.nih.gov), part of the National Institutes of Health, June 2006.

disease (CAD). CAD can cause a heart attack. If atherosclerosis is in the limbs, it also is likely to be in the coronary arteries.

When atherosclerosis affects the major arteries supplying the brain, it is called carotid artery disease. Carotid artery disease can cause a stroke.

PAD (atherosclerosis in the arteries that supply blood to the limbs, especially the legs) is a common, yet serious disease. Men are more likely to have symptoms of PAD, but both men and women can develop the disease. PAD can impair physical health and diminish the ability to walk.

In the advanced stages of PAD, blood flow to one or both legs can be completely or mostly blocked. This is known as chronic critical limb ischemia (CLI). A very severe blockage in the legs and feet means that the legs do not receive the oxygen or nutrition needed for cellular or skin growth and repair. CLI may lead to painful leg or foot sores, and it could eventually lead to gangrene. If this condition is left untreated, the foot or leg may need to be amputated.

Outlook

A person with PAD has a six to seven times greater risk of CAD, heart attack, stroke, or transient ischemic attack ("mini stroke") than the rest of the population. If a person has heart disease, he or she has a 1 in 3 chance of having blocked arteries in the legs. Early diagnosis and treatment of PAD, including screening high-risk individuals, are important to prevent disability and save lives. PAD treatment may stop the disease from progressing and reduce the risk of heart attack, heart disease, and stroke.

Although PAD is serious, it is treatable. The buildup of plaque in the arteries can often be stopped or reversed with dietary changes, exercise, and efforts to lower high cholesterol levels and high blood pressure. In some patients, blood flow in the vessels may be improved by medicines or surgery.

Other Names for Peripheral Arterial Disease

- Atherosclerotic peripheral arterial disease
- Peripheral vascular disease (PVD)
- Vascular disease
- Hardening of the arteries
- Claudication

- Poor circulation
- Leg cramps from poor circulation

What Causes Peripheral Arterial Disease?

The most common cause of peripheral arterial disease (PAD) is atherosclerosis. When atherosclerosis affects the arteries of the limbs, it is called PAD. The exact cause of atherosclerosis is unknown in the majority of cases. In atherosclerosis, the plaque that builds up on artery walls is made up of fat, cholesterol, calcium, and other substances in the blood. Smoking, diabetes, a high blood cholesterol level, and high blood pressure increase the risk of atherosclerosis.

Who Is at Risk for Peripheral Arterial Disease?

Peripheral arterial disease (PAD) affects 8 to 12 million people in the United States. An estimated 5 percent of U.S. adults over age 50 have PAD. Among adults age 65 and older, 12 to 20 percent may have PAD.

Major Risk Factors

Major risk factors for developing PAD include:

- Smoking. Smoking is more closely related to developing PAD than any other risk factor. Smoking increases the risk of developing PAD three to five times. On average, smokers who develop PAD experience symptoms 10 years earlier than nonsmokers who develop PAD. Stopping smoking will slow the progress of PAD. Smoking even one or two cigarettes daily can interfere with the treatment for PAD. Smokers and diabetics have the greatest risk of complications from PAD, including gangrene in the leg from decreased blood flow.

- Chronic or serious illnesses, such as diabetes. One in three people over age 50 with diabetes is likely to have PAD. Anyone over age 50 with diabetes should be screened for PAD.

- Other diseases and conditions, such as:
  - Kidney disease
  - High blood pressure or a family history of it
  - A high cholesterol level or a family history of it
  - Heart disease or a family history of it

199

- A family history of stroke

- Age. Men who are older than age 50 and women who are older than age 55 are at higher risk for PAD.

What Are the Signs and Symptoms of Peripheral Arterial Disease?

At least half of the people who have peripheral arterial disease (PAD) don't have any signs or symptoms of the disease.

People who do have signs or symptoms may have pain when walking or climbing stairs, which may be relieved after resting. This pain is called intermittent claudication. Blood brings oxygen to the muscles, but during exercise, muscles need more blood flow. If there is a blockage in the blood vessels, muscles won't get enough blood. If a person has intermittent claudication and exercises while in pain, his or her muscles may be harmed. When resting, the muscles require less blood flow and the pain goes away. Claudication is more likely in people who also have atherosclerosis in other arteries, such as the heart and brain. About 10 percent of people with PAD have intermittent claudication.

Other signs and symptoms of PAD include:

- pain, numbness, aching, and heaviness in the muscles;

- cramping in the legs, thighs, calves, and feet;

- a weak or absent pulse in the legs or feet;

- sores or wounds on toes, feet, or legs that heal slowly, poorly, or not at all;

- color changes in skin, paleness, or blueness (called cyanosis);

- a decreased temperature in one leg compared to the other leg;

- poor nail growth and decreased hair growth on toes and legs; and

- erectile dysfunction, especially among people with diabetes.

How Is Peripheral Arterial Disease Diagnosed?

Peripheral arterial disease (PAD) is diagnosed based on general medical and family history, history of leg or heart problems, personal risk factors, a physical exam, and test results. An accurate diagnosis is critical, because people with PAD face a six to seven times higher risk of heart disease or stroke than the rest of the population. PAD is often diagnosed after symptoms are reported. If you have PAD, your doctor also may want to look for signs of coronary artery disease (CAD).

Specialists Involved

Mild PAD may be managed by a primary care doctor, internist, or general practitioner. For more advanced PAD, a vascular specialist (a doctor who specializes in treating blood vessel problems) may be involved. A cardiologist (a doctor who specializes in heart diseases) also may be involved in the care of patients with PAD.

Medical and Family History

Medical and family history is important in diagnosing PAD. Your doctor may:

- ask about your family history of cardiovascular disease;
- review your medical history, including high blood pressure or diabetes;
- ask about any symptoms, including any symptoms that occur when walking or exercising;
- ask if you are currently or used to be a smoker;
- ask if you have any symptoms in the legs when sitting, standing, walking, or climbing;
- review your diet; and
- review your current medicines.

Physical Exam

The physical exam may involve:

- checking blood flow in your leg or foot to see if the pulse is either weak or absent.
- checking pulses in your leg arteries for an abnormal whooshing sound called a bruit. A bruit can be heard with a stethoscope and may be a warning of a narrow or blocked section of an artery.
- checking for poor wound healing.

201

- comparing blood pressure between your limbs to see if blood pressure is lower in the affected limb.

- checking hair, skin, and nails for any changes that may indicate PAD.

Diagnostic Tests and Procedures

A simple test called an ankle-brachial index (ABI) can be used to diagnose PAD. The ABI compares blood pressure in the ankle with blood pressure in the arm to see how well blood is flowing. A normal ABI is 1.0 or greater (with a range of 0.90 to 1.30). The test takes about 10–15 minutes to measure both arms and both ankles. It can help the doctor find out if PAD is affecting the legs, but it will not identify which blood vessels are blocked. The ABI can be performed yearly if necessary to see if the disease is getting worse.

A Doppler ultrasound is a test that uses sound waves to tell whether a blood vessel is open or blocked. This test uses a blood pressure cuff and special device to measure blood flow in the veins and arteries in the arms and legs. The Doppler ultrasound can help to determine the level and degree of PAD.

A treadmill test will provide more information on the severity of the symptoms and the level of exercise that provokes symptoms. For this test, you will walk on a treadmill, which will help identify any difficulties that you may have during normal walking.

A magnetic resonance angiogram (MRA) uses radio wave energy to take pictures of blood vessels inside the body. MRA is a type of magnetic resonance imaging (MRI) scan. An MRA can detect problems that may cause reduced blood flow in the blood vessels. It can determine the location and degree of blockage. A patient with a pacemaker, prosthetic joint, stent, surgical clips, mechanical heart valve, or other metallic devices in his or her body might not be eligible for an MRA depending on the type of metallic device.

An arteriogram is a "road map" of the arteries used to pinpoint the exact location of the blockage in a limb. An x-ray is taken after injecting dye through a needle or catheter into an artery. When the dye is injected, the patient may feel mildly flushed. The pictures from the x ray can determine the location, type, and extent of the blockage. Some hospitals are using a newer method that uses tiny ultrasound cameras to take pictures inside the blood vessel.

Blood tests may be done to check the patient's blood sugar level to screen for diabetes. Blood tests also may be used to check the patient's cholesterol levels.

How Is Peripheral Arterial Disease Treated?

Goals of Treatment

The overall goals for treating peripheral arterial disease (PAD) are to reduce symptoms, improve quality of life, and prevent complications. Treatment is based on symptoms, risk factors, physical exam results, and diagnostic tests.

Specific Types of Treatment

Specific treatments for PAD include lifestyle changes, medicines, and surgery or special procedures.

Lifestyle Changes

Treatment often includes making long-lasting lifestyle changes, such as:

- **Quitting smoking.** Smoking increases the risk of developing PAD three to five times. The risk for coronary artery disease (CAD) decreases rapidly if the smoker quits. The risk for CAD decreases 40 percent within 5 years of stopping smoking.

- **Lowering blood pressure.** Lowering blood pressure can help to avoid the risk of stroke, heart attack, congestive heart failure, and kidney disease.

- **Lowering high cholesterol levels.** Lowering cholesterol levels can delay or even reverse the buildup of plaque in the arteries.

- **Lowering blood glucose levels if you have diabetes.** A hemoglobin A1C test—a test that gives an estimate of how well blood sugar has been controlled over the past 3 months—may be performed.

Talk with your doctor about participating in a supervised exercise therapy program. Follow a low-saturated fat, low-cholesterol diet, and eat foods with less salt, total fat, and saturated fat. Eat more fruits, vegetables, and low-fat dairy products. If you are overweight or obese, work with your doctor to develop a reasonable weight-loss plan. If you are diabetic or at risk for critical limb ischemia, have your feet examined regularly.

Medicines

Medicines may be prescribed to:

- lower high cholesterol levels and high blood pressure;
- thin the blood to prevent clots from forming due to low blood flow;
- dissolve blood clots; and
- help improve pain in the legs that is the result of walking or climbing stairs (claudication).

Some medicines lower the level of low density lipoprotein (LDL) cholesterol. LDL is the "bad" cholesterol. The higher the LDL level in the blood, the greater the chance of heart disease. Medicines may include statins, such as lovastatin, simvastatin, pravastatin, fluvastatin, and atorvastatin. Other medicines may include ezetimibe, gemfibrozil, and certain binding agents.

Blood pressure should be lowered if it is too high. Treatment should aim for a blood pressure lower than 130/80 mmHg. Many medicines are available to lower blood pressure, such as angiotensin-converting enzyme (ACE) inhibitors, angiotensin receptor blockers (ARBs), beta-blockers, diuretics ("water pills"), and calcium channel blockers.

Anticoagulants or blood thinners may be prescribed to prevent clots in the arteries. Thrombolytic therapy involves clot-dissolving drugs inserted into an artery to break up a blood clot. To stop platelets from clumping together, antiplatelet drugs such as clopidogrel (Plavix®) and aspirin may be prescribed. To help increase distances walked without pain and help improve claudication, pentoxifylline (Trental®) or cilostazol (Pletal®) may be prescribed.

Surgeries or Special Procedures

Surgery may be necessary if blood flow in a limb is completely or almost completely blocked. In bypass grafting surgery, the doctor uses a blood vessel from another part of your body or a tube made of synthetic (manmade) material to make a graft. This graft bypasses the blockage in the artery, allowing blood to flow around it. Surgery does not cure PAD, but it may increase blood flow to the limb.

Angioplasty may be performed to restore blood flow through a narrowed or blocked artery. During the procedure, a thin tube (catheter) is inserted into a blocked artery and a small balloon on the tip of the catheter is inflated. When the balloon is inflated, plaque is pushed against the artery walls. This causes the artery to widen, restoring blood flow. A stent, a tiny mesh tube that looks like a small spring, is now used in most angioplasties. Some stents are coated with medicine to help prevent the artery from closing again.

Other Types of Treatment

Cell and gene therapies are currently being researched, but are not yet available outside of clinical trials.

How Can Peripheral Arterial Disease Be Prevented?

There are a number of ways to try to prevent peripheral arterial disease (PAD). If you are a smoker, quit smoking. On average, smokers who develop PAD experience symptoms 10 years earlier than nonsmokers who develop PAD. Work to control your blood pressure, cholesterol, and glucose levels. Talk with your doctor about beginning a supervised exercise therapy program. If you are overweight or obese, work with your doctor to develop a reasonable weight-loss plan. Finally, follow a low-fat, low-cholesterol diet and eat more fruits and vegetables.

Living with Peripheral Arterial Disease

Ongoing Health Care Needs

Peripheral arterial disease (PAD) can be treated and controlled.

If you are experiencing pain in calf or thigh muscles after walking (intermittent claudication), try to take a break and allow the pain to ease before walking again. Over time, this should increase the distance that you can walk without pain.

Check your feet and toes regularly for sores or any possible infection. Wear comfortable shoes that fit well. Maintain good foot hygiene and have professional medical treatment for corns, bunions, or calluses.

Be sure to keep your blood pressure, cholesterol, and blood sugar (if diabetic) within normal ranges. Continue to carefully check your feet daily for any sores or infections.

Treatment should decrease pain when walking and allow you to walk longer distances without discomfort. There should be less painful cramping of leg muscles. There may be improvement in the skin's appearance and improvement in ulcers on your legs and feet.

Support Groups

The Peripheral Arterial Disease Coalition is an alliance of leading health organizations, vascular health professional organizations, and government agencies that have united to raise public and health professional awareness about lower extremity PAD. The coalition's Patient Education Workgroup is developing patient education tools.

The Amputee Coalition of America and National Limb Loss Information Center provide support for people with limb loss.

Long-Term Care

For severe cases of chronic clinical limb ischemia (CLI), a patient may be bed-bound and need total supportive care. CLI is a severe blockage of the arteries that seriously decreases blood flow to the hands, legs, and feet. People with severe CLI may experience burning pain in the affected limb, and they can suffer from wounds that do not heal or from tissue death (gangrene).

Chapter 23

Stroke in Pregnancy and Childbirth

Although men are generally more apt to experience stroke than are women, women in their childbearing years are at greater risk for stroke than their male, age-matched counterparts. Indeed, pregnancy, childbirth, and the puerperium [the period of time immediately after the birth of a baby] are the times when women are at particular risk, but there is more to the story. Recent research conducted at Duke University in Durham, North Carolina, demonstrated that not only is the incidence of stroke during pregnancy and the puerperium higher than was previously thought,[1] but women who have had complications during pregnancy are at higher risk for stroke later in life.[2]

The first study,[1] published in the September 2005 issue of *Obstetrics & Gynecology,* looked at data on stroke and pregnancy discharges within the Agency for Healthcare Research and Quality's Nationwide Inpatient Sample from the Healthcare Cost & Utilization Project for years 2000 to 2001. A total of 2,850 discharges for pregnancy complicated by stroke were identified. This translated into a rate of 34.2 strokes for every 100,000 deliveries—a rate higher than was previously deduced in an earlier Canadian study, published in *Stroke* in 2000. That study used similar data and methodology and reported an incidence of 26 strokes for every 100,000 pregnancies.[3]

African Americans were at highest risk. As would be expected, risk also increased with age: women aged 35 years or older were most

"New Findings on Pregnancy and Stroke: Implications and Interventions," by Dee Rapposelli, *Applied Neurology,* January 2006. © CMP Healthcare Media. Reprinted with permission.

vulnerable. The study also confirmed that various cardiovascular and hematologic conditions (heart disease, hypertension, thrombophilia, thrombocytopenia, and sickle cell disease) and complications of pregnancy (postpartum hemorrhage, preeclampsia, and gestational hypertension) raised the stakes for risk. The study also identified migraine, blood transfusion, and lupus as risk factors. The mortality rate was about 4%.

Study coauthor Cheryl D. Bushnell, M.D., MHS, assistant professor of medicine in the Division of Neurology, Department of Medicine, at Duke, noted that new preventive care strategies need to be developed to protect mothers—and their newborns—from stroke and its complications. Prevention and management of hypertension, heart disease, and diabetes are the obvious places to start and have been ongoing campaigns in the general population.

Complicated Pregnancy and Looming Stroke Threat

Preventive strategies won't only decrease the incidence of stroke in young women during and immediately after pregnancy; they also stand to ameliorate the incidence of stroke in older women. A second study by Bushnell and colleagues, reported at the annual meeting of the American Neurological Association (ANA) last fall, found that women who have had complications during pregnancy, specifically preeclampsia and gestational diabetes, are at greater risk for stroke down the line—an average of 13.5 years later.[2]

The researchers combed through the Duke University Medical Center Perinatal and Health Services Outcomes Database and identified 42,263 women who had given birth between 1979 and 2005. They then identified 164 women who had had a stroke after the puerperium and matched them with 311 controls matched by age and by month and year of delivery. What they found was striking: the women who had experienced stroke were 70% more likely to have had a complication of pregnancy than were controls. Average age at the time of stroke was 40 years.

Although a wide range of complications of pregnancy was reviewed, only preeclampsia and gestational diabetes were associated with stroke. When asked what preventive strategies could be put in place to prevent stroke down the road in women at risk, Bushnell told *Applied Neurology* that prevention of preeclampsia might be the key. It's a challenge, however; the causes of preeclampsia are unknown.

Bushnell is developing a set of tests that would assist in predicting preeclampsia. She foresees a long road through NIH [National

Institutes of Health] approval and development. She is also undertaking proof-of-principle studies to confirm that preeclampsia is associated with heart disease and stroke risk.

"We can do that by measuring the thickness of the carotid artery," said Bushnell. "Endothelial dysfunction post-pregnancy is associated with preeclampsia, but it's never been shown as proof of principle that [affected women are] going to be at risk for stroke. That's where I'd like to take this. Once we understand what happens early after pregnancy, we can look at pre-pregnancy and try to prevent preeclampsia altogether."

Although protocols regarding preeclampsia and stroke prevention are relegated to the future, practical steps to prevent stroke in women whose pregnancy complications augur risk are relatively simple but require planning and diligence. These steps include regular monitoring of blood pressure and blood glucose levels and encouraging weight control.

Bushnell noted that these measures generally are not undertaken, but if they became a routine part of postnatal and ongoing care for women who have had complications of pregnancy, the overall incidence of stroke might decline. Indeed, her institution offers a weight management program for women who have recently given birth. "They teach new moms how to incorporate an exercise routine into their lives," explained Bushnell. She added that a woman's knowledge about her stroke risk, based on whether she had preeclampsia or another complication of pregnancy, may act as an incentive to avail herself of postnatal health maintenance programs.

Racial/Socioeconomic Component to Risk

Of particular concern was that an overwhelming majority—73%—of the women affected by stroke were African American. The incidence of hypertension is higher in African Americans than in white persons. This might account for the higher rate of stroke among African American women in the study, according to Bushnell.

When asked whether socioeconomic issues play a role, Bushnell conceded that prenatal care might be suboptimal in low-income minority populations—a circumstance that a colleague of hers, Monique V. Chireau, M.D., assistant professor in the Division of Clinical and Epidemiologic Research in the Department of Obstetrics and Gynecology at Duke, is about to investigate. Chireau also was the lead author of the study presented at the ANA.

The study, funded through a recently awarded grant from the Centers for Medicare & Medicaid Services Historically Black College/University Program, will look at outcomes of complications of pregnancy and patient satisfaction among Medicaid recipients. Among the goals of the study, titled "Shaw-Duke Maternal and Infant Mortality Initiative: Interventions to Improve Outcomes Among Pregnant Medicaid Recipients," are insight into and amelioration of factors that contribute to infant mortality and health care disparities associated with socioeconomic and racial phenomena. The study also will provide recommendations to policymakers in charge of managing Medicaid expenditures.

In addition to shedding light on infant mortality rates and health care quality and access among Medicaid recipients who experience complications of pregnancy, Bushnell said the information gleaned might fortify her own research. "It will be interesting to see, from an observational point, what happens there. That's another cohort where we might be able to do some of these other tests" on preeclampsia and stroke risk, she said.

References

1. James AH, Bushnell CD, Jamison MG, Myers ER. Incidence and risk factors for stroke in pregnancy and the puerperium. *Obstet Gynecol.* 2005;106:509–516.

2. Chireau MV, Bushnell CD, Brown H, et al. Pregnancy complications are associated with stroke risk later in life. Presented at: the 130th Annual Meeting of the American Neurological Association; September 25–28, 2005; San Diego.

3. Jaigobin C, Silver FL. Stroke and pregnancy. *Stroke.* 2000;31:2948–2951.

Chapter 24

Pulmonary Embolism: Artery Blockage That Can Lead to Stroke

What Is Pulmonary Embolism?

A pulmonary embolism, or PE, is a sudden blockage in a lung artery, usually due to a blood clot that traveled to the lung from a vein in the leg. A clot that forms in one part of the body and travels in the bloodstream to another part of the body is called an embolus.

PE is a serious condition that can cause:

- permanent damage to part of your lung from lack of blood flow to lung tissue;

- low oxygen levels in your blood; and

- damage to other organs in your body from not getting enough oxygen.

If the blood clot is large, or if there are many clots, PE can cause death.

Overview

In most cases, PE is a complication of a condition called deep vein thrombosis (DVT). In DVT, blood clots form in the deep veins of the body—most often in the legs. These clots can break free, travel through the bloodstream to the lungs, and block an artery.

"Pulmonary Embolism" is from the National Heart, Lung, and Blood Institute (NHLBI, www.nhlbi.nih.gov), part of the National Institutes of Health, June 2007.

This is unlike clots in the veins close the skin's surface, which remain in place and do not cause PE.

Outlook

At least 100,000 cases of PE occur each year in the United States. PE is the third most common cause of death in hospitalized patients. If left untreated, about 30 percent of patients with PE will die. Most of those who die do so within the first few hours of the event.

What Causes Pulmonary Embolism?

Major Causes

In 9 out of 10 cases, pulmonary embolism (PE) begins as a blood clot in the deep veins of the leg (a condition known as deep vein thrombosis). The clot breaks free from the vein and travels through the bloodstream to the lungs, where it can block an artery.

Clots in the leg can form when blood flow is restricted and slows down. This can happen when you don't move around for long periods of time, such as:

- after some types of surgeries;
- during a long trip in a car or on an airplane; and/or
- if you must stay in bed for an extended time.

Veins damaged from surgery or injured in other ways are more prone to blood clots.

Other Causes

Rarely, an air bubble, part of a tumor, or other tissue travels to the lungs and causes PE. Also, when a large bone in the body (such as the thigh bone) breaks, fat from the marrow inside the bone can travel through the blood to the lungs and cause PE.

Who Is at Risk for Pulmonary Embolism?

Populations Affected

Pulmonary embolism (PE) occurs equally in men and women. Risk increases with age: For each 10 years after age 60, the risk of PE doubles.

Certain inherited conditions, such as factor V Leiden, increase the risk of blood clotting, and, therefore, the risk of PE.

Major Risk Factors

People at high risk for a blood clot that travels to the lungs are those who:

- have deep vein thrombosis (DVT, a blood clot in the leg) or a history of DVT; and/or
- have had PE before.

Other Risk Factors

People who recently have been treated for cancer or who have a central venous catheter (a tube placed in a vein to allow easy access to the bloodstream for medical treatment) are more likely to develop DVT. The same is true for people who have been bedridden or have had surgery or suffered a broken bone in the past few weeks.

Other risk factors for DVT, which can lead to PE, include sitting for long periods of time (such as on long car or airplane rides), pregnancy, and the 6-week period after pregnancy, and being overweight or obese. Women who take hormone therapy or birth control pills also are at increased risk for DVT.

People with more than one risk factor are at higher risk for blood clots.

What Are the Signs and Symptoms of Pulmonary Embolism?

Major Signs and Symptoms

Signs and symptoms of pulmonary embolism (PE) include unexplained shortness of breath, difficulty breathing, chest pain, coughing, or coughing up blood. An arrhythmia (a rapid or irregular heartbeat) also may indicate PE.

In some cases, the only signs and symptoms are related to deep vein thrombosis (DVT). These include swelling of the leg or along the vein in the leg, pain or tenderness in the leg, a feeling of increased warmth in the area of the leg that's swollen or tender, and red or discolored skin on the affected leg. See your doctor at once if you have any symptoms of PE or DVT.

It's possible to have a PE and not have any signs or symptoms of PE or DVT.

Other Signs and Symptoms

Sometimes people who have PE experience feelings of anxiety or dread, lightheadedness or fainting, rapid breathing, sweating, or an increased heart rate.

How Is Pulmonary Embolism Diagnosed?

Specialists Involved

Doctors who treat patients in the emergency room are often the ones to diagnose pulmonary embolism (PE) with the help of a radiologist (a doctor who deals with x-rays and other similar tests).

Medical History and Physical Exam

To diagnose PE, the doctor will ask about your medical history and perform a physical exam to:

- identify your risk factors for deep vein thrombosis (DVT) and PE;
- see how likely it is that you could have PE; and
- rule out other possible causes for your symptoms.

During the physical exam, the doctor will check your legs for signs of DVT. He or she also will check your blood pressure and your heart and lungs.

Diagnostic Tests

There are many different tests that help the doctor determine whether you have PE. The doctor's decision about which tests to use and in which order depends on how you feel when you get to the hospital, your risk factors for PE, available testing options, and other conditions you may have.

You may have one of the following imaging tests:

- **Ultrasound.** Doctors use this test to look for blood clots in your legs. Ultrasound uses high-frequency sound waves to check the flow of blood in your veins. A gel is put on the skin of your leg. A handheld device called a transducer is placed on the leg and moved back and forth over the affected area. The transducer gives off ultrasound waves and detects their echoes after they bounce off the vein walls and blood cells. A computer then turns the echoes of the ultrasound waves into a picture on a computer screen, where your doctor can see the blood flow in your leg. If blood clots are found in the deep veins of your legs, you will begin treatment. DVT and PE are both treated with the same medicines.

- **Spiral CT [computed tomography] scan or CT angiogram.** Doctors use this test to look for blood clots in your lungs and in your legs. Dye is injected into a vein in your arm to make the blood vessels in your lungs and legs more visible on the x-ray image. While you lie on a table, an x-ray tube rotates around you, taking pictures from different angles. This test allows doctors to detect PE in most patients. The test only takes a few minutes. Results are available shortly after the scan is completed.

- **Ventilation-perfusion lung scan (VQ scan).** Doctors use this test to detect PE. The VQ scan uses a radioactive material to show how well oxygen and blood are flowing to all areas of the lungs.

- **Pulmonary angiography** is another test used to diagnose PE. It's not available at all hospitals, and a trained specialist must perform the test. A flexible tube called a catheter is threaded through the groin (upper thigh) or arm to the blood vessels in the lungs. Dye is injected into the blood vessels through the catheter. X-ray pictures are taken to show the blood flow through the blood vessels in the lungs. If a clot is discovered, the doctor may use the catheter to extract it or deliver medicine to dissolve it.

Certain blood tests may help the doctor find out whether you're likely to have PE.

- A D-dimer test measures a substance in the blood that's released when a clot breaks up. High levels of the substance mean there may be a clot. If your test is normal and you have few risk factors, PE isn't likely.

- Other blood tests check for inherited disorders that cause clots and measure the amount of oxygen and carbon dioxide in your blood (arterial blood gas). A clot in a blood vessel in your lung may lower the level of oxygen in your blood.

To rule out other possible causes of your symptoms, the doctor may use one or more of the following tests.

- Echocardiogram uses sound waves to check heart function and to detect blood clots inside the heart.

- EKG (electrocardiogram) measures the rate and regularity of your heartbeat.

- Chest x-ray provides a picture of the lungs, heart, large arteries, ribs, and diaphragm.

- Magnetic resonance imaging (MRI) uses radio waves and magnetic fields to make pictures of organs and structures inside the body. In many cases, an MRI can provide information that can't be seen on an x ray.

How Is Pulmonary Embolism Treated?

Goals of Treatment

The main goals of treating pulmonary embolism (PE) are to:

- stop the blood clot from getting bigger; and
- keep new clots from forming.

Treatment may include medicines to thin the blood and slow its ability to clot. If your symptoms are life threatening, the doctor may give you medicine to dissolve the clot more quickly. Rarely, the doctor may use surgery or another procedure to remove the clot.

Specific Types of Treatment

Medicines. Anticoagulants, which are blood-thinning medicines, decrease your blood's ability to clot. They're used to stop blood clots from getting bigger and to prevent clots from forming. They don't break up blood clots that have already formed. (The body dissolves most clots with time.)

Anticoagulants can be taken as either a pill, an injection, or through a needle or tube inserted into a vein (called intravenous, or IV, injection). Warfarin is given in a pill form. (Coumadin® is a common brand name for warfarin.) Heparin is given as an injection or through an IV tube.

Your doctor may treat you with both heparin and warfarin at the same time. Heparin acts quickly. Warfarin takes 2 to 3 days before it starts to work. Once warfarin starts to work, usually the heparin will be stopped.

Pregnant women usually are treated with heparin only, because warfarin is dangerous for the pregnancy.

If you have deep vein thrombosis, treatment with anticoagulants usually lasts for 3 to 6 months.

If you have had blood clots before, you may need a longer period of treatment. If you're being treated for another illness, such as cancer, you may need to take anticoagulants as long as risk factors for PE are present.

The most common side effect of anticoagulants is bleeding. This happens if the medicine thins your blood too much. This side effect can be life threatening. Sometimes, the bleeding can be internal. This is why people treated with anticoagulants usually receive regular blood tests. These tests are called PT [prothrombin time] and PTT [partial thromboplastin time] tests, and they measure the blood's ability to clot. These tests also help the doctor make sure you're taking the right amount of medicine. Call your doctor right away if you have easy bruising or bleeding.

Thrombin inhibitors are a newer type of anticoagulant medicine. They're used to treat some types of blood clots for patients who can't take heparin.

Emergency Treatment. When PE is life threatening, doctors may use treatments that remove or break up clots in the blood vessels of the lungs. These treatments are given in the emergency room or in the hospital.

Thrombolytics are medicines given to quickly dissolve a blood clot. They're used to treat large clots that cause severe symptoms. Because thrombolytics can cause sudden bleeding, they're used only in life-threatening situations.

In some cases, the doctor may use a catheter to reach the blood clot. A catheter is a flexible tube placed in a vein to allow easy access to the bloodstream for medical treatment. The catheter is inserted into the groin (upper thigh) or arm and threaded through a vein to the clot in the lung. The catheter may be used to extract the clot or deliver medicine to dissolve it.

Rarely, surgery may be needed to remove the blood clot.

Other Types of Treatment

When you can't take medicines to thin your blood, or when you're taking blood thinners but continue to develop clots anyway, the doctor may use a device called a vena cava filter to keep clots from traveling to your lungs. The filter is inserted inside a large vein called the inferior vena cava (the vein that carries blood from the body back to the heart). The filter catches clots before they travel to the lungs. This prevents PE, but it doesn't stop other blood clots from forming.

Graduated compression stockings can reduce the chronic (ongoing) swelling that may occur after a blood clot has developed in a leg. The leg swelling is due to damage to the valves in the leg veins. Graduated compression stockings are worn on the legs from the arch of the foot to just above or below the knee. These stockings are tight at the ankle and become looser as they go up the leg. This causes a gentle compression (or pressure) up the leg. The pressure keeps blood from pooling and clotting.

How Can Pulmonary Embolism Be Prevented?

Preventing pulmonary embolism (PE) begins with preventing deep vein thrombosis (DVT). Knowing whether you're at risk for DVT and taking steps to lower your risk are important.

If you've never had a deep vein clot, but are at risk for it, these are steps you can take to decrease your risk.

- Exercise your lower leg muscles during long car trips and airplane rides.
- Get out of bed and move around as soon as you're able after having surgery or being ill. The sooner you move around, the lower your chance of developing a clot.
- Take medicines to prevent clots after some types of surgery (as directed by your doctor).
- Follow up with your doctor.

If you already have had DVT or PE, you can take additional steps to help keep new blood clots from forming:

- Visit your doctor for regular checkups.
- Use compression stockings to prevent chronic swelling in your legs after DVT (as directed by your doctor).
- Contact your doctor at once if you have any signs or symptoms of DVT or PE.

Living with Pulmonary Embolism

Treatment for PE usually takes place in the hospital. After leaving the hospital you may need to take medicine at home for 6 months or longer. It's important to:

- Take medicines as prescribed.

- Have blood tests done as directed by your doctor.

- Talk to your doctor before taking anticoagulants with any other medicines, including over-the-counter medicines. Over-the-counter aspirin, for example, can thin your blood. Taking two medicines that thin your blood (even if one is over-the-counter) may increase your risk for bleeding.

- Ask your doctor about your diet. Foods that contain vitamin K can affect how well warfarin (Coumadin®) works. Vitamin K is found in green leafy vegetables and some oils, such as canola and soybean oil. It's best to eat a well-balanced, healthy diet.

- Discuss with your doctor what amount of alcohol is safe for you to drink if you're taking medicine.

Medicines used to treat PE can thin your blood too much. This can cause bleeding in the digestive system or the brain. If you have signs or symptoms of bleeding in the digestive system or the brain, get treatment at once.

Signs and symptoms of bleeding in the digestive system include:

- bright red vomit or vomit that looks like coffee grounds;

- bright red blood in your stool or black, tarry stools; and

- pain in your abdomen.

Signs and symptoms of bleeding in the brain include:

- severe pain in your head;

- sudden changes in your vision;

- sudden loss of movement in your legs or arms; and

- memory loss or confusion.

Excessive bleeding from a fall or injury also may mean that your PE medicines have thinned your blood too much. Excessive bleeding is bleeding that will not stop after you apply pressure to a wound for 10 minutes. If you have excessive bleeding from a fall or injury, get treatment at once.

Once you have had PE (with or without deep vein thrombosis [DVT]), you have a greater chance of having another one. During treatment and after, continue to:

- take steps to prevent DVT; and

- check your legs for any signs or symptoms of DVT, such as swollen areas, pain or tenderness, increased warmth in swollen or painful areas, or red or discolored skin.

If you think that you have DVT or are having symptoms of PE, contact your doctor at once.

Chapter 25

Sleep Apnea and Risk for Stroke or Death

Sleep Apnea

Sleep apnea is a common disorder in which you have one or more pauses in breathing or shallow breaths while you sleep.

Breathing pauses can last from a few seconds to minutes. They often occur 5 to 30 times or more an hour. Typically, normal breathing then starts again, sometimes with a loud snort or choking sound.

Sleep apnea usually is a chronic (ongoing) condition that disrupts your sleep 3 or more nights each week. You often move out of deep sleep and into light sleep when your breathing pauses or becomes shallow.

This results in poor sleep quality that makes you tired during the day. Sleep apnea is one of the leading causes of excessive daytime sleepiness.

Overview

Sleep apnea often goes undiagnosed. Doctors usually can't detect the condition during routine office visits. Also, there are no blood tests for the condition.

This chapter includes text excerpted from "Sleep Apnea," by the National Heart, Lung, and Blood Institute (NHLBI, www.nhlbi.nih.gov), part of the National Institutes of Health, February 2006, and "Sleep Apnea and Risk for Stroke or Death," excerpted from the National Institutes of Health (NIH, www.nih.gov), November 9, 2005.

Most people who have sleep apnea don't know they have it because it only occurs during sleep. A family member and/or bed partner may first notice the signs of sleep apnea.

The most common type of sleep apnea is obstructive sleep apnea. This most often means that the airway has collapsed or is blocked during sleep. The blockage may cause shallow breathing or breathing pauses.

When you try to breathe, any air that squeezes past the blockage can cause loud snoring. Obstructive sleep apnea happens more often in people who are overweight, but it can affect anyone.

Central sleep apnea is a less common type of sleep apnea. It happens when the area of your brain that controls your breathing doesn't send the correct signals to your breathing muscles. You make no effort to breathe for brief periods.

Central sleep apnea often occurs with obstructive sleep apnea, but it can occur alone. Snoring doesn't typically happen with central sleep apnea.

This article mainly focuses on obstructive sleep apnea.

Outlook

Untreated sleep apnea can:

- increase the risk for high blood pressure, heart attack, stroke, obesity, and diabetes;
- increase the risk for or worsen heart failure;
- make irregular heartbeats more likely; and
- increase the chance of having work-related or driving accidents.

Lifestyle changes, mouthpieces, surgery, and/or breathing devices can successfully treat sleep apnea in many people.

What Causes Sleep Apnea?

When you're awake, throat muscles help keep your airway stiff and open so air can flow into your lungs. When you sleep, these muscles are more relaxed. Normally, the relaxed throat muscles don't stop your airway from staying open to allow air into your lungs.

But if you have obstructive sleep apnea, your airways can be blocked or narrowed during sleep because:

- Your throat muscles and tongue relax more than normal.

- Your tongue and tonsils (tissue masses in the back of your mouth) are large compared to the opening into your windpipe.

- You're overweight. The extra soft fat tissue can thicken the wall of the windpipe. This causes the inside opening to narrow and makes it harder to keep open.

- The shape of your head and neck (bony structure) may cause a smaller airway size in the mouth and throat area.

- The aging process limits the ability of brain signals to keep your throat muscles stiff during sleep. This makes it more likely that the airway will narrow or collapse.

Not enough air flows into your lungs when your airways are fully or partly blocked during sleep. This can cause loud snoring and a drop in your blood oxygen levels.

When the oxygen drops to dangerous levels, it triggers your brain to disturb your sleep. This helps tighten the upper airway muscles and open your windpipe. Normal breaths then start again, often with a loud snort or choking sound.

The frequent drops in oxygen levels and reduced sleep quality trigger the release of stress hormones. These compounds raise your heart rate and increase your risk for high blood pressure, heart attack, stroke, and irregular heartbeats. The hormones also raise the risk for or worsen heart failure.

Untreated sleep apnea also can lead to changes in how your body uses energy. These changes increase your risk for obesity and diabetes.

Who Is at Risk for Sleep Apnea?

It's estimated that more than 12 million American adults have obstructive sleep apnea. More than half of the people who have this condition are overweight.

Sleep apnea is more common in men. One out of 25 middle-aged men and 1 out of 50 middle-aged women have sleep apnea.

Sleep apnea becomes more common as you get older. At least 1 out of 10 people over the age of 65 has sleep apnea. Women are much more likely to develop sleep apnea after menopause.

African Americans, Hispanics, and Pacific Islanders are more likely to develop sleep apnea than Caucasians.

If someone in your family has sleep apnea, you're more likely to develop it.

People who have small airways in their noses, throats, or mouths also are more likely to have sleep apnea. Smaller airways may be due to the shape of these structures or allergies or other medical conditions that cause congestion in these areas.

Small children often have enlarged tonsil tissues in the throat. This can make them prone to developing sleep apnea.

Other risk factors for sleep apnea include smoking, high blood pressure, and risk factors for stroke or heart failure.

What Are the Signs and Symptoms of Sleep Apnea?

Major Signs and Symptoms. One of the most common signs of obstructive sleep apnea is loud and chronic (ongoing) snoring. Pauses may occur in the snoring. Choking or gasping may follow the pauses.

The snoring usually is loudest when you sleep on your back; it may be less noisy when you turn on your side. Snoring may not happen every night. Over time, the snoring may happen more often and get louder.

You're asleep when the snoring or gasping occurs. You will likely not know that you're having problems breathing or be able to judge how severe the problem is. Your family members or bed partner will often notice these problems before you do.

Not everyone who snores has sleep apnea.

Another common sign of sleep apnea is fighting sleepiness during the day, at work, or while driving. You may find yourself rapidly falling asleep during the quiet moments of the day when you're not active.

Other Signs and Symptoms. Other signs and symptoms of sleep apnea may include:

- morning headaches;
- memory or learning problems and not being able to concentrate;
- feeling irritable, depressed, or having mood swings or personality changes;
- urination at night; and
- a dry throat when you wake up.

In children, sleep apnea can cause hyperactivity, poor school performance, and aggressiveness. Children who have sleep apnea also may have unusual sleeping positions, bedwetting, and may breathe through their mouths instead of their noses during the day.

How Is Sleep Apnea Diagnosed?

Doctors diagnose sleep apnea based on your medical and family histories, a physical exam, and results from sleep studies. Usually, your primary care doctor evaluates your symptoms first. He or she then decides whether you need to see a sleep specialist.

These specialists are doctors who diagnose and treat people with sleep problems. Such doctors include lung, nerve, or ear, nose, and throat specialists. Other types of doctors also can be sleep specialists.

Medical and Family Histories. Your doctor will ask you and your family questions about how you sleep and how you function during the day. To help your doctor, consider keeping a sleep diary for 1 to 2 weeks. Write down how much you sleep each night, as well as how sleepy you feel at various times during the day.

Your doctor also will want to know how loudly and often you snore or make gasping or choking sounds during sleep. Often you're not aware of such symptoms and must ask a family member or bed partner to report them.

If you're a parent of a child who may have sleep apnea, tell your child's doctor about your child's signs and symptoms.

Let your doctor know if anyone in your family has been diagnosed with sleep apnea or has had symptoms of the disorder.

Many people aren't aware of their symptoms and aren't diagnosed.

Physical Exam. Your doctor will check your mouth, nose, and throat for extra or large tissues. The tonsils often are enlarged in children with sleep apnea. A physical exam and medical history may be all that's needed to diagnose sleep apnea in children.

Adults with the condition may have an enlarged uvula or soft palate. The uvula is the tissue that hangs from the middle of the back of your mouth. The soft palate is the roof of your mouth in the back of your throat.

Sleep Studies. A sleep study is the most accurate test for diagnosing sleep apnea. It captures what happens with your breathing while you sleep.

A sleep study is often done in a sleep center or sleep lab, which may be part of a hospital. You may stay overnight in the sleep center.

Polysomnogram. A polysomnogram, or PSG, is the most common study for diagnosing sleep apnea. This test records:

- brain activity;

- eye movement and other muscle activity;

- breathing and heart rate;

- how much air moves in and out of your lungs while you're sleeping; and

- the amount of oxygen in your blood.

A PSG is painless. You will go to sleep as usual, except you will have sensors on your scalp, face, chest, limbs, and finger. The staff at the sleep center will use the sensors to check on you throughout the night.

A sleep specialist reviews the results of your PSG to see whether you have sleep apnea and how severe it is. He or she will use the results to plan your treatment.

How Is Sleep Apnea Treated?

Goals of Treatment. The goals of treating obstructive sleep apnea are to:

- restore regular breathing during sleep; and

- relieve symptoms such as loud snoring and daytime sleepiness.

Treatment may help other medical problems linked to sleep apnea, such as high blood pressure. Treatment also can reduce your risk for heart disease, stroke, and diabetes.

Specific Types of Treatment. Lifestyle changes, mouthpieces, breathing devices, and/or surgery are used to treat sleep apnea. Currently, there are no medicines to treat sleep apnea.

Lifestyle changes and/or mouthpieces may be enough to relieve mild sleep apnea. People who have moderate or severe sleep apnea also will need breathing devices or surgery.

If you have mild sleep apnea, some changes in daily activities or habits may be all that you need.

- Avoid alcohol and medicines that make you sleepy. They make it harder for your throat to stay open while you sleep.

- Lose weight if you're overweight or obese. Even a little weight loss can improve your symptoms.

• Sleep on your side instead of your back to help keep your throat open. You can sleep with special pillows or shirts that prevent you from sleeping on your back.

• Keep your nasal passages open at night with nose sprays or allergy medicines, if needed. Talk to your doctor about whether these treatments might help you.

• Stop smoking.

A mouthpiece, sometimes called an oral appliance, may help some people who have mild sleep apnea. Your doctor also may recommend a mouthpiece if you snore loudly but don't have sleep apnea.

A dentist or orthodontist can make a custom-fit plastic mouthpiece for treating sleep apnea. (An orthodontist specializes in correcting teeth or jaw problems.) The mouthpiece will adjust your lower jaw and your tongue to help keep your airways open while you sleep.

If you use a mouthpiece, it's important that you check with your doctor about discomfort or pain while using the device. You may need periodic office visits so your doctor can adjust your mouthpiece to fit better.

Continuous positive airway pressure (CPAP) is the most common treatment for moderate to severe sleep apnea in adults. A CPAP machine uses a mask that fits over your mouth and nose, or just over your nose. The machine gently blows air into your throat.

The air presses on the wall of your airway. The air pressure is adjusted so that it's just enough to stop the airways from becoming narrowed or blocked during sleep.

Treating sleep apnea may help you stop snoring. But stopping snoring doesn't mean that you no longer have sleep apnea or can stop using CPAP. Sleep apnea will return if CPAP is stopped or not used correctly.

Usually, a technician will come to your home to bring the CPAP equipment. The technician will set up the CPAP machine and adjust it based on your doctor's orders. After the initial setup, you may need to have the CPAP adjusted on occasion for the best results.

CPAP treatment may cause side effects in some people. These side effects include a dry or stuffy nose, irritated skin on your face, sore eyes, and headaches. If your CPAP isn't properly adjusted, you may get stomach bloating and discomfort while wearing the mask.

If you're having trouble with CPAP side effects, work with your sleep specialist, his or her nursing staff, and the CPAP technician. Together, you can take steps to reduce these side effects. These steps include adjusting the CPAP settings or the size/fit of the mask, or adding moisture to the air as it flows through the mask. A nasal spray may relieve a dry, stuffy, or runny nose.

There are many different kinds of CPAP machines and masks. Be sure to tell your doctor if you're not happy with the type you're using. He or she may suggest switching to a different kind that may work better for you.

People who have severe sleep apnea symptoms generally feel much better once they begin treatment with CPAP.

Some people who have sleep apnea may benefit from surgery. The type of surgery and how well it works depend on the cause of the sleep apnea.

Surgery is done to widen breathing passages. It usually involves removing, shrinking, or stiffening excess tissue in the mouth and throat or resetting the lower jaw.

Surgery to shrink or stiffen excess tissue in the mouth or throat is done in a doctor's office or a hospital. Shrinking tissue may involve small shots or other treatments to the tissue. A series of such treatments may be needed to shrink the excess tissue. To stiffen excess tissue, the doctor makes a small cut in the tissue and inserts a small piece of stiff plastic.

Surgery to remove excess tissue is only done in a hospital. You're given medicine that makes you sleep during the surgery. After surgery, you may have throat pain that lasts for 1 to 2 weeks.

Surgery to remove the tonsils, if they're blocking the airway, may be very helpful for some children. Your child's doctor may suggest waiting some time to see whether these tissues shrink on their own. This is common as small children grow.

Living with Sleep Apnea

Obstructive sleep apnea can be very serious. However, following an effective treatment plan can often improve your quality of life quite a bit.

Treatment can improve your sleep and relieve daytime tiredness. It also may make you less likely to develop high blood pressure, heart disease, and other health problems linked to sleep apnea.

Treatment may improve your overall health and happiness as well as your quality of sleep (and possibly your family's quality of sleep).

Ongoing Health Care Needs. Follow up with your doctor regularly to make sure your treatment is working. Tell him or her if the treatment is causing side effects that you can't handle.

This ongoing care is especially important if you're getting continuous positive airway pressure (CPAP) treatment. It may take a while before you adjust to using CPAP.

If you aren't comfortable with your CPAP device or it doesn't seem to be working, let your doctor know. You may need to switch to a different device or mask. Or, you may need treatment to relieve CPAP side effects.

Try not to gain weight. Weight gain can worsen sleep apnea and require adjustments to your CPAP device. In contrast, weight loss may relieve your sleep apnea.

Until your sleep apnea is properly treated, know the dangers of driving or operating heavy machinery while sleepy.

If you're having any type of surgery that requires medicine to put you to sleep, let your surgeon and doctors know you have sleep apnea. They might have to take extra steps to make sure your airway stays open during the surgery.

How Can Family Members Help?

Often, people with sleep apnea don't know they have it. They're not aware that their breathing stops and starts many times while they're sleeping. Family members or bed partners usually are the first to notice signs of sleep apnea.

Family members can do many things to help a loved one who has sleep apnea.

- Let the person know if he or she snores loudly during sleep or has breathing stops and starts.

- Encourage the person to get medical help.

- Help the person follow the doctor's treatment plan, including CPAP.

- Provide emotional support.

Sleep Apnea and Risk for Stroke and Death

An observational study of more than 1,000 patients at the Yale Center for Sleep Medicine found that obstructive sleep apnea significantly increases the risk of stroke or death from any cause, and that the risk is linked to sleep apnea severity. The researchers found the increased risk to be independent of other factors, including hypertension. Participants were over age 50 without a history of heart attack or stroke at the start of the study. They were followed for an average of just under 3.5 years. The report cites support from the National Heart, Lung, and Blood Institute (NHLBI) of the National Institutes of Health, the Yale Center for Sleep Medicine, and the Veterans Affairs Health Services Research and Development Service.

Chapter 26

Trauma or Infection Can Increase Stroke Risk

Chapter Contents

Section 26.1

Traumatic Brain Injury

"Traumatic Brain Injury Information Page" is from the National Institute of Neurological Disorders and Stroke (NINDS, www.ninds.nih.gov), part of the National Institutes of Health, October 17, 2007.

What Is Traumatic Brain Injury?

Traumatic brain injury (TBI), also called acquired brain injury or simply head injury, occurs when a sudden trauma causes damage to the brain. TBI can result when the head suddenly and violently hits an object, or when an object pierces the skull and enters brain tissue. Symptoms of a TBI can be mild, moderate, or severe, depending on the extent of the damage to the brain. A person with a mild TBI may remain conscious or may experience a loss of consciousness for a few seconds or minutes. Other symptoms of mild TBI include headache, confusion, lightheadedness, dizziness, blurred vision or tired eyes, ringing in the ears, bad taste in the mouth, fatigue or lethargy, a change in sleep patterns, behavioral or mood changes, and trouble with memory, concentration, attention, or thinking. A person with a moderate or severe TBI may show these same symptoms, but may also have a headache that gets worse or does not go away, repeated vomiting or nausea, convulsions or seizures, an inability to awaken from sleep, dilation of one or both pupils of the eyes, slurred speech, weakness or numbness in the extremities, loss of coordination, and increased confusion, restlessness, or agitation.

Is There Any Treatment?

Anyone with signs of moderate or severe TBI should receive medical attention as soon as possible. Because little can be done to reverse the initial brain damage caused by trauma, medical personnel try to stabilize an individual with TBI and focus on preventing further injury. Primary concerns include insuring proper oxygen supply to the brain and the rest of the body, maintaining adequate blood flow, and controlling blood pressure. Imaging tests help in determining the diagnosis and prognosis of a TBI patient. Patients with mild to moderate injuries may receive skull and neck X-rays to check for bone fractures or spinal instability. For moderate to severe cases, the imaging test is a computed tomography (CT) scan. Moderately to severely injured patients receive rehabilitation that involves individually tailored treatment programs in the areas of physical therapy, occupational therapy, speech/language therapy, physiatry (physical medicine), psychology/psychiatry, and social support.

What Is the Prognosis?

Approximately half of severely head-injured patients will need surgery to remove or repair hematomas (ruptured blood vessels) or contusions (bruised brain tissue). Disabilities resulting from a TBI depend upon the severity of the injury, the location of the injury, and the age and general health of the individual. Some common disabilities include problems with cognition (thinking, memory, and reasoning), sensory processing (sight, hearing, touch, taste, and smell), communication (expression and understanding), and behavior or mental health (depression, anxiety, personality changes, aggression, acting out, and social inappropriateness). More serious head injuries may result in stupor, an unresponsive state, but one in which an individual can be aroused briefly by a strong stimulus, such as sharp pain; coma, a state in which an individual is totally unconscious, unresponsive, unaware, and unarousable; vegetative state, in which an individual is unconscious and unaware of his or her surroundings, but continues to have a sleep-wake cycle and periods of alertness; and a persistent vegetative state (PVS), in which an individual stays in a vegetative state for more than a month.

What Research Is Being Done?

The National Institute of Neurological Disorders and Stroke (NINDS) conducts TBI research in its laboratories at the National Institutes of Health (NIH) and also supports TBI research through grants to major medical institutions across the country. This research involves studies in the laboratory and in clinical settings to better understand TBI and the biological mechanisms underlying damage to the brain. This research will allow scientists to develop strategies and interventions to limit the primary and secondary brain damage that occurs within days of a head trauma, and to devise therapies to treat brain injury and improve long-term recovery of function.

Section 26.2

Chiropractic Neck Manipulation and the Risk of Stroke

"Chiropractic's Dirty Secret: Neck Manipulation and Strokes," by
Stephen Barrett, M.D., © 2006 Quackwatch. Reprinted with permission.

Stroke from chiropractic neck manipulation occurs when an artery
to the brain ruptures or becomes blocked as a result of being stretched.
The injury often results from extreme rotation in which the practitioner's hands are placed on the patient's head in order to rotate the
cervical spine by rotating the head.[1] The vertebral artery is vulnerable because it winds around the topmost cervical vertebra (atlas) to
enter the skull, so that any abrupt rotation may stretch the artery
and tear its delicate lining. The anatomical problem is illustrated on
page 7 of *The Chiropractic Report,* July 1999. A blood clot formed over
the injured area may subsequently be dislodged and block a smaller
artery that supplies the brain. Less frequently, the vessel may be
blocked by blood that collects in the vessel wall at the site of the dissection.[2]

Chiropractors would like you to believe that the incidence of stroke
following neck manipulation is extremely small. Speculations exist
that the odds of a serious complication due to neck manipulation are
somewhere between one in 40,000 and one in 10 million manipulations. No one really knows, however, because (a) there has been little
systematic study of its frequency; (b) the largest malpractice insurers won't reveal how many cases they know about; and (c) a large
majority of cases that medical doctors see are not reported in scientific journals.

Published Reports

In 1992, researchers at the Stanford Stroke Center asked 486 California members of the American Academy of Neurology how many patients they had seen during the previous two years who had suffered
a stroke within 24 hours of neck manipulation by a chiropractor. The

survey was sponsored by the American Heart Association. A total of 177 neurologists reported treating 56 such patients, all of whom were between the ages of 21 and 60. One patient had died, and 48 were left with permanent neurologic deficits such as slurred speech, inability to arrange words properly, and vertigo (dizziness). The usual cause of the strokes was thought to be a tear between the inner and outer walls of the vertebral arteries, which caused the arterial walls to balloon and block the flow of blood to the brain. Three of the strokes involved tears of the carotid arteries.[3] In 1991, according to circulation figures from Dynamic Chiropractic, California had about 19% of the chiropractors practicing in the United States, which suggests that about 147 cases of stroke each year were seen by neurologists nationwide. Of course, additional cases could have been seen by other doctors who did not respond to the survey.

A 1993 review concluded that potential complications and unknown benefits indicate that children should not undergo neck manipulation.[4]

Louis Sportelli, DC, NCMIC president and a former ACA board chairman contends that chiropractic neck manipulation is quite safe. In an 1994 interview reported by the Associated Press, he reacted to the American Heart Association study by saying, "I yawned at it. It's old news." He also said that other studies suggest that chiropractic neck manipulation results in a stroke somewhere between one in a million and one in three million cases.[5] The one-in-a-million figure could be correct if California's chiropractors had been averaging about 60 neck manipulations per week. Later that year, during a televised interview with *"Inside Edition,"* Sportelli said the "worst-case scenario" was one in 500,000 but added: "When you weigh the procedure against any other procedure in the health-care industry, it is probably the lowest risk factor of anything." According to the program's narrator, Sportelli said that 90% of his patients receive neck manipulation.

In 1996, RAND issued a booklet that tabulated more than 100 published case reports and estimated that the number of strokes, cord compressions, fractures, and large blood clots was 1.46 per million neck manipulations. Even though this number appears small, it is significant because many of the manipulations chiropractors do should not be done. In addition, as the report itself noted, neither the number of manipulations performed nor the number of complications has been systematically studied.[6] Since some people are more susceptible than others, it has also been argued that the incidence should be expressed as rate per patient rather than rate per adjustment.

In 1996, the National Chiropractic Mutual Insurance Company (NCMIC), which is the largest American chiropractic malpractice insurer, published a report called "Vertebrobasilar Stroke Following Manipulation," written by Allen G.J. Terrett, an Australian chiropractic educator/researcher. Terrett based his findings on 183 cases of vertebrobasilar strokes (VBS) reported between 1934 and 1994. He concluded that 105 of the manipulations had been administered by a chiropractor, 25 were done by a medical practitioner, 31 had been done by another type of practitioner, and that the practitioner type for the remaining 22 was not specified in the report. He concluded that VBS is "very rare," that current pretesting procedures are seldom able to predict susceptibility, and that in 25 cases serious injury might have been avoided if the practitioner had recognized that symptoms occurring after a manipulation indicated that further manipulations should not be done.[7]

A 1999 review of 116 articles published between 1925 and 1997 found 177 cases of neck injury associated with neck manipulation, at least 60% of which was done by chiropractors.[8]

In 2001, NCMIC published a second edition of Terrett's book, titled, "Current Concepts: Vertebrobasilar Complications following Spinal Manipulation," which covered 255 cases published between 1934 and 1999.[9] NCMIC's web site claims that the book "includes an analysis of every known case related to this subject." That description is not true. It does not include many strokes that resulted in lawsuits against NCMIC policyholders but were not published in scientific journals. And it does not include the thoroughly documented case of Kristi Bedenbauer whose autopsy report I personally mailed to Terrett after speaking with him in 1995.

In 2001, Canadian researchers published a report about the relationships between chiropractic care and the incidence of vertebrovascular accidents (VBAs) due to vertebral artery dissection or blockage in Ontario, Canada, between 1993 and 1998. Using hospital records, each of 582 VBA cases was age- and sex-matched to four controls with no history of stroke. Health insurance billing records were used to document use of chiropractic services. The study found that VBA patients under age 45 were five times more likely than controls to (a) have visited a chiropractor within a week of the VBA and (b) to have had three or more visits with neck manipulations. No relationship was found after age 45. The authors discuss possible shortcomings of the study and urge that further research be done.[10] An accompanying editorial states that the data correspond to an incidence of 1.3 cases of vertebral artery dissection or blockage per 100,000 individuals receiving chiropractic neck manipulation, a number higher than most chiropractic estimates.[11]

In 2001, British researchers reported on a survey in which all members of the Association of British Neurologists were asked to report cases referred to them of neurological complications occurring within 24 hours of neck manipulation over a 12-month period. The 35 reported cases included 7 strokes involving the vertebrobasilar artery and 2 strokes involving a carotid artery. None of the 35 cases were reported to medical journals.[12] Edzard Ernst, professor of complementary medicine at the University of Exeter School of Sport and Health Sciences, believes that these results are very significant. In a recent commentary, he stated:

"One gets the impression that the risks of spinal manipulation are being played down, particularly by chiropractors. Perhaps the best indication that this is true are estimates of incidence rates based on assumptions, which are unproven at best and unrealistic at worse. One such assumption, for instance, is that 10% of actual complications will be reported. Our recent survey, however, demonstrated an underreporting rate of 100%. This extreme level of underreporting obviously renders estimates nonsensical."[13]

In 2002, researchers representing the Canadian Stroke Consortium reported on 98 cases in which external trauma ranging from "trivial" to "severe" was identified as the trigger of strokes caused by blood clots formed in arteries supplying the brain. Chiropractic-style neck manipulation was the apparent cause of 38 of the cases, 30 involving vertebral artery dissection and 8 involving carotid artery dissection. Other Canadian statistics indicate the incidence of ischemic strokes in people under 45 is about 750 a year. The researchers believe that their data indicate that 20% are due to neck manipulation, so there may be "gross underreporting" of chiropractic manipulation as a cause of stroke.[14]

In 2003, another research team reviewed the records of 151 patients under age 60 with cervical arterial dissection and ischemic stroke or transient ischemic attack (TIA) from between 1995 and 2000 at two academic stroke centers. After an interview and a blinded chart review, 51 patients with dissection and 100 control patients were studied. Patients with dissection were more likely to have undergone spinal manipulation within 30 days (14% vs 3%). The authors concluded that spinal manipulation is associated with vertebral arterial dissection and that a significant increase in neck pain following neck manipulation warrants immediate medical evaluation.[15]

In 2006, the *Journal of Neurology* published a German Vertebral Artery Dissection Study Group report about 36 patients who had experienced vertebral artery dissection associated with neck manipulation.[16] Twenty-six patients developed their symptoms within 48 hours after a manipulation, including five patients who got symptoms at the time of manipulation and four who developed them within the next hour. In 27 patients, special imaging procedures confirmed that blood supply had decreased in the areas supplied by the vertebral arteries as suggested by the neurological examinations. In all but one of the 36 patients, the symptoms had not previously occurred and were clearly distinguishable from the complaints that led them to seek manipulative care. This report is highly significant but needs careful interpretation. Although it is titled "Vertebral dissections after chiropractic neck manipulation . . . " only four of the patients were actually manipulated by chiropractors. Half were treated by orthopedic surgeons, five by a physiotherapist, and the rest by a neurologist, general medical practitioner, or homeopath. It is possible—although unlikely—that the nonchiropractors used techniques that were more dangerous than chiropractors use in North America. The authors suggested that the orthopedists' treatment was safer, but there is no way to determine this from their data. Regardless, the study supports the assertion that neck manipulation can cause strokes—which many chiropractors deny.

Are Complications Predictable?

Although some chiropractors advocate "screening tests" with the hope of detecting individuals prone to stroke due to neck manipulation.[17,18] These tests, which include holding the head and neck in positions of rotation to see whether the patient gets dizzy, are not reliable,[19] partly because manipulation can rotate the neck further than can be done with the tests.[19] Listening over the neck arteries with a stethoscope to detect a murmur, for example, has not been proven reliable, though patients that have one should be referred to a physician. Vascular function tests in which the patient's head is briefly held in the positions used during cervical manipulation are also not reliable as a screen for high-risk patients because a thrust that further stretches the vertebral artery could still damage the vessel wall." In a chapter in the leading chiropractic textbook, Terrett and a coauthor have stated:

"Even after performing the relevant case history, physical examination, and vertebrobasilar function tests, accidents may still occur. There is no conclusive, foolproof screening procedure to eliminate patients at risk. Most victims are young, without [bony] or vascular pathology, and do not present with vertebrobasilar symptoms. The screening procedures described cannot detect those patients in whom [manipulation] may cause an injury. They give a false sense of security to the practitioner.[20]

Several medical reports have described chiropractic patients who, after neck manipulation, complained of dizziness and other symptoms of transient loss of blood supply to the brain but were manipulated again and had a full-blown stroke. During a workshop I attended at the 1995 Chiropractic Centennial Celebration, Terrett said such symptoms are ominous and that chiropractors should abandon rotational manipulations that overstretch the vertebral arteries. But, as far as I know, his remarks have not been published and have had no impact on his professional colleagues.

The lack of predictability has been supported by data published by Scott Haldeman, D.C., M.D., Ph.D., a chiropractor who has served as an expert witness (usually for the defense) in many court cases involving chiropractic injury. In 1995, he published an abstract summarizing his review of 53 cases that had not been previously reported in medical or chiropractic journals. His report stated:

"These cases represent approximately a 45% increase in the number of such cases reported in the English language literature over the past 100 years. . . . No clear cut risk factors can be elicited from the data. Previously proposed risk factors such as migraine headaches, hypertension, diabetes, history of cardiovascular disease, oral contraceptives, recent head or neck trauma, or abnormalities on x-rays do not appear to be significantly greater in patients who have cerebrovascular complications of manipulation than that noted in the general population."[21]

Haldeman's main point was he could not identify any factor that could predict that a particular patient was prone to cerebrovascular injury from neck manipulation. This report was published in the proceedings of 1995 Chiropractic Centennial Celebration and was not cited in either the RAND or NCMIC reports.

In 2001, Haldeman and two colleagues published a more detailed analysis that covered 64 cases involving malpractice claims filed between 1978 and 1994.[22] They reported that 59 (92%) came to treatment with a history of head or neck symptoms. However, the report provides insufficient information to judge whether manipulation could have been useful for treating their condition. Of course, malpractice claims don't present the full story, because most victims of professional negligence do not take legal action. Even when serious injury results, some are simply not inclined toward suing, some don't blame the practitioner, some have an aversion to lawyers, and some can't find an attorney willing to represent them.

What Should Be Done?

Chiropractors cannot agree among themselves whether the problem is significant enough to inform patients that vertebrobasilar stroke is a possible complication of manipulation.[19,23] In 1993, the Canadian Chiropractic Association published a consent form which stated, in part:

"Doctors of chiropractic, medical doctors, and physical therapists using manual therapy treatments for patients with neck problems such as yours are required to explain that there have been rare cases of injury to a vertebral artery as a result of treatment. Such an injury has been known to cause stroke, sometimes with serious neurological injury. The chances of this happening are extremely remote, approximately 1 per 1 million treatments.

Appropriate tests will be performed on you to help identify if you may be susceptible to that kind of injury. . . . [24]

This notice is a step in the right direction but does not go far enough. A proper consent should disclose that (a) the risk is unknown; (b) alternative treatments may be available; (c) in many cases, neck symptoms will go away without treatment; (d) certain types of neck manipulation carry a higher risk than others; and (e) claims that spinal manipulation can remedy systemic diseases, boost immunity, improve general health, or prolong life have neither scientific justification nor a plausible rationale.

In 2003, a coroner's jury concluded that Lana Dale Lewis of Toronto, Canada, was killed in 1996 by a chiropractic neck manipulation. Among other things, the jury recommended that all patients for whom neck manipulation is recommended be informed that risk exists and that the Ontario Ministry of Health establish a database for chiropractors and other health professionals to report on neck adjustments.[25]

The Bottom Line

As far as I know, most chiropractors do not warn their patients that neck manipulation entails risks. I believe they should and that the profession should implement a reporting system that would enable this matter to be appropriately studied. This might be achieved if (a) state licensing boards required that all such cases be reported, and

(b) chiropractic malpractice insurance companies, which now keep their data secret, were required to disclose them to an independently operated database that has input from both medical doctors and chiropractors.

Meanwhile, since stroke is such a devastating event, every effort should be made to stop chiropractors from manipulating necks without adequate reason. Many believe that all types of headaches might be amenable to spinal manipulation even though no scientific evidence supports such a belief. Many include neck manipulation as part of "preventative maintenance" that involves unnecessarily treating people who have no symptoms. Even worse, some chiropractors—often referred to as "upper cervical specialists"—claim that most human ailments are the result of misalignment of the topmost vertebrae (atlas and axis) and that every patient they see needs neck manipulation. Neck manipulation of children under age 12 should be outlawed.[26]

For Additional Information

- Neck911USA.com (http://www.neck911usa.com): Dangers of neck manipulation

- Chiropractors Angry about bus ad (http://www.chirobase.org/08Legal/bus_ad.html)

Reader Comment

From a former chiropractor: I have been doing a vascular surgery rotation for the past month, which is part of my postgraduate medical education. During my chiropractic training, when the subject of manipulation-induced stroke was brought up, we were reassured that "millions of chiropractic adjustments are made each year and only a few incidents of stroke have been reported following neck manipulation." I recently found that two of the patients on my vascular service that suffered a cerebrovascular accident (stroke) had undergone neck manipulation by a chiropractor, one the day that symptoms had begun and the other four days afterward. If indeed the incidence of stroke is rare, one M.D. would see a case of manipulation-induced CVA [cerebrovascular accident] about every 10 years. But I believe I have seen two in the past month! I therefore urge my medical colleagues to question their patients regarding recent visits to a chiropractor/neck manipulation when confronted with patients that present with the neurologic symptoms of stroke. I also urge potential chiropractic patients to not allow their necks to be manipulated in any way. The

risk-to-benefit ratio is much too high to warrant such a procedure.—
Rob Alexander, M.D.

References

1. Homola S. *Inside Chiropractic: A Patient's Guide.* Amherst,
   NY: Prometheus Books, 1999.

2. Norris JW and others. Sudden neck movement and cervical
   artery dissection. *Canadian Medical Journal* 163:38–40,
   2000.

3. Lee KP and others. Neurologic complications following chiropractic manipulation: A survey of California neurologists.
   Neurology 45:1213–1215, 1995.

4. Powell FC and others. A risk/benefit analysis of spinal manipulation therapy for relief of lumbar or cervical pain. *Neurosurgery* 33:73–79, 1993.

5. Haney DQ. Twist of the neck can cause stroke warn doctors.
   Associated Press news release, Feb 19, 1994.

6. Coulter I and others. *The Appropriateness of Manipulation
   and Mobilization of the Cervical Spine.* Santa Monica, CA:
   RAND, 1996, pp. 18–43.

7. Di Fabio R. Manipulation of the cervical spine: Risks and benefits. *Physical Therapy* 79:50–65, 1999.

8. Terrett AGJ. *Current Concepts in Vertebrobasilar Stroke following Manipulation.* West Des Moines, IA: National Chiropractic Mutual Insurance Company, Inc., 2001.

9. Terrett AGJ. *Current Concepts: Vertebrobasilar Complications
   following Spinal Manipulation.* West Des Moines, IA: NCMIC
   Group, Inc., 2001.

10. Rotherwell DAM and others. Chiropractic manipulation and
    stroke. *Stroke* 32:1054–1059, 2001.

11. Bousser MG. Editorial comment. *Stroke* 32:1059–1060, 2001.

12. Stevinson C and others. Neurological complications of cervical
    spine manipulation. *Journal of the Royal Society of Medicine*
    94:107–110, 2001.

13. Ernst E. Spinal manipulation: Its safety is uncertain. *Cana-
    dian Medical Association Journal* 166:40–41, 2002.

14. Beletsky V. Chiropractic manipulation may be underestimated as cause of stroke. Presented at the American Stroke Association's 27th International Stroke Conference, San Antonio, TX Feb 7–8, 2002.

15. Smith WS and others. Spinal manipulative therapy is an independent risk factor for vertebral artery dissection. *Neurology* 60:1424–1428, 2003.

16. Reuter U and others. Vertebral artery dissections after chiropractic neck manipulation in Germany over three years. *Journal of Neurology* 256:724–730, 2006.

17. George PE and others. Identification of high-risk pre-stroke patient. *ACA Journal of Chiropractic* 15:S26–S28, 1981.

18. Sullivan EC. Prevent strokes: Screening can help. *The Chiropractic Journal,* May 1989, p 27.

19. Chapman-Smith D. Cervical adjustment: Rotation is fine, pre-testing is out, but get consent. *The Chiropractic Report* 13(4):1–3, 6–7, 1999.

20. Terrett AGJ, Kleynhans AM. Cerebrovascular complications of manipulation. In Haldeman S (ed). *Principles and Practice of Chiropractic,* Second Edition. East Norwalk, CT: Appleton and Lange, 1992.

21. Haldeman S, Kohlbeck F, McGregor M. Cerebrovascular complications following cervical spine manipulation therapy: A review of 53 cases. Conference Proceedings of the Chiropractic Centennial, July 6–8, 1995, 282–283. Davenport IA: Chiropractic Centennial Foundation, 1995.

22. Haldeman S and others. Unpredictability of cerebrovascular ischemia associated with cervical spine manipulation therapy. *Spine* 27:49–55, 2001.

23. Magner G. Informed consent is needed. In Magner G. *Chiropractic: The Victim's Perspective.* Amherst, NY: Prometheus Books, 1995, pp 177–184.

24. Henderson D et al. *Clinical Guidelines for Chiropractic Practice in Canada.* Toronto: Canadian Chiropractic Association, 1994, p 4.

25. Coroner's jury concludes that neck manipulation killed Canadian woman. *Chirobase,* Jan 22, 2004.

26.   Stewart B and others. Statement of concern to the Canadian
       public from Canadian neurologists regarding the debilitating
       and fatal damage manipulation of the neck may cause to the
       nervous system, February 2002.

Section 26.3

Stroke Caused by Syphilis

"Stroke secondary to syphilis"
© 2008 A.D.A.M., Inc. Reprinted with permission.

Definition

Stroke is life-threatening complication of a long-term syphilis infection.

Causes

Untreated, late-stage tertiary syphilis can cause inflammation and
blockage of the arteries that supply the brain. A stroke is an interruption of the blood supply to any part of the brain. Stroke can lead
to brain tissue damage.

Symptoms

The following symptoms may occur about 1–4 weeks before the
stroke:

- Headache
- Vertigo (abnormal sensation of movement)
- Behavioral changes
- Irritability

Symptoms of stroke include:

- Weakness or the total inability to move a body part

- Numbness, tingling, or other abnormal sensations
- Decreased or lost vision, partial or temporary
- Language difficulties (aphasia)
- Inability to recognize or identify sensory stimuli (agnosia)
- Loss of memory
- Vertigo (abnormal sensation of movement)
- Loss of coordination
- Swallowing difficulties
- Personality changes
- Mood and emotion changes
- Urinary incontinence (lack of control over bladder)
- Lack of control over the bowels
- Consciousness changes
  - Drowsiness
  - Fatigue
  - Loss of consciousness

Exams and Tests

The doctor will ask if you have a history of syphilis. Blood tests can be done to check for substances in the blood produced by the bacteria that causes syphilis. These include:

- Venereal disease research laboratory test (VDRL)
- Rapid plasma reagin test (RPR)

If tests are positive, other tests are done to confirm the diagnosis. A spinal tap may be done to check for syphilis-related substances in the CSF (cerebrospinal fluid).

The following tests may be used to determine the location and severity of the stroke:

- Head CT scan
- Head MRI scan
- Angiography of the head or neck

Treatment

Antibiotics are used in high doses to treat the syphilis infection. Pain killers may be needed to control severe headaches.

Outlook (Prognosis)

The outcome depends on the extent of damage to the brain, the presence of other complications of late syphilis, and other factors.

When to Contact a Medical Professional

Go to the emergency room or call the local emergency number (such as 911) if you have any symptoms of a stroke.

Prevention

Stroke secondary to syphilis may be prevented by receiving prompt treatment and follow-up care for syphilis.

Chapter 27

Substance Use and Stroke

Chapter Contents

Section 27.1

Smoking

Stroke is largely a preventable disease. Research has identified primary risk factors for stroke: high blood cholesterol, elevated blood glucose, carotid artery bruits, atrial fibrillation, high blood pressure, and transient ischemic attacks.

If you smoke, stop.

Smoking and Stroke

The U.S. Surgeon General has stated, "Smoking cessation (stopping smoking) represents the single most important step that smokers can take to enhance the length and quality of their lives." Quitting smoking is not easy, but it can be done. To have the best chance of quitting successfully, you need to know what you're up against, what your options are, and where to go for help.

Why Quit?

Your Health

Health concerns usually top the list of reasons people give for quitting smoking. Nearly everyone knows that smoking can cause lung cancer, but few people realize it is also a risk factor for many other kinds of cancer as well, including cancer of the mouth, voice box (larynx), throat (pharynx), esophagus, bladder, kidney, pancreas, liver, cervix, stomach, colon and rectum, and some leukemias.

Smoking Doubles the Risk for Stroke

You already know what smoking does to your heart and lungs. But do you know what it does to your brain?

Smoking puts you at risk for having a brain attack or stroke, which can damage the areas of your brain that control everything you do—from speaking, writing, and reading to walking and even breathing. Imagine not being able to go to the bathroom by yourself, or speak or walk upstairs to your bedroom to dress yourself. Every time you smoke, you increase your chances of having a disabling or even deadly stroke. How can smoking cause that kind of damage? When you smoke, you reduce the amount of oxygen in your blood, causing your heart to work harder and allowing clots to form more easily. Smoking also increases the amount of fat buildup in your arteries, which may block brain-nourishing blood from getting through; causing a stroke.

Smoking increases the risk of lung diseases such as emphysema and chronic bronchitis. They can cause chronic illness and disability and can be eventually fatal.

Smokers are twice as likely to die from heart attacks as are non-smokers and smoking is a major risk factor for peripheral vascular disease, a narrowing of the blood vessels that carry blood to the leg and arm muscles.

Smoking also causes premature wrinkling of the skin, bad breath, bad smelling clothes and hair, and yellow fingernails.

For women, there are unique risks. Women over 35 who smoke and use "the pill" (oral contraceptives) are in a high-risk group for heart attack, stroke, and blood clots of the legs. Women who smoke while they are pregnant are more likely to have a miscarriage or a lower birth-weight baby.

Based on data collected from 1995 to 1999, the U.S. Centers for Disease Control (CDC) recently estimated that adult male smokers lost an average of 13.2 years of life and female smokers lost 14.5 years of life because of smoking.

No matter what your age or how long you've smoked, quitting will help you live longer. People who stop smoking before age 35 avoid 90% of the health risks attributable to tobacco. Even those who quit later in life can significantly reduce their risk of dying at a younger age.

Ex-smokers also enjoy a higher quality of life with fewer illnesses from cold and flu viruses, better self-reported health status, and reduced rates of bronchitis and pneumonia.

For decades the Surgeon General has reported the health risks associated with smoking. Regardless of your age or smoking history, there are advantages to quitting smoking. Benefits apply whether you are healthy or you already have smoking-related diseases. In 1990, the Surgeon General concluded:

- Quitting smoking has major and immediate health benefits for men and women of all ages. Benefits apply to people with and without smoking-related disease.

- Former smokers live longer than continuing smokers. For example, people who quit smoking before age 50 have one-half the risk of dying in the next 15 years compared with continuing smokers.

- Quitting smoking decreases the risk of lung cancer, other cancers, heart attack, stroke, and chronic lung disease.

- Women who stop smoking before pregnancy or during the first 3 to 4 months of pregnancy reduce their risk of having a low birth-weight baby to that of women who never smoked.

- The health benefits of quitting smoking far exceed any risks from the average 5-pound weight gain or any adverse psychological effects that may follow quitting.

When Smokers Quit—What Are the Benefits over Time?

- **20 minutes** after quitting: Your blood pressure drops to a level close to that before the last cigarette. The temperature of your hands and feet increases to normal.

- **8 hours** after quitting: The carbon monoxide level in your blood drops to normal.

- **24 hours** after quitting: Your chance of a heart attack decreases.

- **2 weeks to 3 months** after quitting: Your circulation improves and your lung function increases up to 30%.

- **1 to 9 months** after quitting: Coughing, sinus congestion, fatigue, and shortness of breath decrease; cilia (tiny hair like structures that move mucus out of the lungs) regain normal function in the lungs, increasing the ability to handle mucus, clean the lungs, and reduce infection.

- **1 year** after quitting: The excess risk of coronary heart disease is half that of a smoker's.

- **5 years** after quitting: Your stroke risk is reduced to that of a nonsmoker 5–15 years after quitting.

- **10 years** after quitting: The lung cancer death rate is about half that of a continuing smoker's. The risk of cancer of the mouth, throat, esophagus, bladder, kidney, and pancreas decreases.

- **15 years** after quitting: The risk of coronary heart disease is that of a nonsmoker's.

Source: U.S. Surgeon General's Report, 1988, 1990.

Visible and Immediate Rewards of Quitting

Quitting helps stop the damaging effects of tobacco on your appearance including:

- premature wrinkling of the skin
- bad breath
- stained teeth
- gum disease
- bad smelling clothes and hair
- yellow fingernails

Kicking the tobacco habit also offers benefits that you'll notice immediately and some that will develop gradually in the first few weeks. These rewards can improve your day-to-day life substantially:

- Food tastes better.
- Sense of smell returns to normal.
- Ordinary activities no longer leave you out of breath (climbing stairs, light housework, etc.)

The prospect of better health is a major reason for quitting, but there are others as well. Smoking is expensive. The economic costs of smoking are estimated to be about $3,391 per smoker per year. Do you really want to continue burning up your money with nothing to show for it except possible health problems?

Cost

Smoking is expensive. It isn't hard to figure out how much you spend on smoking: multiply how much money you spend on tobacco every day by 365 (days per year). The amount may surprise you. Now

251

multiply that by the number of years you have been using tobacco and that amount will probably astound you.

Multiply the cost per year by 10 (for the upcoming 10 years) and ask yourself what you would rather do with that much money. If you smoke 2 packs per day, that's nearly $18,000 in 10 years! And this doesn't include the higher costs for health and life insurance, as well as the possible health care costs due to tobacco-related conditions.

Social Acceptance

Smoking is less socially acceptable now than it was in the past. While decisions may not be based entirely on social acceptance, most workplaces have some type of smoking restrictions. Some employers prefer to hire nonsmokers.

Studies show smoking employees cost businesses more to employ because they are "out sick" more frequently. Employees who are ill more often than others can raise an employer's need for expensive temporary replacement workers. They can increase insurance costs both for other employees and for the employer, who typically pays part of the workers' insurance premiums. Smokers in a building also typically increase the maintenance costs of keeping odors at an acceptable level, since residue from cigarette smoke clings to carpets, drapes, and other fabrics.

Landlords, also, may choose not to rent to smokers since maintenance costs and insurance rates may rise when smokers occupy buildings.

Friends may ask you not to smoke in their houses or cars. Public buildings, concerts, and even sporting events are largely smoke-free. And more and more communities are restricting smoking in all public places, including restaurants and bars. Like it or not, finding a place to smoke can be a hassle. Smokers may find their opportunities for dating or romantic involvement, including marriage, are largely limited to only other smokers, who make up only about 1/4th of the population.

Health of Others

Smoking not only harms your health but the health of those around you. Exposure to secondhand smoke (also called environmental tobacco smoke or passive smoking) includes exhaled smoke as well as smoke from burning cigarettes.

Studies have shown that secondhand smoke causes thousands of deaths each year from lung cancer and heart disease in healthy nonsmokers.

Smoking by mothers is linked to a higher risk of their babies developing asthma in childhood, especially if the mother smokes while pregnant. It is also associated with sudden infant death syndrome (SIDS) and low-birth weight infants. Babies and children raised in a household where there is smoking have more ear infections, colds, bronchitis, and other respiratory problems than children from non-smoking families. Secondhand smoke can also cause eye irritation, headaches, nausea, and dizziness.

Setting an Example

If you have children, you want to set a good example for them. When asked, nearly all smokers say they don't want their children to smoke, but children whose parents smoke are more likely to start smoking themselves. You can become a good role model for them by quitting now.

Help Is Available

With the wide array of counseling services, self-help materials, and medicines available today, smokers have more tools than ever before to help them quit successfully. For most people, the best way to quit will be some combination of medicine, a method to change personal habits, and emotional support. The following sections describe these tools and how they may be helpful for you.

Tips for Quitting

The urge to smoke a cigarette will pass in three short minutes. Common concerns will probably go along with your decision to quit. You can address them and succeed.

"I'll gain weight if I quit smoking."

Weight gain varies from person to person. The average person gains less than 10 pounds. Exercise and a low fat diet can help prevent weight gain. Eat plenty of fruits and vegetables and whole grain cereals. Low-sugar candy might also help. Get enough sleep. Talk with your doctor about how to quit smoking while maintaining your weight.

"What do I do when I get the urge to smoke?"

When possible, stay away from places where others may be smoking. Ask others not to smoke around you. When you do feel an urge to smoke, distract yourself and keep busy. If you just wait three minutes, the urge will go away. You can also check with your doctor about prescription medications or nicotine replacement therapy, including over-the-counter patches or gum.

"Smoking relaxes me. I get too nervous and anxious if I don't smoke."

Take it easy. Warn those around that you have quit. Get enough rest. Relax. Exercise helps relieve tension. Go for a walk.

"I blew it. What do I do now?"

Smoking cigarettes again doesn't mean that you've failed. You've had some success. You got through a number of minutes, days, or months without smoking. Don't let relapses serve as excuses to start smoking again. You are an ex-smoker and can continue to be an ex-smoker.

"I've tried to quit smoking before. What makes this time different?"

You can choose to be a non-smoker and be successful. It's important enough to make another attempt. Set a goal for yourself. Think about why you smoke and different methods to handle those situations without smoking. Help is out there if you ask for it! Talk to your doctor, pharmacist, or local support group for more information. There are over 46.5 million ex-smokers in the United States and you can be one of them!

You Can Quit Smoking

Follow these six tips:

1. Set a Quit Date; mark your calendars at work and home.

2. Tell your family, friends, and co-workers that you are going to quit. Ask for their support and understanding.

3. Talk with your doctor about nicotine replacement therapy or medications that can help you quit. Both can help control your urges to smoke.

4. Throw away all cigarettes, ashtrays, lighters, and matches in your home and workplace before your Quit Date.

5. When you feel the urge to smoke, think about something else, chew gum, drink water, take a walk, and keep busy. The urge to smoke will go away in three to four minutes.

6. Reward yourself for doing well. Go the movies, rent a video or DVD, or buy yourself something nice.

Stroke is the third leading cause of death and a leading cause of adult disability in this country. When you stop smoking, you greatly reduce your chances of having a stroke. Be smoke-free three minutes at a time. Soon, you'll be a non-smoker for good.

Source: National Stroke Association

Section 27.2

Heavy Drinking

"Researchers Say Heavy Drinking May Cause Stroke," August 21, 2007, reprinted with permission from Join Together, www.jointogether.org.

Heavy drinkers increase their risk of stroke by up to 22 percent, according to researchers who studied a group of more than 64,000 Chinese men ages 40 and older.

HealthDay News reported Aug. 20 [2007] that Lydia Bazzano of Tulane University and colleagues found that among the men—who had no history of stroke when previously surveyed—the relative stroke risk was 0.92 for those who consumed one to six drinks weekly, 1.02 for those consuming 7–20 drinks weekly, and 1.22 for those who had 21 or more drinks weekly.

"At the top level of alcohol consumption (at least 35 drinks per week), risk of stroke incidence was 22 percent higher, and risk of mortality was 30 percent higher than among nondrinkers," the study noted.

The research was published online in the *Annals of Neurology.*

Reference: Bazzano, L.A., et al. (2007) Alcohol consumption and risk for stroke among Chinese men. *Annals of Neurology,* published online 20 Aug 2007; doi: 10.1002/ana.21194.

Section 27.3

Amphetamine and Cocaine Use

This section includes text from "Study Finds That Methamphetamine Use Can Increase Stroke-Related Brain Damage," by the National Institute on Drug Abuse (NIDA), March 19, 2001, and from "Cocaine's Effect on Blood Components May Be Linked to Heart Attack and Stroke," from NIDA, *NIDA Notes*, by Patrick Zickler, Vol. 17, No. 6, March 2003. Both documents were reviewed by David A. Cooke, M.D., April 5, 2008.

Methamphetamine Use Can Increase Stroke-Related Brain Damage

Researchers from the National Institute on Drug Abuse (NIDA) found that methamphetamine use prior to stroke increases damage to the brain. Methamphetamine appears to inhibit factors that occur naturally within the brain and that help protect it from neuronal damage following trauma such as stroke or other injury.

NIDA researchers, joined by scientists from the Tri-Service General Hospital, National Defense Medical Center, Taipei, Taiwan, used mice to ascertain the effects of methamphetamine on the brain following stroke. The researchers pretreated mice with either methamphetamine or a saline solution, temporarily blocked the blood flow through the animals' right middle cerebral artery and bilateral carotid arteries (mimicking an ischemic stroke), and observed the effects.

The researchers found more extensive brain damage in the mice pretreated with methamphetamine than in those treated with the saline solution.

Dr. Yun Wang, head of the research team, says that their experiments found at least one possible mechanism to explain this effect. They observed that methamphetamine pretreatment decreased glial-cell-line-derived neurotrophic factor (GDNF) in the mice brain; when GDNF was administered into the brains of the mice before their arteries were blocked, the effects of methamphetamine-facilitated stroke were reduced.

This result, Dr. Wang says, indicates that methamphetamine may act to exacerbate brain damage following stroke by inhibiting GDNF pathways.

What It Means: Scientists knew that methamphetamine, an addictive stimulant drug, increases heart rate and blood pressure and can cause irreversible damage to blood vessels in the brain, resulting in strokes. This evidence that methamphetamine can increase stroke-related damage to the brain further illustrates the danger of this drug.

Cocaine's Effect on Blood Components May Be Linked to Heart Attack and Stroke

Cocaine use increases the risk of sudden heart attack and may also trigger stroke, even in users who otherwise are not at high risk for these sometimes fatal cardiovascular events. The risk is related to narrowing of blood vessels and increases in blood pressure and heart rate. Recently, NIDA-supported researchers at the Alcohol and Drug Abuse Research Center at McLean Hospital in Belmont, Massachusetts, have identified changes in blood components that may also play a role in cocaine-related heart attack and stroke. Cocaine users who reported heavy use (6 to 20 times per week) show higher levels of C-reactive protein, von Willebrand factor, and fibrinogen—blood components that contribute to clotting—than do less frequent users (2 to 6 times per month).

Dr. Arthur Siegel and his colleagues studied the effect of cocaine on blood factors that respond to inflammation by promoting clotting to initiate repair. They found that a component that promotes clotting—von Willebrand factor (vWF)—increases and remains elevated for hours after a single exposure to cocaine. They also found that, compared with less frequent users, heavy users of cocaine have elevated levels of vWF, fibrinogen (a clotting factor), and C-reactive protein (CRP), a blood protein that increases in concentration in response to inflammation and is a reliable indicator of risk for heart attack.

"These findings suggest that cocaine creates a temporary risk for heart attack or stroke by increasing clotting factors," Dr. Siegel explains. "Elevated CRP levels could indicate that long-term use of the drug is triggering inflammation in the cardiovascular system."

Participants in the study were 20 individuals (10 women and 10 men, average age 26 years) who used cocaine 2 to 6 times per month but were drug free at the time of the study. They received injections of low (0.2 mg/kg) or moderate (0.4 mg/kg) doses of cocaine or of saline solution, and their clotting-related blood components were measured every 30 minutes for 4 hours. In participants who received moderate doses of cocaine, but not those receiving low-dose cocaine or saline, levels of vWF increased by roughly 40 percent and remained elevated for 4 hours.

"With healthy subjects, it's not unusual to see a temporary increase in vWF after normal activity such as exercise," Dr. Siegel says. "But the increase is balanced by higher levels of factors that control clotting. The increases that followed cocaine administration were not accompanied by compensatory increases in protective factors."

The researchers also compared the blood factor levels of the original study participants to those of 10 other individuals (6 women, 4 men, average age 41 years) who used the drug far more heavily—6 to 20 times per week, on average—when both groups were drug free. The heavy cocaine users had higher levels of vWF, fibrinogen, and CRP.

"Elevated levels of CRP and clotting factors that we see in the heavy users suggest that repeated use of cocaine poses an exposure-related and cumulative risk for heart attack or stroke," Dr. Siegel says. "The fact that neither group showed any compensatory increase in anticlotting mechanisms suggests that cocaine use upsets the body's ability to maintain a balance between risk and protective factors and tips the scale toward increased risk for heart attack or stroke."

The findings are preliminary, Dr. Siegel cautions, and based on a relatively small sample of cocaine users. "Other factors certainly play a role in CRP levels, and cocaine alone is probably not responsible for the elevated levels we found. For example, age is a factor but does not account for all of the difference. Smoking also may be a factor. In our study, cocaine users who smoked had higher CRP levels than those who did not. On the whole, these findings suggest that cocaine compounds the effects of other risk factors."

If larger studies confirm the relationship between elevated CRP levels and cumulative cocaine exposure, the blood component may serve as a marker for damage, Dr. Siegel says. Moreover, he adds, "measuring CRP is simple and inexpensive, and could be used as a test for the effects of cocaine in much the same way as blood composition is used to test for diabetes. It could serve as an objective measure of risk for heart attack and stroke and provide a way for patients and treatment providers to assess progress during drug treatment."

Sources

Siegel, A.J., et al. Cocaine-induced erythrocytosis and increase in von Willebrand factor. *Archives of Internal Medicine* 159:1925–1930, 1999. [Abstract]

Siegel, A.J., et al. Effect of cocaine usage on C-reactive protein, von Willebrand factor, and fibrinogen. *American Journal of Cardiology* 89:1133–1135, 2002. [Abstract]

Chapter 28

Stopping Stroke before It Occurs: Prevention Strategies

Chapter Contents

Section 28.1

Ten Strategies to Reduce Stroke Risk

"Stroke Prevention Guidelines," Copyright © 2007 National Stroke
Association. Reprinted with permission.

1. Know your blood pressure.

Have it checked at least annually. If it is elevated, work with your
doctor to keep it under control.

High blood pressure (hypertension) is a leading cause of stroke.

You can check your blood pressure at your doctor's office, at health
fairs, at home with an automatic blood pressure machine, or at your
local pharmacy or supermarket.

If the higher number (your systolic blood pressure) is consistently
above 120 or if the lower number (your diastolic blood pressure) is
consistently over 80, talk to your doctor.

If your doctor decides that you have high blood pressure, s/he may
recommend some changes in your diet, regular exercise, or medicine.

Blood pressure drugs have improved. Once you and your doctor find
the right medicine for you, it will almost never cause side effects or
interfere with your quality of life.

2. Find out if you have atrial fibrillation.

Atrial fibrillation (AF) is an irregular heartbeat that changes how your
heart works and allows blood to collect in the chambers of your heart.

This blood, which is not moving through your body, tends to clot.

The beating of your heart can move one of these blood clots into
your blood stream, and can cause a stroke.

Your doctor can diagnose AF by carefully taking your pulse.

AF can be confirmed or ruled out with an electrocardiogram (ECG)
(a recording of the electrical activity of the heart) which can probably
be done in your doctor's office.

If you have AF, your doctor may choose to lower your risk for stroke
by prescribing medicines called blood thinners. Aspirin and warfarin
(Coumadin®) are the most commonly prescribed treatments.

3. If you smoke, stop.

Smoking doubles the risk for stroke.

If you stop smoking today, your risk for stroke will immediately begin to drop.

Quitting smoking today can significantly reduce your risk of stroke from this factor.

4. If you drink alcohol, do so in moderation.

Studies now show that drinking up to two alcoholic drinks per day can reduce your risk for stroke by about half. More alcohol than this each day can increase your risk for stroke by as much as three times and can also lead to liver disease, accidents, and more. If you drink, we recommend no more than two drinks each day, and if you don't drink, don't start!

Remember that alcohol is a drug and it can interact with some drugs. It's a good idea to ask your doctor or pharmacist if any of the medicines you are taking could interact with alcohol.

5. Find out if you have high cholesterol (a soft, waxy fat [lipid] in the bloodstream and in all body cells).

Know your cholesterol number.

If your total cholesterol level (LDL and HDL) is over 200, talk to your doctor. You may be at increased risk for stroke. LDL, known as the "bad" cholesterol, is the form that builds up and causes plaque which may narrow arteries and limit or stop blood flow. LDL can be inherited from your family members or be a result of your body chemistry. It can also be the result of a diet high in saturated fats, lack of exercise, or diabetes. HDL is the "good" cholesterol that sweeps the blood and removes plaque. Lowering your cholesterol (if elevated) may reduce your risk for stroke.

High cholesterol can be controlled in many individuals with diet and exercise.

Some individuals with high cholesterol may require medicine.

6. If you are diabetic . . .

Follow your doctor's advice carefully to control your diabetes.

Often, diabetes may be controlled through careful attention to what you eat.

Work with your doctor and your dietitian (a health care professional who helps promote good health through proper eating) to develop a healthy eating program that fits your lifestyle.

Your doctor can prescribe lifestyle changes and medicine that can help control your diabetes.

Having diabetes puts you at an increased risk for stroke; by controlling your diabetes, you may lower your risk for stroke.

7. Exercise.

Include exercise in your daily activities.

A brisk walk for as little as 30 minutes a day can improve your health in many ways, and may reduce your risk for stroke.

Try walking with a friend; this will make it more likely that you'll make it a habit.

If you don't enjoy walking, choose another exercise or activity that you do enjoy, such as biking, swimming, golf, tennis, dance, or aerobics.

Make time each day to take care of yourself by exercising.

8. Enjoy a lower sodium (salt), lower fat diet.

By cutting down on sodium and fat in your diet, you may be able to lower your blood pressure and, most importantly, lower your risk for stroke.

Work towards a balanced diet each day with plenty of fruits, vegetables, grains, and a moderate amount of protein (meat, fish, eggs, milk, nuts, tofu, and some beans).

Adding fiber, such as whole grain bread and cereal products, raw, unpeeled fruits and vegetables and dried beans, to the diet can reduce cholesterol levels by 6 to 19 percent.

9. Circulation (movement of the blood through the heart and blood vessels) problems: Ask your doctor if you have circulation problems which increase your risk for stroke.

Strokes can be caused by problems with your heart (pump), arteries and veins (tubes), or the blood which flows through them. Together, they are your circulation. Your doctor can check to see if you have problems in the circulation supplying blood to your brain.

Fatty deposits—caused by atherosclerosis (a hardening or buildup of cholesterol plaque and other fatty deposits in the arteries) or other diseases—can block the arteries which carry blood from your heart to your brain. These arteries, located on each side of your neck, are called carotid and vertebral arteries.

This kind of blockage, if left untreated, can cause stroke.

You can be tested for this problem by your doctor. Your doctor can listen to your arteries just as s/he listens to your heart, or look at x-rays called ultrasound or MRI images.

If you have blood problems such as sickle cell disease, severe anemia (lower than normal number of red blood cells), or other diseases, work with your doctor to manage these problems. Left untreated, these can cause stroke.

Circulation problems can usually be treated with medicines. If your doctor prescribes aspirin, warfarin (Coumadin®), ticlopidine (Ticlid®), clopidogrel (Plavix®), dipyridamole (Aggrenox®), or other medicine for circulation problems, take it exactly as prescribed.

Occasionally, surgery is necessary to correct circulation problems such as a blocked artery.

10. Symptoms.

If you have any stroke symptoms, seek immediate medical attention. These include:

- Sudden numbness or weakness of face, arm or leg—especially on one side of the body.

- Sudden confusion, trouble speaking, or understanding.

- Sudden trouble seeing in one or both eyes.

- Sudden trouble walking, dizziness, loss of balance or coordination.

- Sudden severe headache with no known cause.

If you have experienced any of these symptoms, you may have had a TIA [transient ischemic attack] or mini-stroke. Ask your doctor if you can lower your risk for stroke by taking aspirin, or by other means.

If you think someone may be having a stroke, **act F.A.S.T.** and do this simple test:

- **FACE:** Ask the person to smile. Does one side of the face droop?

- **ARMS:** Ask the person to raise both arms. Does one arm drift downward?

- **SPEECH:** Ask the person to repeat a simple sentence. Are the words slurred? Can he/she repeat the sentence correctly?

- **TIME:** If the person shows any of these symptoms, time is important.

Call 911 or get to the hospital fast. Brain cells are dying.

Section 28.2

Preconditioning the Brain May Protect against Stroke

From the National Institute of Neurological Disorders and Stroke (NINDS, www.ninds.nih.gov), part of the National Institutes of Health, January 13, 2004.

Scientists studying an animal model of stroke have learned that the brain reacts to the trauma caused by a mild stroke in a way that serves to protect it from a subsequent injurious attack. The discovery may aid in the development of medications for persons at risk of stroke.

Stroke is the nation's third largest killer. There are as many as 700,000 strokes in the United States per year and 150,000 deaths as a result. The majority of strokes are ischemic, caused when a clot suddenly blocks blood flow to a vein or artery. Disabilities that can result from stroke include paralysis, cognitive deficits, speech problems, emotional difficulties, daily living problems, and pain.

Researchers Mary Stenzel-Poore, Ph.D., Oregon Health & Science University School of Medicine, and Roger Simon, M.D., Legacy Health Systems, led colleagues in testing the hypothesis that "ischemic preconditioning" naturally provides protection against a later, prolonged ischemic stroke. This preconditioning is based on a model which states that an organism, if given time to adjust to a trauma, will become stronger and more able to resist later trauma that might otherwise be lethal. The study was funded by the National Institute of Neurological Disorders and Stroke (NINDS) and published in *The Lancet*.

The researchers studied gene expression and cellular mechanisms in normal mice and in a mouse model of stroke that was preconditioned (these mice had their cerebral artery blocked for 15 minutes, resulting in small protective strokes called transient ischemic attacks or TIA). The preconditioned mice showed an innate reprogramming of certain gene expression that led to a 70 percent decrease in brain damage during a second larger stroke.

"These results show that the body is able to reprogram or change its genetic response in anticipation of a future, larger stroke," said Dr. Simon. "Several systems were found to adapt to TIA insult and either increase or decrease gene expression in a way that protects the body." The most striking changes in gene profiles were in response to ischemic injury following preconditioning. In response to an induced stroke, the genetic activity in preconditioned animals was found to slow metabolism, conserve cellular energy, and prevent blood clotting. Other changes seen in preconditioned mice included decreased blood flow and limited glucose and oxygen intake similar to that seen in hibernation.

"The genetic changes that occur in animals preconditioned for stroke are very similar to those that occur in hibernating animals, providing an evolutionary basis for this neuroprotective response," noted Dr. Stenzel-Poore. "Our findings link preconditioning in the brain with systemic effects of longer blood clotting times, which would be an important neuroprotective strategy against ischemic stroke."

Ischemic tolerance studies led by John Hallenbeck, M.D., NINDS intramural stroke branch chief, are revealing a cellular mechanism in hibernating ground squirrels that may protect the nervous system from being damaged during the profound reduction in organ blood flow, greatly reduced capacity to delivery oxygen, and extremely cold temperatures (hypothermic stress) that characterize hibernation. "A better understanding of the body's naturally occurring neuroprotective mechanisms may lead to new therapies and/or preventive measures for persons at high risk of ischemia and other neurological disorders," said Dr. Hallenbeck.

The findings may lead to preventive medicines that target certain genes and/or a combination therapy to address the many aspects of stroke.

Reference: "Effect of ischaemic preconditioning on genomic response to cerebral ischaemia: similarity to neuroprotective strategies in hibernation and hypoxia-tolerant states." Stenzel-Poore, Mary P; Stevens, Susan L.; Xiong, Zhigang; Lessov, Nikola S.; Harrington, Christina A.; Mori, Motomi; Meller, Robert; Rosenzweig, Holly L.; Tobar, Eric; Shaw, Tatyana E.; Chu, Xiangping; Simon, Roger P. *The Lancet,* Vol. 362, September 27, 2003, pp. 1028–1037.

Section 28.3

Community Health Center and Workplace Strategies to Reduce Stroke Risk

From "Preventing Heart Disease and Stroke," by the Department of Health and Human Services (HHS, www.hhs.gov), July 2005.

The Reality

- Heart disease and stroke—the principal components of cardiovascular disease—are the first and third leading causes of death in the United States, accounting for nearly 40% of all deaths.

- Nearly 930,000 Americans die of cardiovascular diseases each year, which amounts to one death every 33 seconds.

- About 70 million Americans (almost one-fourth of the population) have some form of cardiovascular disease, which is responsible for more than 6 million hospitalizations each year.

- Much of the burden of heart disease and stroke could be eliminated by reducing their major risk factors: high blood pressure, high blood cholesterol, tobacco use, diabetes, physical inactivity, and poor nutrition.

- About 90% of middle-aged Americans will develop high blood pressure in their lifetime, and nearly 70% of those who have it now do not have it under control.

- In 2002, more than 106 million people were told that they had total blood cholesterol levels that were above normal or high (200 mg/dL or higher).

The Cost of Heart Disease and Stroke

- In 2005, the cost of heart disease and stroke in the United States is projected to exceed $394 billion: $242 billion for health care expenditures and $152 billion for lost productivity from death and disability.

- In 2001, the cost of hospitalization for cardiovascular problems among Medicare beneficiaries topped $29 billion.

- In 2005, $60 billion in health care spending was attributed to high blood pressure.

Reducing Risk Factors for Heart Disease Saves Lives and Money

- An average reduction of just 12–13 mm Hg in systolic blood pressure over 4 years of follow-up is associated with a 21% reduction in coronary heart disease, a 37% reduction in stroke, a 25% reduction in total cardiovascular disease deaths, and a 13% reduction in overall death rates.

- A 10% reduction in serum cholesterol levels can result in a 30% reduction in the incidence of heart attacks and strokes.

- U.S. adults substantially lowered their blood pressure, high cholesterol levels, and other heart disease risk factors during the 1980s. As a result, U.S. costs associated with coronary heart disease declined by an estimated 9%—from about $240 billion in 1981 to about $220 billion in 1990.

Effective Strategies

Community health centers and other health care settings need to have systems in place that will improve the quality of care that high-risk patients receive. For example, community health centers and private clinics and doctor's offices can use electronic reminder messages to alert doctors to patients' follow-up needs. In Utah, community health centers have used such a system to substantially increase the proportion of patients who have their blood pressure under control. Before the system was in place, 33% of patients had their blood pressure under control, compared with 58% of patients just 6 months after the centers began using the system.

Work sites are an ideal place to promote the cardiovascular health of millions of people. For example, employers can offer health screenings and follow-up services to help employees control their blood pressure and cholesterol levels. These services are proven effective in the workplace. In addition, employees can be trained to recognize the signs of a heart attack and stroke and how to respond. Another strategy is for work sites to offer adequate insurance coverage for health services that aim to prevent heart disease and stroke.

Educating the public about signs of a heart attack and stroke and the importance of calling 911 quickly is an important step to improving the chances for survival and minimizing the damage that can occur following a heart attack or stroke. Research indicates that 47% of deaths from heart attack occur before a person can be admitted to a hospital, and about 48% of stroke victims die before emergency medical personnel arrive. Only 11% of adults in this country know both the signs of a heart attack and the urgency of calling 911.

Other important strategies to reduce people's risk for heart disease and stroke are to avoid tobacco use, eat healthier foods, control diabetes, and be more physically active.

Hope for the Future

The prevention and control of the major risk factors for heart disease and stroke are critical to achieving a heart-healthy and stroke-free America. Health agencies at the federal, state, and local levels are working to reduce these risk factors and to eliminate disparities in health as well as those in the delivery of health care services.

Whether you are a citizen, health care provider, employer, school administrator, or elected official, there are things you can do to improve the health of your heart. For suggestions, check out CDC's Moving Into Action, available at http://www.cdc.gov/cvh.

Chapter 29

A Vaccine to Prevent Stroke: Is It Possible?

A vaccine that interferes with inflammation inside blood vessels greatly reduces the frequency and severity of strokes in spontaneously hypertensive, genetically stroke-prone rats, according to a study from the NIH's National Institute of Neurological Disorders and Stroke (NINDS). If the vaccine works in humans, it could prevent many of the strokes that occur each year.

In the study, researchers used a nasal spray to deliver a protein that, under normal circumstances, contributes to inflammation of the cells that line the inner walls of blood vessels. Exposing rats to this substance, called E-selectin, programs blood cells called lymphocytes to monitor the blood vessel lining for the inflammatory protein. When these lymphocytes detect E-selectin, they produce substances that suppress inflammation.

The vaccine is the first treatment to target inflammation in blood vessels as a possible means of preventing stroke, says senior author John M. Hallenbeck, M.D., chief of the Stroke Branch at NINDS. "Clinically, stroke is hard to treat. If we can prevent it from happening, that's clearly the way to go," he adds. The study appears in the September 2002 issue of the journal *Stroke*.[1]

Stroke is the third leading cause of death in the United States and the most common cause of disability in adults. Each year more than

Excerpted from "Vaccine Prevents Stroke in Rats," by the National Institute of Neurological Disorders and Stroke (NINDS, www.ninds.nih.gov), part of the National Institutes of Health (NIH), September 5, 2002. This document was reviewed and revised by David A. Cooke, M.D., March 3, 2008.

500,000 Americans have a stroke, and about 150,000 die from stroke-related causes. A stroke occurs when the blood supply to the brain is suddenly interrupted, as with a blood clot (ischemic stroke), or when a blood vessel in the brain bursts, spilling blood into the spaces surrounding brain cells (hemorrhagic stroke). Current stroke prevention strategies include reducing risk factors, such as high blood pressure (hypertension), or blocking the formation of blood clots using drugs such as aspirin and warfarin.

Animal studies have shown that blood vessels undergo periodic cycles of inflammation. These cycles are more frequent and intense in stroke-prone animals. In rats with stroke risk factors, such as hypertension, diabetes, or advanced age, a single dose of a substance found in bacteria can provoke inflammation that leads to a blood clot or a blood vessel hemorrhage.

Researchers believe inflammation also contributes to stroke in humans. In the new study, Dr. Hallenbeck and colleagues tested human E-selectin and two other substances (used as controls) in a total of 113 stroke-prone rats with genetically induced hypertension. Some of the rats received a single course of E-selectin every other day for 10 days, while others received the 10-day course of treatment every 3 weeks until they died or until the study was complete.

The results of the investigation were dramatic. During more than a year of study, the rats that received repeated E-selectin vaccine treatment had 16 times fewer ischemic strokes than those given repeated treatment with a control substance. Furthermore, none of the rats given repeated vaccine treatment had a hemorrhagic stroke, while the other groups had two to three hemorrhagic strokes on average during the study period. Strokes that did occur in the rats with repeated vaccine treatment caused much less brain damage than strokes in the control rats. The researchers also found that lymphocytes from rats treated with the E-selectin vaccine produced a type of chemical called a cytokine that blocked inflammation in blood vessels.

The single course of vaccine treatment did not maintain the animals' resistance to stroke; repeated treatment with the vaccine was required for long-term stroke prevention, the researchers say.

The vaccine did not have any effect on the rats' blood pressure. This shows that its beneficial effects are not linked to reduction of high blood pressure, a proven means of reducing the risk of stroke, Dr. Hallenbeck notes. If the vaccine proves effective in people, it would be used in conjunction with control of high blood pressure and other risk factors, he adds.

"We think the E-selectin vaccine works by reducing immune and inflammatory reactions in vessels that threaten either to become blocked or to rupture and bleed," Dr. Hallenbeck says. This contrasts with many other vaccines, such as flu shots, which work by increasing the immune system's reactions to specific viruses or bacteria.

Since the study described above, Dr. Hallenbeck's group has performed additional studies with their E-selectin vaccine. These have confirmed the results of their first study and expanded somewhat upon them. For example, a 2003 study found that pre-treating rats with the vaccine significantly reduced the degree of brain damage that occurred after a major brain artery was tied off. This shows that not only does the vaccine prevent strokes, it also limits damage if a stroke occurs. They have continued to explore how the vaccine provides its benefits and to look at factors influencing its effectiveness.

1. Takeda H, Spatz M, Ruetzler C, McCarron R, Becker K, Hallenbeck J. "Induction of mucosal tolerance to E-selectin prevents ischemic and hemorrhagic stroke in spontaneously hypertensive genetically stroke-prone rats." *Stroke: Journal of the American Heart Association,* Vol. 33, No. 9, September 2002, pp. 2156–2164.

2. Chen Y, Ruetzler C, Pandipati S, Spatz M, McCarron RM, Becker K, Hallenbeck JM. "Mucosal tolerance to E-selectin provides cell-mediated protection against ischemic brain injury." *Proceedings of the National Academy of Sciences of the United States of America,* Vol. 100, No. 25, December 9, 2003, pp. 15107–12.

3. Illoh K, Campbell C, Illoh O, Diehl J, Cherry J, Elkhaloun A, Hallenbeck J. "Mucosal tolerance to E-selectin and response to systemic inflammation." *Journal of Cerebral Blood Flow & Metabolism,* Vol. 26, No. 12, December 2006, pp. 1538–1550.

Part Three

Diagnosing and Treating Stroke

Chapter 30

Stroke Warning Signs

Chapter Contents

Section 30.1

Identifying the Signs of Stroke

"Know Stroke. Know the Signs. Act in Time" is by the National Institute of Neurological Disorders and Stroke (NINDS, www.ninds.nih.gov), part of the National Institutes of Health, NIH Publication No. 08-4872, January 2008.

Know Stroke

Stroke is the third leading cause of death in the United States and a leading cause of serious, long-term disability in adults. About 600,000 new strokes are reported in the United States each year. The good news is that treatments are available that can greatly reduce the damage caused by a stroke. However, you need to recognize the symptoms of a stroke and get to a hospital quickly. Getting treatment within 60 minutes can prevent disability.

What is a stroke?

A stroke, sometimes called a "brain attack," occurs when blood flow to the brain is interrupted. When a stroke occurs, brain cells in the immediate area begin to die because they stop getting the oxygen and nutrients they need to function.

What causes a stroke?

There are two major kinds of stroke.

The first, called an ischemic stroke, is caused by a blood clot that blocks or plugs a blood vessel or artery in the brain. About 80 percent of all strokes are ischemic. The second, known as a hemorrhagic stroke, is caused by a blood vessel in the brain that breaks and bleeds into the brain. About 20 percent of strokes are hemorrhagic.

What disabilities can result from a stroke?

Although stroke is a disease of the brain, it can affect the entire body. The effects of a stroke range from mild to severe and can include paralysis, problems with thinking, problems with speaking, and emotional problems. Patients may also experience pain or numbness after a stroke.

Know the Signs

Because stroke injures the brain, you may not realize that you are having a stroke. To a bystander, someone having a stroke may just look unaware or confused. Stroke victims have the best chance if someone around them recognizes the symptoms and acts quickly.

What are the symptoms of a stroke?

The symptoms of stroke are distinct because they happen quickly:

- Sudden numbness or weakness of the face, arm, or leg (especially on one side of the body)
- Sudden confusion, trouble speaking or understanding speech
- Sudden trouble seeing in one or both eyes
- Sudden trouble walking, dizziness, loss of balance or coordination
- Sudden severe headache with no known cause

Act in Time

Stroke is a medical emergency. Every minute counts when someone is having a stroke. The longer blood flow is cut off to the brain, the greater the damage. Immediate treatment can save people's lives and enhance their chances for successful recovery.

What can I do to prevent a stroke?

The best treatment for stroke is prevention. There are several risk factors that increase your chances of having a stroke:

- High blood pressure
- Heart disease
- Smoking
- Diabetes
- High cholesterol

If you smoke—quit. If you have high blood pressure, heart disease, diabetes, or high cholesterol, getting them under control—and keeping them under control—will greatly reduce your chances of having a stroke.

Section 30.2

Stroke: Tips and Information for Bystanders

Excerpted from "Stroke FAQs," by the Centers for Disease Control and Prevention (CDC, www.cdc.gov), October 2007.

What are the symptoms of stroke?

The National Institute of Neurological Disorders and Stroke notes these major signs of stroke:

- Sudden numbness or weakness of the face, arms, or legs
- Sudden confusion or trouble speaking or understanding others
- Sudden trouble seeing in one or both eyes
- Sudden trouble walking, dizziness, or loss of balance or coordination
- Sudden severe headache with no known cause

All of the major symptoms of stroke appear suddenly, and often there is more than one symptom at the same time.

What should a bystander do?

If you think someone is having a stroke, you should call 911 or emergency medical services right away.

Why is there a need to act fast?

Death or permanent disability can result from a stroke. With timely treatment, however, the risk of death and disability from stroke can be lowered. It is very important to know the symptoms of a stroke and act right away.

Chapter 31

Overview of Neurological Diagnostic Tests and Procedures

Diagnostic tests and procedures are vital tools that help physicians confirm or rule out the presence of a neurological disorder or other medical condition. A century ago, the only way to make a positive diagnosis for many neurological disorders was by performing an autopsy after a patient had died. But decades of basic research into the characteristics of disease, and the development of techniques that allow scientists to see inside the living brain and monitor nervous system activity as it occurs, have given doctors powerful and accurate tools to diagnose disease and to test how well a particular therapy may be working.

Perhaps the most significant changes in diagnostic imaging over the past 20 years are improvements in spatial resolution (size, intensity, and clarity) of anatomical images and reductions in the time needed to send signals to and receive data from the area being imaged. These advances allow physicians to simultaneously see the structure of the brain and the changes in brain activity as they occur. Scientists continue to improve methods that will provide sharper anatomical images and more detailed functional information.

Researchers and physicians use a variety of diagnostic imaging techniques and chemical and metabolic analyses to detect, manage, and treat neurological disease. Some procedures are performed in specialized settings, conducted to determine the presence of a

"Neurological Diagnostic Tests and Procedures" is from the National Institute of Neurological Disorders and Stroke (NINDS, www.ninds.nih.gov), part of the National Institutes of Health, October 16, 2007.

particular disorder or abnormality. Many tests that were previously conducted in a hospital are now performed in a physician's office or at an outpatient testing facility, with little if any risk to the patient. Depending on the type of procedure, results are either immediate or may take several hours to process.

What are some of the more common screening tests?

Laboratory screening tests of blood, urine, or other substances are used to help diagnose disease, better understand the disease process, and monitor levels of therapeutic drugs. Certain tests, ordered by the physician as part of a regular checkup, provide general information, while others are used to identify specific health concerns. For example, blood and blood product tests can detect brain and/or spinal cord infection, bone marrow disease, hemorrhage, blood vessel damage, toxins that affect the nervous system, and the presence of antibodies that signal the presence of an autoimmune disease. Blood tests are also used to monitor levels of therapeutic drugs used to treat epilepsy and other neurological disorders. Genetic testing of DNA extracted from white cells in the blood can help diagnose Huntington disease and other congenital diseases. Analysis of the fluid that surrounds the brain and spinal cord can detect meningitis, acute and chronic inflammation, rare infections, and some cases of multiple sclerosis. Chemical and metabolic testing of the blood can indicate protein disorders, some forms of muscular dystrophy and other muscle disorders, and diabetes. Urinalysis can reveal abnormal substances in the urine or the presence or absence of certain proteins that cause diseases including the mucopolysaccharidoses.

Genetic testing or counseling can help parents who have a family history of a neurological disease determine if they are carrying one of the known genes that cause the disorder or find out if their child is affected. Genetic testing can identify many neurological disorders, including spina bifida, in utero (while the child is inside the mother's womb). Genetic tests include the following:

- **Amniocentesis,** usually done at 14-16 weeks of pregnancy, tests a sample of the amniotic fluid in the womb for genetic defects (the fluid and the fetus have the same DNA). Under local anesthesia, a thin needle is inserted through the woman's abdomen and into the womb. About 20 milliliters of fluid (roughly 4 teaspoons) is withdrawn and sent to a lab for evaluation. Test results often take 1–2 weeks.

280

- **Chorionic villus sampling,** or CVS, is performed by removing and testing a very small sample of the placenta during early pregnancy. The sample, which contains the same DNA as the fetus, is removed by catheter or fine needle inserted through the cervix or by a fine needle inserted through the abdomen. It is tested for genetic abnormalities and results are usually available within 2 weeks. CVS should not be performed after the tenth week of pregnancy.

- **Uterine ultrasound** is performed using a surface probe with gel. This noninvasive test can suggest the diagnosis of conditions such as chromosomal disorders.

What is a neurological examination?

A neurological examination assesses motor and sensory skills, the functioning of one or more cranial nerves, hearing and speech, vision, coordination and balance, mental status, and changes in mood or behavior, among other abilities. Items including a tuning fork, flashlight, reflex hammer, ophthalmoscope, and needles are used to help diagnose brain tumors, infections such as encephalitis and meningitis, and diseases such as Parkinson disease, Huntington disease, amyotrophic lateral sclerosis (ALS), and epilepsy. Some tests require the services of a specialist to perform and analyze results.

X-rays of the patient's chest and skull are often taken as part of a neurological work-up. X-rays can be used to view any part of the body, such as a joint or major organ system. In a conventional x-ray, also called a radiograph, a technician passes a concentrated burst of low-dose ionized radiation through the body and onto a photographic plate. Since calcium in bones absorbs x-rays more easily than soft tissue or muscle, the bony structure appears white on the film. Any vertebral misalignment or fractures can be seen within minutes. Tissue masses such as injured ligaments or a bulging disk are not visible on conventional x-rays. This fast, noninvasive, painless procedure is usually performed in a doctor's office or at a clinic.

Fluoroscopy is a type of x-ray that uses a continuous or pulsed beam of low-dose radiation to produce continuous images of a body part in motion. The fluoroscope (x-ray tube) is focused on the area of interest and pictures are either videotaped or sent to a monitor for viewing. A contrast medium may be used to highlight the images. Fluoroscopy can be used to evaluate the flow of blood through arteries.

What are some diagnostic tests used to diagnose neurological disorders?

Based on the result of a neurological exam, physical exam, patient history, x-rays of the patient's chest and skull, and any previous screening or testing, physicians may order one or more of the following diagnostic tests to determine the specific nature of a suspected neurological disorder or injury. These diagnostics generally involve either nuclear medicine imaging, in which very small amounts of radioactive materials are used to study organ function and structure, or diagnostic imaging, which uses magnets and electrical charges to study human anatomy.

The following list of available procedures—in alphabetical rather than sequential order—includes some of the more common tests used to help diagnose a neurological condition.

Angiography is a test used to detect blockages of the arteries or veins. A cerebral angiogram can detect the degree of narrowing or obstruction of an artery or blood vessel in the brain, head, or neck. It is used to diagnose stroke and to determine the location and size of a brain tumor, aneurysm, or vascular malformation. This test is usually performed in a hospital outpatient setting and takes up to 3 hours, followed by a 6- to 8-hour resting period. The patient, wearing a hospital or imaging gown, lies on a table that is wheeled into the imaging area. While the patient is awake, a physician anesthetizes a small area of the leg near the groin and then inserts a catheter into a major artery located there. The catheter is threaded through the body and into an artery in the neck. Once the catheter is in place, the needle is removed and a guide wire is inserted. A small capsule containing a radiopaque dye (one that is highlighted on x-rays) is passed over the guide wire to the site of release. The dye is released and travels through the bloodstream into the head and neck. A series of x-rays is taken and any obstruction is noted. Patients may feel a warm to hot sensation or slight discomfort as the dye is released.

Biopsy involves the removal and examination of a small piece of tissue from the body. Muscle or nerve biopsies are used to diagnose neuromuscular disorders and may also reveal if a person is a carrier of a defective gene that could be passed on to children. A small sample of muscle or nerve is removed under local anesthetic and studied under a microscope. The sample may be removed either surgically, through a slit made in the skin, or by needle biopsy, in which a thin hollow needle is inserted through the skin and into the muscle. A small piece of muscle or nerve remains in the hollow needle when it is removed from the body. The biopsy is usually performed at an outpatient testing facility. A brain biopsy, used to determine tumor type, requires surgery to remove a small piece of the brain or tumor. Performed in a hospital, this operation is riskier than a muscle biopsy and involves a longer recovery period.

Brain scans are imaging techniques used to diagnose tumors, blood vessel malformations, or hemorrhage in the brain. These scans are used to study organ function or injury or disease to tissue or muscle. Types of brain scans include computed tomography, magnetic resonance imaging, and positron emission tomography.

Cerebrospinal fluid analysis involves the removal of a small amount of the fluid that protects the brain and spinal cord. The fluid is tested to detect any bleeding or brain hemorrhage, diagnose infection to the brain and/or spinal cord, identify some cases of multiple sclerosis and other neurological conditions, and measure intracranial pressure.

The procedure is usually done in a hospital. The sample of fluid is commonly removed by a procedure known as a lumbar puncture, or spinal tap. The patient is asked to either lie on one side, in a ball position with knees close to the chest, or lean forward while sitting on a table or bed. The doctor will locate a puncture site in the lower back, between two vertebrate, then clean the area and inject a local anesthetic. The patient may feel a slight stinging sensation from this injection. Once the anesthetic has taken effect, the doctor will insert a special needle into the spinal sac and remove a small amount of fluid (usually about three teaspoons) for testing. Most patients will feel a sensation of pressure only as the needle is inserted.

A common after-effect of a lumbar puncture is headache, which can be lessened by having the patient lie flat. Risk of nerve root injury or infection from the puncture can occur but it is rare. The entire procedure takes about 45 minutes.

Computed tomography, also known as a CT scan, is a noninvasive, painless process used to produce rapid, clear two-dimensional images of organs, bones, and tissues. Neurological CT scans are used to view the brain and spine. They can detect bone and vascular irregularities, certain brain tumors and cysts, herniated disks, epilepsy, encephalitis, spinal stenosis (narrowing of the spinal canal), a blood clot or intracranial bleeding in patients with stroke, brain damage from head injury, and other disorders. Many neurological disorders share certain characteristics and a CT scan can aid in proper diagnosis by differentiating the area of the brain affected by the disorder.

Scanning takes about 20 minutes (a CT of the brain or head may take slightly longer) and is usually done at an imaging center or hospital on an outpatient basis. The patient lies on a special table that slides into a narrow chamber. A sound system built into the chamber allows the patient to communicate with the physician or technician. As the patient lies still, x-rays are passed through the body at various angles and are detected by a computerized scanner. The data is processed and displayed as cross-sectional images, or "slices" of the internal structure of the body or organ. A light sedative may be given to patients who are unable to lie still and pillows may be used to support and stabilize the head and body. Persons who are claustrophobic may have difficulty taking this imaging test.

Occasionally a contrast dye is injected into the bloodstream to highlight the different tissues in the brain. Patients may feel a warm or cool sensation as the dye circulates through the bloodstream or they may experience a slight metallic taste.

Although very little radiation is used in CT, pregnant women should avoid the test because of potential harm to the fetus from ionizing radiation.

Discography is often suggested for patients who are considering lumbar surgery or whose lower back pain has not responded to conventional treatments. This outpatient procedure is usually performed at a testing facility or a hospital. The patient is asked to put on a metal-free hospital gown and lie on an imaging table. The physician numbs the skin with anesthetic and inserts a thin needle, using x-ray guidance, into the spinal disk. Once the needle is in place, a small amount of contrast dye is injected and CT scans are taken. The contrast dye outlines any damaged areas. More than one disk may be imaged at the same time. Patient recovery usually takes about an hour. Pain medicine may be prescribed for any resulting discomfort.

An intrathecal contrast-enhanced CT scan (also called cisternography) is used to detect problems with the spine and spinal nerve roots. This test is most often performed at an imaging center. The patient is asked to put on a hospital or imaging gown. Following application of a topical anesthetic, the physician removes a small sample of the spinal fluid via lumbar puncture. The sample is mixed with a contrast dye and injected into the spinal sac located at the base of the lower back. The patient is then asked to move to a position that will allow the contrast fluid to travel to the area to be studied. The dye allows the spinal canal and nerve roots to be seen more clearly on a CT scan. The scan may take up to an hour to complete. Following the test, patients may experience some discomfort and/or headache that may be caused by the removal of spinal fluid.

Electroencephalography, or EEG, monitors brain activity through the skull. EEG is used to help diagnose certain seizure disorders, brain tumors, brain damage from head injuries, inflammation of the brain and/or spinal cord, alcoholism, certain psychiatric disorders, and metabolic and degenerative disorders that affect the brain. EEGs are also used to evaluate sleep disorders, monitor brain activity when a patient has been fully anesthetized or loses consciousness, and confirm brain death.

This painless, risk-free test can be performed in a doctor's office or at a hospital or testing facility. Prior to taking an EEG, the person must avoid caffeine intake and prescription drugs that affect the nervous system. A series of cup-like electrodes are attached to the patient's scalp, either with a special conducting paste or with extremely fine needles. The electrodes (also called leads) are small devices that are attached to wires and carry the electrical energy of the brain to a machine for reading. A very low electrical current is sent through the electrodes and the baseline brain energy is recorded. Patients are then exposed to a variety of external stimuli—including bright or flashing light, noise or certain drugs—or are asked to open and close the eyes, or to change breathing patterns. The electrodes transmit the resulting changes in brain wave patterns. Since movement and nervousness can change brain wave patterns, patients usually recline in a chair or on a bed during the test, which takes up to an hour. Testing for certain disorders requires performing an EEG during sleep, which takes at least 3 hours.

In order to learn more about brain wave activity, electrodes may be inserted through a surgical opening in the skull and into the brain to reduce signal interference from the skull.

Electromyography, or EMG, is used to diagnose nerve and muscle dysfunction and spinal cord disease. It records the electrical activity from the brain and/or spinal cord to a peripheral nerve root (found in the arms and legs) that controls muscles during contraction and at rest.

During an EMG, very fine wire electrodes are inserted into a muscle to assess changes in electrical voltage that occur during movement and when the muscle is at rest. The electrodes are attached through a series of wires to a recording instrument. Testing usually takes place at a testing facility and lasts about an hour but may take longer, depending on the number of muscles and nerves to be tested. Most patients find this test to be somewhat uncomfortable.

An EMG is usually done in conjunction with a nerve conduction velocity (NCV) test, which measures electrical energy by assessing the nerve's ability to send a signal. This two-part test is conducted most often in a hospital. A technician tapes two sets of flat electrodes on the skin over the muscles. The first set of electrodes is used to send small pulses of electricity (similar to the sensation of static electricity) to stimulate the nerve that directs a particular muscle. The second set of electrodes transmits the responding electrical signal to a recording machine. The physician then reviews the response to verify any nerve damage or muscle disease. Patients who are preparing to take an EMG or NCV test may be asked to avoid caffeine and not smoke for 2 to 3 hours prior to the test, as well as to avoid aspirin and non-steroidal anti-inflammatory drugs for 24 hours before the EMG. There is no discomfort or risk associated with this test.

Electronystagmography (ENG) describes a group of tests used to diagnose involuntary eye movement, dizziness, and balance disorders, and to evaluate some brain functions. The test is performed at an imaging center. Small electrodes are taped around the eyes to record eye movements. If infrared photography is used in place of electrodes, the patient wears special goggles that help record the information. Both versions of the test are painless and risk-free.

Evoked potentials (also called evoked response) measure the electrical signals to the brain generated by hearing, touch, or sight. These tests are used to assess sensory nerve problems and confirm neurological conditions including multiple sclerosis, brain tumor, acoustic neuroma (small tumors of the inner ear), and spinal cord injury. Evoked potentials are also used to test sight and hearing (especially in infants and young children), monitor brain activity among coma patients, and confirm brain death.

Testing may take place in a doctor's office or hospital setting. It is painless and risk-free. Two sets of needle electrodes are used to test for nerve damage. One set of electrodes, which will be used to measure the electrophysiological response to stimuli, is attached to the patient's scalp using conducting paste. The second set of electrodes is attached to the part of the body to be tested. The physician then records the amount of time it takes for the impulse generated by stimuli to reach the brain. Under normal circumstances, the process of signal transmission is instantaneous.

Auditory evoked potentials (also called brain stem auditory evoked response) are used to assess high-frequency hearing loss, diagnose any damage to the acoustic nerve and auditory pathways in the brainstem, and detect acoustic neuromas. The patient sits in a soundproof room and wears headphones. Clicking sounds are delivered one at a time to one ear while a masking sound is sent to the other ear. Each ear is usually tested twice, and the entire procedure takes about 45 minutes.

Visual evoked potentials detect loss of vision from optic nerve damage (in particular, damage caused by multiple sclerosis). The patient sits close to a screen and is asked to focus on the center of a shifting checkerboard pattern. Only one eye is tested at a time; the other eye is either kept closed or covered with a patch. Each eye is usually tested twice. Testing takes 30-45 minutes.

Somatosensory evoked potentials measure response from stimuli to the peripheral nerves and can detect nerve or spinal cord damage or nerve degeneration from multiple sclerosis and other degenerating diseases. Tiny electrical shocks are delivered by electrode to a nerve in an arm or leg. Responses to the shocks, which may be delivered for more than a minute at a time, are recorded. This test usually lasts less than an hour.

Magnetic resonance imaging (MRI) uses computer-generated radio waves and a powerful magnetic field to produce detailed images of body structures including tissues, organs, bones, and nerves. Neurological uses include the diagnosis of brain and spinal cord tumors, eye disease, inflammation, infection, and vascular irregularities that may lead to stroke. MRI can also detect and monitor degenerative disorders such as multiple sclerosis and can document brain injury from trauma.

The equipment houses a hollow tube that is surrounded by a very large cylindrical magnet. The patient, who must remain still during the test, lies on a special table that is slid into the tube. The patient will be asked to remove jewelry, eyeglasses, removable dental work, or other items that might interfere with the magnetic imaging. The patient should wear a sweatshirt and sweatpants or other clothing free of metal eyelets or buckles. MRI scanning equipment creates a magnetic field around the body strong enough to temporarily realign water molecules in the tissues. Radio waves are then passed through the body to detect the "relaxation" of the molecules back to a random alignment and trigger a resonance signal at different angles within the body. A computer processes this resonance into either a three-dimensional picture or a two-dimensional "slice" of the tissue being scanned, and differentiates between bone, soft tissues and fluid-filled spaces by their water content and structural properties. A contrast dye may be used to enhance visibility of certain areas or tissues. The patient may hear grating or knocking noises when the magnetic field is turned on and off. (Patients may wear special earphones to block out the sounds.) Unlike CT scanning, MRI does not use ionizing radiation to produce images. Depending on the part(s) of the body to be scanned, MRI can take up to an hour to complete. The test is painless and risk-free, although persons who are obese or claustrophobic may find it somewhat uncomfortable. (Some centers also use open MRI machines that do not completely surround the person being tested and are less confining. However, open MRI does not currently provide the same picture quality as standard MRI and some tests may not be available using this equipment). Due to the incredibly strong magnetic field generated by an MRI, patients with implanted medical devices such as a pacemaker should avoid the test.

Functional MRI (fMRI) uses the blood's magnetic properties to produce real-time images of blood flow to particular areas of the brain. An fMRI can pinpoint areas of the brain that become active and note how long they stay active. It can also tell if brain activity within a region occurs simultaneously or sequentially. This imaging process is used to assess brain damage from head injury or degenerative disorders such as Alzheimer disease and to identify and monitor other neurological disorders, including multiple sclerosis, stroke, and brain tumors.

Myelography involves the injection of a water- or oil-based contrast dye into the spinal canal to enhance x-ray imaging of the spine. Myelograms are used to diagnose spinal nerve injury, herniated disks, fractures, back or leg pain, and spinal tumors.

The procedure takes about 30 minutes and is usually performed in a hospital. Following an injection of anesthesia to a site between two vertebrae in the lower back, a small amount of the cerebrospinal fluid is removed by spinal tap and the contrast dye is injected into the spinal canal. After a series of x-rays is taken, most or all of the contrast dye is removed by aspiration. Patients may experience some pain during the spinal tap and when the dye is injected and removed. Patients may also experience headache following the spinal tap. The risk of fluid leakage or allergic reaction to the dye is slight.

Positron emission tomography (PET) scans provide two- and three-dimensional pictures of brain activity by measuring radioactive isotopes that are injected into the bloodstream. PET scans of the brain are used to detect or highlight tumors and diseased tissue, measure cellular and/or tissue metabolism, show blood flow, evaluate patients who have seizure disorders that do not respond to medical therapy and patients with certain memory disorders, and determine brain changes following injury or drug abuse, among other uses. PET may be ordered as a follow-up to a CT or MRI scan to give the physician a greater understanding of specific areas of the brain that may be involved with certain problems. Scans are conducted in a hospital or at a testing facility, on an outpatient basis. A low-level radioactive isotope, which binds to chemicals that flow to the brain, is injected into the blood-stream and can be traced as the brain performs different functions. The patient lies still while overhead sensors detect gamma rays in the body's tissues. A computer processes the information and displays it on a video monitor or on film. Using different compounds, more than one brain function can be traced simultaneously. PET is painless and relatively risk-free. Length of test time depends on the part of the body to be scanned. PET scans are performed by skilled technicians at highly sophisticated medical facilities.

A polysomnogram measures brain and body activity during sleep. It is performed over one or more nights at a sleep center. Electrodes are pasted or taped to the patient's scalp, eyelids, and/or chin. Through-out the night and during the various wake/sleep cycles, the electrodes record brain waves, eye movement, breathing, leg and skeletal muscle activity, blood pressure, and heart rate. The patient may be videotaped to note any movement during sleep. Results are then used to identify any characteristic patterns of sleep disorders, including restless legs syndrome, periodic limb movement disorder, insomnia, and breathing disorders such as obstructive sleep apnea. Polysomnograms are non-invasive, painless, and risk-free.

Single photon emission computed tomography (SPECT), a nuclear imaging test involving blood flow to tissue, is used to evaluate certain brain functions. The test may be ordered as a follow-up to an MRI to diagnose tumors, infections, degenerative spinal disease, and stress fractures. As with a PET scan, a radioactive isotope, which binds to chemicals that flow to the brain, is injected intravenously into the body. Areas of increased blood flow will collect more of the isotope. As the patient lies on a table, a gamma camera rotates around the head and records where the radioisotope has traveled. That information is converted by computer into cross-sectional slices that are stacked to produce a detailed three-dimensional image of blood flow and activity within the brain. The test is performed at either an imaging center or a hospital.

Thermography uses infrared sensing devices to measure small temperature changes between the two sides of the body or within a specific organ. Also known as digital infrared thermal imaging, thermography may be used to detect vascular disease of the head and neck, soft tissue injury, various neuromusculoskeletal disorders, and the presence or absence of nerve root compression. It is performed at an imaging center, using infrared light recorders to take thousands of pictures of the body from a distance of 5 to 8 feet. The information is converted into electrical signals which results in a computer-generated two-dimensional picture of abnormally cold or hot areas indicated by color or shades of black and white. Thermography does not use radiation and is safe, risk-free, and noninvasive.

Ultrasound imaging, also called ultrasound scanning or sonography, uses high-frequency sound waves to obtain images inside the body. Neurosonography (ultrasound of the brain and spinal column) analyzes blood flow in the brain and can diagnose stroke, brain tumors, hydrocephalus (build-up of cerebrospinal fluid in the brain), and vascular problems. It can also identify or rule out inflammatory processes causing pain. It is more effective than an x-ray in displaying soft tissue masses and can show tears in ligaments, muscles, tendons, and other soft tissue masses in the back. Transcranial Doppler ultrasound is used to view arteries and blood vessels in the neck and determine blood flow and risk of stroke.

During ultrasound, the patient lies on an imaging table and removes clothing around the area of the body to be scanned. A jelly-like lubricant is applied and a transducer, which both sends and receives high-frequency sound waves, is passed over the body. The sound wave echoes are recorded and displayed as a computer-generated real-time visual image of the structure or tissue being examined. Ultrasound is painless, noninvasive, and risk-free. The test is performed on an outpatient basis and takes between 15 and 30 minutes to complete.

What lies ahead?

Scientists funded by the NINDS seek to develop additional and improved screening methods to more accurately and quickly confirm a specific diagnosis and allow scientists to investigate other factors that might contribute to disease. Technological advances in imaging will allow researchers to better see inside the body, at less risk to the patient. These diagnostics and procedures will continue to be important clinical research tools for confirming a neurological disorder, charting disease progression, and monitoring therapeutic effect.

Chapter 32

Diagnosing Stroke

Chapter Contents

Section 32.1

How a Stroke Is Diagnosed

If you have had a stroke, or have had stroke warning signs or risk factors, it is very important to seek prompt medical attention. Your doctor will work with you to find the cause of your problem and determine the best treatment. Even if your symptoms resolve without treatment, you should still discuss them with your doctor. Don't assume that a problem is unimportant if it goes away on its own. Never try to make a diagnosis by yourself.

Important: If you or someone you know is having stroke symptoms now, call 911! Stroke is a medical emergency. Read about the warning signs of stroke at http://www.strokecenter.org/patients/warning .htm.

The first step in understanding your problem is to obtain a careful medical history. Your doctor or health care provider will ask questions about your situation. If you can't communicate, a family member or friend will be asked to provide this information. Your doctor will ask about the symptoms you are having now and have had in the past, previous medical problems or operations, and any illnesses which run in your family. Be sure to bring a current list of all the medicines you take (prescription and non-prescription). If your symptoms lasted only a while, your doctor might also want to talk with someone else who was with you at the time.

The next step is a thorough physical examination. Your doctor will check your pulse and blood pressure and examine the rest of your body (heart, lungs, etc.). The neurologic examination includes detailed tests of your muscles and nerves. The doctor will check your strength, sensation, coordination, and reflexes. In addition, you will be asked questions to check your memory, speech, and thinking.

Depending on the results of your evaluation, your doctor may need additional tests to fully understand your problem.

You may also be referred to a medical specialist in brain disorders (neurologist), brain surgery (neurosurgery), or another area.

Be patient. Sometimes it takes a while to discover the cause of stroke symptoms, and sometimes the cause of a stroke cannot be determined.

Be sure to discuss any questions or concerns with your doctor or health care provider.

Section 32.2

Blood Tests and Procedures Used for Stroke Diagnosis

If you are being evaluated for stroke, it is likely that your doctor will order some blood tests. Stroke cannot be diagnosed by a blood test alone. However, these tests can provide information about stroke risk factors and other medical problems which may be important.

Please note that the first set of tests are commonly used for routine or emergency evaluation of stroke, while the others are used only in very specific situations. Unless otherwise noted, each of these tests require just one tube of blood (a few teaspoons) drawn from a vein.

Commonly Used Blood Tests

CBC (Complete blood count). This is a routine test to determine the number of red blood cells, white blood cells, and platelets in your blood. Hematocrit and hemoglobin are measures of the number of red blood cells. A complete blood count might be used to diagnose anemia (too little blood) or infection (shown by too many white blood cells).

Coagulation tests (PT [Prothrombin time], PTT [Partial thromboplastin time], INR [International normalized ratio]). These tests measure how quickly your blood clots. An abnormality could result in excessive bleeding or excessive clotting (which is difficult to measure). If you have been prescribed a blood-thinning medicine such as warfarin (Coumadin or similar drugs), the INR is used to be sure that you receive the correct dose. It is very important that you obtain regular checks. If you are taking heparin, the PT (or a PTT) test is used to determine the correct dose.

Blood chemistry tests. These tests measure the levels of normal chemical substances in your blood. The most important test in emergency stroke evaluation is glucose (or blood sugar), because levels of blood glucose which are too high or too low can cause symptoms which may be mistaken for stroke. A fasting blood glucose is used to help in the diagnosis of diabetes, which is a risk factor for stroke. Other blood chemistry tests measure serum electrolytes, the normal ions in your blood (sodium, potassium, calcium) or check the function of your liver or kidneys.

Blood lipid tests (Cholesterol, total lipids, HDL [high-density lipoprotein], and LDL [low-density lipoprotein]). Elevated cholesterol (particularly "bad" cholesterol, or LDL) is a risk factor for heart disease and stroke. Learn more about cholesterol and cardiovascular risks from the National Institutes of Health (http://www.nhlbi.nih.gov/health/public/heart/chol/wyntk.htm).

Blood Tests for Specific Situations

This is a partial list of less common blood tests sometimes ordered for specific stroke situations, or where the cause of stroke is unclear (for example, in a young person without known stroke risk factors). Abnormal results may suggest a cause for the stroke.

- Antinuclear antibodies (ANA)
- Antiphospholipid antibodies (APL), Anticardiolipin antibodies (ACL), Lupus anticoagulant (LA)
- Blood culture
- Cardiac enzymes: Troponin, Creatine kinase (CPK, CK), LDH [lactate dehydrogenate] isoenzymes
- Coagulation factors: Antithrombin III, Protein C, Protein S; Factor VIII; activated Protein C resistance (Factor V Leiden)
- Erythrocyte sedimentation rate (ESR)

- Hemoglobin electrophoresis

- Homocysteine

- Syphilis serology (VDRL [venereal disease research laboratory], FTA [fluorescent treponemal antibody], others)

- Toxicology screen (serum or urine)

Please note that this information applies only to the use of these tests for stroke diagnosis. Be sure to discuss any questions or concerns with your doctor or health care provider.

Section 32.3

Lab Tests and Procedures Used for Stroke Diagnosis

If you have had a stroke or stroke warning signs, your doctor may need additional information to fully understand your problem or plan the best treatment. In addition to blood tests, you may need to schedule special tests or procedures to examine your brain, heart, or blood vessels.

Here are the tests doctors use most often in stroke diagnosis.

Tests That View the Brain, Skull or Spinal Cord

CT scan (CAT Scan, Computed axial tomography). CT scan uses x-rays to produce a 3-dimensional image of your head. A CT scan can be used to diagnose ischemic stroke, hemorrhagic stroke, and other problems of the brain and brainstem.

MRI scan (Magnetic resonance imaging, MR). MR uses magnetic fields to produce a 3-dimensional image of your head. The MR scan shows the brain and spinal cord in more detail than CT. MR can be

295

used to diagnose ischemic stroke, hemorrhagic stroke, and other problems involving the brain, brainstem, and spinal cord.

Tests That View the Blood Vessels That Supply the Brain

Carotid Doppler (Carotid duplex, Carotid ultrasound). Painless ultrasound waves are used to take a picture of the carotid arteries in your neck, and to show the blood flowing to your brain. This test can show if your carotid artery is narrowed by arteriosclerosis (cholesterol deposition).

Transcranial Doppler (TCD). Ultrasound waves are used to measure blood flow in some of the arteries in your brain.

MRA (Magnetic resonance angiogram). This is a special type of MRI scan which can be used to see the blood vessels in your neck or brain.

Cerebral arteriogram (Cerebral angiogram, Digital subtraction angiography [DSA]). A catheter is inserted in an artery in your arm or leg, and a special dye is injected into the blood vessels leading to your brain. X-ray images show any abnormalities of the blood vessels, including narrowing, blockage, or malformations (such as aneurysms or arteriovenous malformations). Cerebral arteriogram is a more difficult test than carotid Doppler or MRA, but the results are the most accurate.

Tests That View the Heart or Check Its Function

Electrocardiogram (EKG, ECG). This is a standard test to show the pattern of electrical activity in your heart. Three to 10 electrical leads are attached to your chest, arms, and legs. Sometimes the EKG is recorded continuously over days, with the signals sent to a portable recorder (Holter monitor) or by radio to a hospital monitoring station (telemetry).

Echocardiogram (2-d echo, Cardiac echo, TTE, TEE). Painless ultrasound waves are used to take a picture of your heart and the circulating blood. The ultrasound probe may be placed on your chest (trans-thoracic echocardiogram, TTE) or deep in your throat (trans-esophageal echocardiogram, TEE).

Routine Screening Tests

Chest x-ray (CXR). An x-ray of the heart and lungs is a standard test for patients with acute medical problems. Abnormalities may alert your doctor to important problems such as pneumonia or heart failure.

Urinalysis (UA). A urine sample is often obtained to screen for bladder infection or kidney problems. If infection is suggested, a urine culture test may be required.

Pulse oximetry (Blood oxygen). This painless test is sometimes done in the emergency room or hospital to determine if your blood is receiving enough oxygen from the lungs. A small probe with a red light is usually attached to one finger.

Other Neurologic Tests

Electroencephalogram (EEG). The EEG measures your brain waves through several electrical leads painlessly attached to your head. EEG is not routinely used for stroke diagnosis, but would be ordered if your doctor thinks that you may have had a seizure.

Lumbar puncture (LP, spinal tap). A needle is inserted in your lower back to obtain a sample of the fluid (cerebrospinal fluid, CSF) which surrounds your brain and spinal cord. LP is not routinely used for diagnosis of ischemic stroke. However, LP is often required if subarachnoid hemorrhage (bleeding from a cerebral aneurysm) is suspected. LP may also be needed if your doctor suspects a nervous system infection (such as meningitis) or inflammation.

Electromyogram/Nerve conduction test (EMG/NCV). This test records the electrical activity of the nerves and muscles. EMG is not used for stroke diagnosis, but might be needed if your doctor suspects a problem with the nerves in your arms or legs.

Brain biopsy. This is a surgical procedure in which a small piece of the brain is removed for microscopic examination. Biopsy is used to diagnose lesions (such as tumors) which cannot be identified by CT or MRI scan. It is very rarely used for stroke diagnosis, when cerebral vasculitis is suspected.

Section 32.4

Brain Imaging May Identify High-Risk Stroke Patients

From the National Institute of Neurological Disorders and Stroke (NINDS, www.ninds.nih.gov), part of the National Institutes of Health, October 7, 2004.

By using sophisticated magnetic resonance imaging (MRI) technology, researchers have been able to study early changes in the blood-brain barrier (BBB), a semi-permeable membrane that surrounds and protects the brain, to predict a stroke patient's outcome. This study showed that the patients who had disruption in the BBB were more likely to experience bleeding in the brain and have a poor clinical outcome. The researchers say this technique could help identify patients who are most likely to do the best with thrombolytic therapy, and to help clinicians offer additional therapies to those who might suffer complications.

The only Food and Drug Administration approved treatment for acute stroke is a "clot-busting" drug called tPA, which helps to restore blood flow in the brain. This "reperfusion" of the brain can sometimes result in too much blood flow and cause hemorrhagic bleeds. tPA is given to patients with the most common type of stroke, ischemic, which is caused by a clot in the brain, and must be given to the patient within 3 hours of the onset of symptoms.

The standard imaging tool for stroke assessment is a computed tomography (CT) scan. MRI scans, which are also used in the study of stroke, provide more information than CT about brain blood flow, water movement, and chemical abnormalities. For this study, Steven Warach, M.D., Ph.D., and his team at the National Institute of Neurological Disorders and Stroke (NINDS), looked at MRI scans of the brains of 144 patients who had suffered an ischemic stroke and had the MRI within 24 hours after their stroke. The majority of patients received their MRI within 6 hours of the onset of the stroke. The patients were seen between June 2000 and March 2002 at the National Institutes of Health Stroke Center at Suburban Hospital in Bethesda, Maryland, home to the NIH Stroke Team. The study appears in the October [2004] issue of the *Annals of Neurology*.[1]

The research team tested a hypothesis, based on animal studies, that there was a connection between disruption of the BBB and subsequent bleeding in the brain. Patients received injections of a paramagnetic contrast agent which allowed the researchers to visualize a leak in the BBB as a bright enhancement in the MRI scans. The contrast agent does not cross an intact BBB, so when the researchers observed image enhancement on the scan, they knew that a part of the BBB was no longer intact.

The study authors found BBB disruption in 47, or 33 percent of the 144 patients in the study. They also found hemorrhages in 22 patients, or 72 percent, of those who had early BBB disruption. Thrombolytic therapy had been given to 38 of the 144 patients. Fifteen of the tPA-treated patients showed evidence of early BBB disruption on the MRI. Eight of the nine tPA treated patients who bled had BBB disruption. However, the results showed a link between BBB disruption and poor clinical outcome, independent of whether patients had treatment with tPA, successful reperfusion, or bleeding. In addition to leaking in the BBB, another strong indicator of poor outcome was the patient's score on the NIH Stroke Scale, a clinical tool that allows doctors to evaluate the severity of a stroke. If the stroke was severe, and the BBB was disrupted early, the doctors found that the patient was more likely to suffer subsequent hemorrhage.

"Using this simple tool may help us broaden the arsenal of weapons we have to fight stroke, as well as the time we have to do so," said Dr. Warach. "Watching for these significant changes in the brain may help us target which patients may need additional therapies to fight the complications of the thrombolytic therapies and ultimately improve outcomes for all stroke patients."

The researchers do not know precisely at what time the BBB disruption occurred, because they could not see the contrast agent until a second, follow-up MRI was done. Therefore, the researchers could only estimate that on average the opening of the BBB occurred at 3.8 hours after the onset of the stroke, which is beyond the targeted 3-hour window of opportunity for tPA treatment. But the researchers are now exploring ways to have the contrast agent administered earlier, and to look for markers on the MRI that could help them identify which patients are at the highest risk of bleeding. Since this study was done, they have learned that they can detect BBB disruption as early as 15 minutes after the contrast agent is injected. They also say this finding may identify which patients would benefit from so-called adjunctive therapies that are given in combination with tPA, to prevent reduce the risk of bleeding. Preliminary studies are now looking at these possibilities.

The NINDS is a component of the National Institutes of Health within the Department of Health and Human Services and is the nation's primary supporter of biomedical research on the brain and nervous system.

1. Early blood-brain barrier disruption in human focal brain ischemia," Latour L, Kang D-W, Ezzeddine M, Chalela J, Warach S. *Annals of Neurology,* Vol. 56, pp. 468–477.

Chapter 33

Treating Stroke: The Importance of Rapid Action

Chapter Contents

Section 33.1

Early Treatment Confirmed as Key to Stroke Recovery

Excerpted from a press release by the National Institute of
Neurological Disorders and Stroke (NINDS, www.ninds.nih.gov),
part of the National Institutes of Health, March 4, 2004.

A study in the March 6, 2004, issue of *The Lancet*[1] confirms the
benefits of getting stroke patients to the hospital quickly for rapid
thrombolytic treatment. The study provides the results of an extensive analysis of more than 2,700 stroke patients in six controlled clinical trials who were randomized for treatment with thrombolytic tPA
or a placebo.

While physicians have known since a breakthrough study in 1995
that early treatment with thrombolytics can improve a stroke patient's
chance of a full recovery, only an estimated 2 to 5 percent of all eligible acute stroke patients in the United States are being treated with
thrombolytics.

Stroke patients who were treated within 90 minutes of the onset
of their symptoms showed the most improvement. The study suggests
that tPA given up to 4 hours after the onset of symptoms may be of
benefit, but the authors caution that as time goes on there is a diminishing effect of treatment, and there is estimated to be almost no
benefit when treatment is at 6 hours.

"Once again we learn that time is brain," said John R. Marler, M.D.,
one of the study authors and associate director for clinical trials at
the National Institute of Neurological Disorders and Stroke (NINDS),
a part of the National Institutes of Health (NIH). "Although rapid
stroke treatment presents a great challenge to physicians and may
require substantial change in many health care systems, we now have
stronger evidence that rapid early treatment offers the best chance
of recovery for acute ischemic stroke patients."

Thrombolytics work as "clot busters," breaking up the clot that
appears in the brain during an ischemic stroke, and allowing blood
to flow freely again in the occluded or blocked artery. Patients must

have computerized tomography (CT) scans of the brain taken before treatment begins to confirm that the stroke is caused by a clot. Seventy-five percent of patients who were treated within 60 minutes of stroke onset had the best chance of having a complete or partial reopening of the occluded artery.

Another significant finding reported by the authors is that severe stroke patients tend to present to the hospital earlier than patients with milder strokes, and those who were treated had much better recoveries than patients who were given a placebo. This means that the greatest effect of early treatment was seen in the group with the most to gain in terms of reducing long-term disability.

"This study confirms that door-to-needle time is just as critical in stroke as it is in heart attack. We need to work on breaking down the current barriers to rapid stroke treatment," said Story C. Landis, Ph.D., NINDS director.

The pooled data from the trials—two of which were sponsored by pharmaceutical companies and one that was by the NIH—represent the work of 16 teams of researchers and several statisticians around the world. "This scientific work is a good example of a cooperative effort between the federal government and the pharmaceutical industry," said NIH Director Elias A. Zerhouni, M.D. "By sharing these important data, the scientists have advanced our understanding of stroke treatment, which we hope will lead to significant improvements in treating this major disease."

In 1995, the NINDS tPA Study Group published the results of two randomized clinical trials with more than 600 patients that showed a clear benefit of tPA in stroke patients treated within 3 hours of onset and a diminishing effect for patients treated later than that. [The U.S. Food and Drug Administration (FDA) approved tPA as a treatment for acute stroke in June of 1996, with the restriction that treatment begin within 3 hours of the stroke onset.]

Two other groups have conducted large randomized trials of tPA for stroke, using longer windows of treatment. The European Cooperative Acute Stroke Study (ECASS) conducted two trials using a 6-hour window and the Alteplase ThromboLysis for Acute Noninterventional Therapy in Ischemic Stroke (ATLANTIS) investigators conducted two trials with treatment windows of 5 and 6 hours each. The investigators from the three studies collaborated to test the hypothesis that pooling their patient data would show the importance of time to treatment, and their results appear in *The Lancet*.

To measure favorable outcome at 3 months, investigators used various neurological scales to measure poststroke disability. They also looked at the occurrence of hemorrhage, the primary risk of tPA use. The final analysis included 2,775 patients treated at 300 hospitals from 18 countries. The median age was 68 years and the median time of "onset to treatment" was 243 minutes. Substantial intracerebral hemorrhage occurred in 5.9% of the treated patients as compared to 1.1% of placebo patients.

Although the data in *The Lancet* paper suggest that the beneficial effect of tPA may extend beyond 3 hours (from 181 to 270 minutes), the authors caution that large prospective randomized trials would be required to confirm this finding and that this does not justify any delays in treatment. The ATLANTIS trial enrolled 79% of patients in the 4–5 hour window and failed to demonstrate efficacy.

"The most appropriate interval for beginning thrombolytic treatment remains to be clarified," the authors write in *The Lancet*; however they urge those in the health care system, from paramedics to physicians, to set a target of 1 hour after arrival in the emergency room to begin intravenous thrombolytic treatment for patients with acute ischemic stroke.

The ATLANTIS trial was funded by Genentech, Inc., the makers of tPA. The ECASS trial was funded by Boehringer Ingelheim Pharmaceuticals, which markets tPA in Europe. The NINDS trials were funded by the NIH. Genentech provided the study drug and additional study monitoring as required by the FDA.

The NINDS is a component of the National Institutes of Health within the Department of Health and Human Services and is the nation's primary supporter of biomedical research on the brain and nervous system.

1. Association of outcome with early stroke treatment: pooled analysis of ATLANTIS, ECASS, and NINDS rtPA stroke trials." Authors: The ATLANTIS, ECASS and NINDS r-tPA Study Group Investigators. *The Lancet*, March 6, 2004, Vol. 363, pp. 768–774.

Section 33.2

Understanding the Enzyme Contributing to Stroke Damage

From "Double-Agent MMP-9: Timing Is Everything in Stroke Treatment," by the National Institute of Neurological Disorders and Stroke (NINDS, www.ninds.nih.gov), part of the National Institutes of Health, August 3, 2006.

In a surprise twist, researchers have learned that a type of enzyme that contributes to brain damage immediately after a stroke also plays a role in brain remodeling and movement of neurons days after stroke. Understanding the secondary role for this enzyme in healing stroke damage may lead to new treatments for stroke and offer a longer window of time for treatment.

Previous studies have shown that enzymes called matrix metalloproteinases (MMPs) contribute to stroke damage by chewing up and degrading the supporting material between the cells, called the cellular matrix. This can result in bleeding or cell death. Now, Eng Lo, Ph.D., and colleagues from the departments of radiology and neurology at Massachusetts General Hospital and the Harvard Medical School show that, days after a stroke, one of the MMPs, called MMP-9, moves into the stroke-affected area and helps repair damaged tissue. This new finding suggests that MMP-9 may be a double agent, meaning the same enzyme may cause good or bad results in the brain.

The study results were reported in *The Journal of Neuroscience* and *Nature Medicine*. Both studies were funded in part by the National Institute of Neurological Disorders and Stroke (NINDS).

MMP-9 is an enzyme which naturally exists in the brain. Currently tPA (tissue Plasminogen Activator), the only FDA [U.S. Food and Drug Administration]-approved treatment for stroke, must be used within 3 hours of the onset of symptoms. While tPA helps to dissolve clots in blood vessels that cause strokes, it also increases levels of MMP-9, which can cause bleeding complications. MMP inhibitors seem to supplement the positive effects of tPA, and this has prompted researchers to propose that these drugs would be good candidates for stroke treatment. However, Dr. Lo's research shows that inhibition of

MMPs during the later time period after stroke actually hinders brain repair and may paradoxically increase the risk of bleeding in the brain.

"We need to think about the role of MMP-9 in stroke and its treatments as having two phases—an acute phase, which is damage producing, and a later phase, which helps with repair," says Dr. Lo. "Treatments that affect MMP-9 will have different consequences depending on when they are given."

"Early on in the developing brain, MMPs have a role to play in structuring and modeling. We have assumed that this beneficial role didn't reoccur in the mature brain. However, we now know that the brain's plasticity allows this initial remodeling to happen again," says Dr. Lo.

Both studies used rodent models of stroke to examine the role of MMP-9 after brain injury. After stroke, neuroblasts (cells from which nerve tissue is formed) swerve away from their designated path and move toward damaged areas. This cellular migration requires help from special enzymes. *The Journal of Neuroscience* study shows that the migration of these cells through the tangle of damaged brain tissue uses MMPs. Researchers injected markers into the mouse brain to monitor the movement of the cells and examined their final location 14 days after the stroke. MMP-9 co-localized with these markers of neuroblast migration, and inhibiting MMP stopped the movement of these neurons to the damaged site. This is the first study to show that MMPs are required for neuroblast migration as the brain attempts to heal itself.

In the *Nature Medicine* study, Dr. Lo and his colleagues examined the action of MMPs with respect to timing after stroke damage. In rats, an MMP inhibitor was administered at different times after an induced stroke. When the injection was given immediately following the stroke, rats showed smaller areas of brain damage. Injections given at 3 days had no effect, while blocking MMPs at 7 days or 14 days led to more extensive brain damage in the treated rats. These findings highlight the time-dependent nature of MMP activity. Delayed inhibition of MMPs after a stroke seems to have negative effects, while early inhibition of MMPs may help protect the brain.

The scientists also examined the role MMPs play in remodeling within the brains of rats following stroke. Researchers located the enzymes in the damaged areas of the brain at 1 and 3 days after the stroke. However, 7 to 14 days after the stroke, high levels of MMPs were found instead in the region surrounding the initial damage, called the peri-infarct cortex. The peri-infarct cortex is the location where newly born immature neurons migrate and where axons sprout new connections after a stroke. The reorganization in the peri-infarct area is correlated with functional recovery after stroke. The increased presence of MMPs in this area suggests that it has a beneficial role in remodeling after brain injury.

"We need to think carefully about the use of MMP inhibitors after stroke and about their possible effects. Our current research shows that the brain is actively trying to heal itself after stroke," says Dr. Lo. "This dynamic state of remodeling in the brain signals us to not give up hope after the initial stroke event and to recognize that the therapeutic window may be longer than we assumed."

Previous studies have shown that MMPs contribute to blood vessel growth, as well as proliferation, differentiation, and movement of cells. These diverse and important functions may explain the paradoxical positive and negative effects of MMPs. Future studies in Dr. Lo's lab will examine the effects of low-dose and slow-release treatments with MMP-9 and MMP inhibitors. Dr. Lo hypothesizes that to achieve the biggest impact on stroke therapies, scientists must take into account the timing and specific brain area placement of MMP activity.

"It is a powerful lesson to learn that the same molecule can do very different things. Learning how to manipulate the system will be the key to developing improved treatments," say Dr. Lo. "Combination therapy using tPA and short-term inhibitor MMPs would be invaluable for targeting acute treatment, while some way of modulating MMPs or controlling neurovascular proteolysis days later may provide a new approach for poststroke therapy and could extend the narrow treatment time that we currently race against."

1. Lee S-R, Kim H-Y, Rogowska J, Zhao B-Q, Bhide P, Parent JM, and Lo EH. "Involvement of Matrix Metalloproteinase in Neuroblast Cell Migration from the Subventricular Zone after Stroke." *The Journal of Neuroscience,* March 29, 2006, Vol. 26, pp. 3491–3495.

2. Zhao B-Q, Wang S, Kim H-Y, Storrie H, Rosen BR, Mooney DJ, Wang X, and Lo, EH. "Role of Matrix Metalloproteinases in Delayed Cortical Responses after Stroke." *Nature Medicine,* April 2006, Vol. 12, pp. 441–445.

Chapter 34

Medicare Changes Allow Hospitals to Adopt New Stroke Treatment Protocols

Neurologists have a saying about stroke patients: "Time lost is brain lost." During an all-too-brief period of only one to three hours after the onset of stroke symptoms, aggressive and appropriate treatments can spare patients' more extensive brain damage and disability.

But for many patients, that window slams shut without intervention. Studies have found, for example, that less than 5% of ischemic stroke patients receive tissue-plasminogen activator (tPA), a powerful thrombolytic approved for treating acute ischemic stroke. And in North Carolina—the heart of the so-called "stroke belt"—a 2003 study found that entire regions of the state lacked either a basic or advanced stroke prevention and treatment center.

That's not unique to North Carolina, said neurologist James C. Grotta, M.D., director of the stroke program at the University of Texas Medical School at Houston. "The percentage of patients treated appropriately for acute stroke in the country overall is very small," he said.

Why does stroke remain undertreated? In part, it's a problem of patient education. While patients have been taught to recognize the signs of a heart attack, they're less aware of what a stroke feels like, so don't quickly get medical help.

Undertreatment is also due to hospital and emergency services limitations. Medicare reimbursement has historically been low for stroke care—a factor that may be turning around with new Medicare tPA coverage that took effect last month.

But money is not the only issue. Many emergency physicians and hospital-based internists, who are often the physicians who first see stroke patients, are uncomfortable administering tPA because of the drug's potentially deadly downside of increasing hemorrhage risk. And according to Dr. Grotta, "You can finish an emergency medicine or internal medicine residency without having had any exposure to neurology and without ever having taken care of a stroke patient."

That may be changing. More hospitals are developing protocols that target the use of appropriate therapies and create new staffing and communication models. And a growing trend to certify designated hospitals as stroke centers is another factor working to improve the speed and effectiveness of stroke care.

Reimbursement and Certification

Although tPA was first approved in 1996, Medicare didn't change its reimbursement policies for stroke treatment until last month. Hospitals that administer the thrombolytic therapy will receive a base rate of about $6,000 more per stroke case—approximately double the previous reimbursement.

"Before, there was no way to break even on a patient treated with tPA and hospitals ended up losing money," said neurologist Larry B. Goldstein, M.D., director of the stroke program at Duke University Medical Center in Durham, N.C., and chair of the stroke council of the American Stroke Association (ASA).

Recommendations for administering tPA are showing up in stroke protocols being increasingly adopted by hospitals. Many protocols are based on recommendations published in 1996 by the ASA, the American Academy of Neurology and the Brain Attack Coalition, a coalition of stroke experts that includes the National Institute of Neurological Disorders and Stroke (NINDS).

Those recommendations are also being used in a new primary stroke center certification program established by the Joint Commission on Accreditation of Healthcare Organizations last year. The program has already certified more than 150 primary stroke centers in 30 states, while states—including New York and Massachusetts—are likewise moving to create designated stroke centers. (See "More Hospitals Get Stroke Center Designation.")

tPA: Raising the Comfort Level

A central element of acute stroke care, tPA poses significant challenges. The use of tPA increases the chance of converting an ischemic stroke to a bleeding stroke tenfold (from 0.6% to 6%), even when patients with contraindications are excluded. To offer tPA, a hospital must have expert consults and imaging—usually CT [computed tomography] scanning—available around the clock to rule out hemorrhagic stroke and other contraindications.

Even with such resources, some emergency physicians remain wary of the drug. "I'm concerned that public expectation is going to be that this has become the standard of care, and it's not," said J. Brian Hancock, M.D., immediate past president of the American College of Emergency Physicians and regional vice president of Ohio's Sterling Healthcare, a clinical staffing company that places emergency physicians and intensivists. "It remains controversial in the medical and scientific literature, and I'm concerned the system isn't in place to support widespread use of tPA."

Claiborne Johnston, M.D., Ph.D., director of the stroke service at the University of California, San Francisco, acknowledged these concerns. Typically, he said, two trials are needed to demonstrate a new agent's effectiveness. However, tPA was approved based on only one trial: the NINDS study, with findings published in the Dec. 14, 1995, issue of *New England Journal of Medicine*.

"That trial demonstrated a very powerful treatment effect," he said. "Findings from European studies are very consistent when you look at the same time range of treatment." A post hoc analysis of the NINDS trial data published in the April 2005 issue of *Annals of Emergency Medicine* confirmed the earlier findings.

At Valley Medical Center in Renton, Wash., stroke protocols adopted over the past year have changed how tPA is administered—and boosted physicians' comfort level with the therapy. "The decision to treat or not to treat with tPA is completely in the ER," explained Lawrence Dell Isola, M.D., Valley Medical's chief hospitalist and a member of the committee that drafted the new protocols. "As hospitalists, we don't actually get called until that treatment decision has been made." (See "Stroke Protocol Resources.")

The new protocols spell out the diagnostic sequence in which the drug is used. Suspected stroke patients receive a CT scan within 30 minutes of arrival, looking for an intercranial bleed or other tPA contraindications. Most Valley Medical stroke patients also receive a CT angiogram to fine-tune diagnosis.

"A thrombotic stroke doesn't appear on a CT for a couple of days, so usually a diagnosis of stroke is made on physical examination and presenting symptoms," Dr. Dell Isola said. "With the CT angiogram, we can see the thrombus." (According to Dr. Goldstein, CT angiography is not a necessary part of standard tPA treatment recommendations as the test shows only clots in relatively large cerebral arteries.)

In cases of middle cerebral artery or internal carotid artery thrombus, Dr. Dell Isola added, neurosurgeons may be called in to deliver tPA intra-arterially.

"Injecting the drug right into the artery involves much less systemic risk and more effectiveness," he said. "This can be done outside the usual three-hour time frame for tPA, if an interventional neurologist is available." He made it clear, however, that intra-arterial tPA is used only for patients who aren't candidates for intravenous tPA—and only after an appropriate discussion of risks and benefits.

Beyond tPA

New care models aren't just about tPA, explained the ASA's Dr. Goldstein. "Many other components of the stroke center protocol should lead to improved patient outcomes, whether [patients] receive tPA or not," he said.

At Valley Medical, for instance, other stroke protocol components address blood pressure management, as well as tight glucose control and the use of angiotensin-converting enzyme inhibitors, aspirin, and statins.

"Blood pressure management for stroke patients is tricky, because you can cause damage either way," said Dr. Dell Isola. "You don't want to let their blood pressure get too high, but if you bring down their blood pressure too rapidly, you can increase the size of the stroke."

Prior to the new protocols being adopted, he said, caring for stroke patients was frustrating. "You would have people who didn't do anything about blood pressure," he explained. "tPA would be administered based on who happened to be on call. Nothing was formalized, but now we have a rational plan for what we're doing and that makes an enormous difference."

Protocols being adopted also include:

- **Creating an acute care stroke team.** A team does not have to be led by a neurologist or neurosurgeon, but should include personnel with expertise in cerebrovascular disease. At a minimum, a stroke team should include a physician and another health care professional—a nurse, physician assistant, or nurse practitioner—who can be available around the clock. A team member should be at the patient's bedside within 15 minutes of being called.

- **Establishing written care protocols.** These should include protocols for the emergency care of patients with ischemic and hemorrhagic stroke, including stabilization of vital functions; initial diagnostic testing, including 24-hour CT scanning and lab service availability; and use of medications, including but not limited to tPA. Studies have shown that clear protocols reduce tPA-related complications and improve stroke care in general.

- **Directing emergency medical services (EMS).** Hospital staff should be able to communicate effectively with EMS personnel while they're transporting a stroke patient—and should have written plans and cooperative educational activities in place.

- **Creating a stroke unit.** European studies show that patients cared for in multidisciplinary stroke units that include rehabilitative services have a 17% lower death rate and a 7% increase in being able to live at home compared to those treated on general wards. Stroke units do not have to be distinct wards but should include expert staff and written care protocols.

- **Offering neurosurgical services.** Not all hospitals have on-site access to a neurosurgeon. But hospitals treating stroke patients should be able to get neurosurgical care for these patients within two hours—either by transfer to another facility or through an on-call neurosurgeon.

Increasing Patient Awareness

Then there's the X factor: the patient. State-of-the-art protocols will be less effective if people don't dial 911 at the first sign of a stroke.

Dr. Johnston led a study that examined tPA treatment in the San Francisco metropolitan area and found that, much like the national average, only between 4% and 5% of patients got the drug. The researchers then modeled what would happen if tPA candidates who arrived within three hours of the onset of symptoms all received it—and found that treatment rates would go up to only 8%.

"But if everyone called 911 at the moment they had a stroke symptom and was taken to a stroke center, treatment rates would rise to about 50%," said Dr. Grotta. How to make that happen, he said, is the million-dollar question, particularly when public education efforts on stroke awareness haven't to date had much effect.

Meanwhile, Dr. Goldstein said that new interventions on the horizon—including new thrombolytic drugs, endovascular and experimental intra-arterial approaches—make the stroke center concept an idea whose time has come.

"Stroke isn't what it was a decade ago," he said. "Before, we had nothing that had proven efficacy to manage patients with acute stroke." He pointed out, however, that "it does no good to have these new options if you don't have systems in place to be able to implement them safely."

Stroke Protocol Resources

The Brain Attack Coalition's web site offers practical tools to help hospitals establish guidelines for stroke care, including sample physician checklists, standing order sheets, and step-by-step clinical pathways. More information is at www.stroke-site.org.

More Hospitals Get Stroke Center Designation

According to the Joint Commission on Accreditation of Healthcare Organizations (JCAHO), a major step forward in providing stroke care is designating certain hospitals as stroke centers.

More and more states seem to agree, with New York, Massachusetts, and Florida establishing state stroke-center programs. Emergency responders in those states are required to take stroke patients directly to a state-designated stroke service.

This year, Texas passed legislation establishing a mechanism for identifying regional stroke centers. And "Colorado is also moving in this direction," said neurologist Larry B. Goldstein, M.D., chair of the American Stroke Association's stroke council.

Although more stroke centers—both JCAHO-designated and others—are being created, gaps in care still remain. Some experts advocate regional stroke care systems much like the trauma networks that have been set up for victims of violence and accidents.

At the same time, the stroke center model is meeting some resistance. Richard Stennes, M.D., a past president of the American College of Emergency Physicians (ACEP), told the Sept. 21, 2005, *San Diego Union-Tribune* that for every patient who did have a stroke, paramedics might divert as many as 10 patients with migraines, seizures, metabolic problems, drug reactions, or hypoglycemia—all conditions with symptoms that can mimic stroke—to stroke center hospitals unnecessarily.

"To the extent that stroke centers help emergency physicians do what needs to be done as part of an overall system approach, that's something we can support," said J. Brian Hancock, M.D., ACEP's immediate past president. "But if it's confusing to the public, or if it causes delays in care because people drive further than they should to get to a stroke center, then that could be a problem." According to Dr. Hancock, not every patient who has a stroke needs to go to a stroke center—"and I don't think every hospital needs to be a stroke center."

The information included herein should never be used as a substitute for clinical judgment and does not represent an official position of ACP.

Gina Shaw is a freelance health care writer based in Montclair, N.J.

Chapter 35

Medications for Acute Stroke Treatment

Chapter Contents

Section 35.1

Commonly Used Stroke Medicines

"Information about Specific Medications," by Chad Mosely and Susan Fagan, University of Georgia College of Pharmacy. © 2007 Internet Stroke Center at Washington University in St. Louis. Reprinted with permission.

The medications in Table 35.1 are among the most commonly prescribed for stroke treatment and prevention. U.S. trade names are provided—these drugs may have different names in other countries.

In addition to the medications shown here, many stroke patients also receive medications to treat high blood pressure, diabetes, or high cholesterol. If you do not find the information you are seeking, you may want to visit the drug information area of Medline Plus from the National Library of Medicine.

The choice of medication for stroke depends on your individual condition. Remember: if you have questions about your medications, ask your doctor.

Table 35.1. Commonly Used Medications for Stroke Treatment and Prevention

Drug Name	Other Names	Used For	Drug Type
Aspirin	acetylsalicylic acid, ASA	Stroke prevention	Antiplatelet
Clopidogrel	Plavix®	Stroke prevention	Antiplatelet
Dipyridamole	Aggrenox®, Persantine®, others	Stroke prevention	Antiplatelet
Heparin	Calciparine®, Liquaemin®	Stroke prevention	Anticoagulant
Ticlopidine	Ticlid®	Stroke prevention	Antiplatelet
Tissue Plasminogen Activator	tPA, Activase®	Acute stroke treatment	Thrombolytic
Warfarin	Coumadin®, others	Stroke prevention	Anticoagulant

Section 35.2

Antiplatelets

"Antiplatelets," by Chad Mosely and Susan Fagan, University of Georgia College of Pharmacy. © 2007 Internet Stroke Center at Washington University in St. Louis. Reprinted with permission.

Platelets are blood cells that help the blood clot (stick together) and prevent bleeding. When the body has a cut, scratch, bruise, or bleed, platelets go into action and begin to work. They can be thought of as materials (like bricks or blocks) that aggregate (link together or stack up) to form this clot. These platelet cells need thromboxane A2 and adenosine, vitamin K specific clotting factors (chemicals produced by the body) to make them stick together. These chemicals are essentially the glue that holds the blocks together to make the clot. However, in patients who have had a TIA [transient ischemic attack] or stroke, the blocks don't need to stick together as much because this causes the blood to be too thick (like adding flour to milk when making a cake batter) and possibly form a clot that can't fit through the vessels.

Doctors often place stroke and TIA patients on blood thinners to decrease the possibility of the body forming another clot in the blood, which may lead to another stroke and TIA. Below is information on specific types of antiplatelets used for stroke prevention:

Aspirin (Acetylsalicylic Acid, ASA)

Besides relieving pain, fever, and inflammation, aspirin has many other uses. Aspirin is also used as an antiplatelet/platelet aggregation inhibitor (to keep your blood from sticking together) in patients who have had a TIA or stroke. It can also reduce the risk of having another TIA or stroke. Different doses are used for this purpose, ranging from 50 mg to 325 mg/day, depending on the patient's condition and the doctor's decision.

The idea that "if one is good for me, two or three must be better" is wrong. Do not adjust your dose without first talking to the pharmacist or doctor that dispensed or prescribed the medication. The dose is not the same for everyone. The usual dose for stroke/TIA prevention is 30–325 mg a day. Take the medication the way the doctor instructs you to. So, even though you may be taking an 81 mg (baby aspirin) a day, someone else who had a stroke may be taking 325 mg of aspirin a day or may be on a different medicine for stroke prevention. So don't rely on what you hear from other stroke patients, and don't take more or less of the drug without first talking to the doctor who prescribed it.

Since aspirin can irritate the stomach, it is best to take it with food or a full glass of water or milk to help avoid or lessen possible stomach problems.

This medication will help prevent platelets (glue like particles) from making the blood too thick, thereby risking a clot. Therefore, it will lessen your body's ability to stop bleeding when you are cut, scratched, or bruised. Your doctor wants the aspirin to thin the blood (decrease the body's ability to form a clot) just enough to help prevent a future TIA or stroke. Watch for blood in the urine, stools, or around the gums when eating and brushing teeth; bleeding from the nose; or easy bruising. If you notice abnormal or excessive bleeding, let your pharmacist and doctor know, and talk with them before you change or take any new medicines.

Abdominal (stomach area) pain that will not go away and ringing in the ears are other signs that there might be a problem with the medication. Let the pharmacist or doctor know if you have any of these warning signs.

Talk with your pharmacist or doctor before taking any other aspirin products, anti-inflammatory agents (Aleve, Naprosyn, Ibuprofen, etc.) or any other medications.

Clopidogrel (Plavix®)

Clopidogrel (Plavix®) is an antiplatelet/platelet aggregation inhibitor drug that is used to help prevent another stroke. It does this by decreasing the blood's ability to clot (clump together). This means that when you get a cut or scratch it will take a little longer to stop bleeding. Watch for blood in the urine, blood in the stools, bleeding around the gums when eating and brushing teeth, bleeding from the nose, or bruising easily. If you notice abnormal or excessive bleeding, let your pharmacist and doctor know, and talk with them before you change or take any new medicines.

You will take one 75 mg tablet once a day in the morning (can be taken with or without food), or when and how your pharmacist and doctor tell you. Do not adjust the dose without first talking to the pharmacist or doctor that dispensed or prescribed the mediation, and be sure to talk with your pharmacist or doctor before taking any other medications.

Dipyridamole (Aggrenox®, Persantine®, and Others)

Aggrenox is the combination of, aspirin (25 mg) and extended release dipyridamole (200 mg), two antiplatelet/platelet aggregation inhibitors. Each of these medications work together in a similar way (but on separate chemicals in the blood) to help prevent a future TIA or stroke. Do not adjust the dose without first talking to the pharmacist or doctor that dispensed or prescribed the medication. The aspirin portion of the combination works in the same way as above, but the dipyridamole helps prevent platelets, blood cells, and the vessels from using adenosine (another chemical that helps the bricks and glue form a clot). Dipyridamole also has the potential to vasodilate the vessels that carry the blood to allow a more blood and particles to flow through (like a water hose expanding in the summer sun).

The combination capsule Aggrenox® (aspirin and dipyridamole) cannot be substituted by taking each drug separately. Taking the two separately does not have the desired effect as the combination capsule does.

Take one capsule in the morning (with or without food) and take one capsule in the evening (with or without food) for a total of two capsules a day. Swallow the capsule. Do not chew it or crush it. It must be swallowed whole. Take the medication the way the pharmacist and doctor told you.

Many patients starting on Aggrenox® develop a severe headache due to the vessels in the brain vasodilating (expanding). This headache tends to decrease and go away as the body gets used to the medicine. In the meantime use an over-the-counter pain reliever and call the pharmacist or doctor to inform them of the headache.

The combination of aspirin and dipyridamole is a stronger blood thinner than either drug alone. So, watch for blood in the urine, blood in the stools, bleeding around the gums when eating and brushing teeth, bleeding from the nose, or bruising easily. If you notice abnormal or excessive bleeding, let your pharmacist and doctor know, and talk with them before you change or take any new medicines.

Talk with your pharmacist or doctor before taking any other aspirin products, anti-inflammatory agents (Aleve, Naprosyn, Ibuprofen, etc.) or any other medications.

Ticlopidine (Ticlid®)

Ticlid® is used to help prevent another stroke. You will take a 250 mg tablet two times a day (one in the morning and one in the evening) with food. Take the medicines like the pharmacist and doctor told you, and do not adjust the dose without first talking to the pharmacist or doctor that dispensed or prescribed the medications. Be especially observant of any excessive bleeding such as blood in the urine, blood in the stools, bleeding around the gums when eating and brushing teeth, bleeding from the nose, or bruising easily. If you notice abnormal or excessive bleeding, let your pharmacist and doctor know, and talk with them before you change or take any new medicines.

You will have to have lab work done every two weeks for the first three months of treatment to check your blood levels. Talk with your pharmacist or doctor before taking any other aspirin products, anti-inflammatory agents (Aleve, Naprosyn, Ibuprofen, etc.) or any other medications.

Section 35.3

Anticoagulants

"Anticoagulants," by Chad Mosely and Susan Fagan, University of Georgia College of Pharmacy. © 2007 Internet Stroke Center at Washington University in St. Louis. Reprinted with permission.

Anticoagulants are a class of drugs commonly used to prevent the blood from forming dangerous clots that could result in a stroke. Often called "blood thinners," anticoagulants are often the first medication prescribed by doctors following a stroke. By reducing the ability of the blood to clot—and thereby reducing the likelihood of coronary or vascular emboli—anticoagulants are frequently used in patients that are already at high-risk for stroke. Below is information on specific types of anticoagulants used for stroke prevention:

Heparin

Heparin is an anticoagulant drug ("blood thinner"). It can be given intravenously or subcutaneously, but not by mouth. Heparin is sometimes used to reduce acute stroke damage or stroke risk in hospitalized patients. In addition, heparin may be used in hospitalized stroke patients to reduce the risk of blood clots forming in leg veins.

322

Warfarin (Coumadin® and Others)

Warfarin is an anticoagulant drug ("blood thinner") which is taken by mouth. Daily use of warfarin can reduce the risk of stroke in certain patients. For example, many patients with atrial fibrillation (a heart irregularity) should be prescribed warfarin. Use of warfarin requires careful monitoring, and you should closely follow your doctor's recommendations, including regular blood tests. Let your doctor know if you're taking any other medications.

Your doctor will start you on a low dose of Coumadin® and will have you see him or someone else to check your blood weekly. You want your blood levels to be within a certain range (think of it as keeping your car between the yellow line on the left side of the road and the white line on the right side of the road). The doctor wants you to be right in the middle, so you will have your blood drawn and the doctor will increase or decrease your dose based on the blood values and where he or she wants you to be.

Patients receiving Coumadin® also need to be very careful about their diet and activities to prevent problems while taking the medication. The levels of the drug in the body can be affected by the amount of vitamin K in your diet. Foods high in vitamin K include: leafy green vegetables, green teas, as well as pork and beef liver. Patients should avoid large amounts of alfalfa, broccoli, asparagus, Brussels sprouts, cauliflower, cabbage, kale, spinach, watercress, lettuce, and turnip greens. You can still eat these items, but eat the same amount regularly. For example, don't eat a plateful of turnips every day for a week and then decide to stop eating them the next week. Keep relatively the same diet foods high in vitamin K. Large changes in the amount you eat can cause problems with your treatment.

Also, since Coumadin® is a fairly strong blood thinner, you have a chance of bleeding more than usual with common cut, scrapes, and falls. Use caution walking and with activities that place you at risk to fall or get hurt. Be careful while shaving, because a common cut may take longer to stop bleeding. Watch for blood in the urine, in the stools, or around the gums when eating and brushing teeth; bleeding from the nose; or bruising easily. If you notice abnormal or excessive bleeding, let your pharmacist and doctor know, and talk with them before you change or take any new medicines. Lastly, get an identification bracelet or necklace to let people, doctors, and dentist know you are taking Coumadin®.

Section 35.4

Thrombolytics

"Thrombolytics," by Chad Mosely and Susan Fagan, University of Georgia College of Pharmacy. © 2007 Internet Stroke Center at Washington University in St. Louis. Reprinted with permission.

Thrombolytic therapy is the use of drugs to break up the clot that is causing the disruption in blood flow to the brain.

It is crucial, imperative, and very important that you immediately go to the hospital when you first notice the warning signs of a stroke. The length of time between the first warning signs and the time you get to a hospital may be the difference between a good or poor outcome. Patients who present to the hospital within 3 hours of the first sign of a stroke have the possibility to receive alteplase (tPA, Activase®). Alteplase is a clot-buster. It breaks up the clot to restore blood flow to the area of the stroke.

There are many factors that determine whether or not a patient is able to receive thrombolytic therapy. One of these factors, that you have control of, is the amount of time between the onset of symptoms and presentation to the hospital. If you get to the hospital within the 3 hour time frame and the doctor determines you are able to receive this clot-buster, you may have a better recovery.

Tissue Plasminogen Activator (tPA, Activase®)

Tissue plasminogen activator is a thrombolytic drug (a "clot-buster"). It can reduce the severity of ischemic stroke if it is given within three hours of stroke onset. This drug can be given intravenously or by arterial catheter, but not by mouth.

Section 35.5

Ultrasound and Thrombolytic Therapy Work Better Than Drugs Alone

From "Ultrasound-aided Therapy Better Than Stroke Drug Alone, Trials Find," a press release by the National Institute of Neurological Disorders and Stroke (NINDS, www.ninds.nih.gov), part of the National Institutes of Health, November 17, 2004.

Using ultrasound in combination with the drug tPA can improve response to an ischemic stroke, according to a study involving 126 patients. This first-of-its-kind human trial compared the safety and efficacy of ultrasound and tPA versus use of tPA alone. The trial was funded in part by the National Institute of Neurological Disorders and Stroke (NINDS), a component of the National Institutes of Health (NIH). The finding appears in the November 18, 2004, issue of the *New England Journal of Medicine*.

Since 1996, the clot-busting drug tPA (tissue plasminogen activator) has been the only FDA-approved therapy for acute ischemic stroke. Previous studies have shown that tPA, when administered within 3 hours of onset of ischemic stroke, can greatly improve a patient's chance for a full recovery. tPA cannot be used to treat the less common hemorrhagic stroke.

Researchers wanted to test the effectiveness of using transcranial Doppler ultrasound (TCD) in combination with tPA, and to ensure that ultrasound did not cause bleeding into the brain. Ultrasound is a safe, non-invasive, FDA-approved diagnostic test that uses sound waves to measure blood flow velocity in large arteries. An international team led by Andrei Alexandrov, M.D., associate professor of neurology at the University of Texas-Houston School of Medicine, examined 126 patients who suffered an ischemic stroke. All patients received intravenous tPA within 3 hours of stroke onset. The 63 patients in the control group received tPA alone, while the other 63 patients received tPA in combination with continuous TCD monitoring that started shortly before the patients received the drug. A small device attached to a head frame was used to deliver the ultrasound.

Results showed that 49 percent of patients who received continuous ultrasound and tPA showed dramatic clinical improvement and little or no blockage within 2 hours after therapy began compared to 30 percent who received tPA alone. Notably, 38 percent of the patients who received continuous ultrasound and tPA showed no blockage within two hours, compared to 13 percent who received tPA alone. In all, 73 percent of patients who received the combined therapy showed complete or partial clearance of the clot, compared to 50 percent in the control group. Bleeding into the brain was experienced by 4.8 percent of patients in both groups. This early improvement of blood flow to the brain resulted in a trend that 13.5 percent more patients who received continuous ultrasound and tPA had recovered completely by 3 months after stroke.

The team also found that patients who experienced complete clearance of their clot within 2 hours following treatment had the greatest likelihood of regaining body strength, speech, and other functions affected by stroke. Researchers named the trial CLOTBUST (Combined Lyses Of Thrombus in Brain ischemia Using transcranial ultrasound and Systemic tPA).

"In the past 30 years, scientists around the world have shown that ultrasound is fast, gentle, and effective in helping tPA to break up clots. For the first time, we have demonstrated this benefit in patients. This approach enhances flow to the brain and augments clinical recovery within minutes of treatment initiation," said Dr. Alexandrov.

"Stroke can be devastating for patients and their caregivers," said Story C. Landis, Ph.D., NINDS director. "These initial findings suggest that patients who receive the combined therapy are able to leave the hospital with a greater chance for recovery following an ischemic stroke. This is an excellent example of improving on an existing therapy and providing better outcomes."

Ultrasound causes vibrations among the molecules on and within clot structures, which in turn creates more binding sites for tPA interaction and subsequent clot breakdown. The researchers think that this "jiggle" improves drug transport to and around the clot and helps to open more blocked vessels faster than can be expected with tPA therapy alone.

Stroke is the nation's third leading cause of death, behind heart disease and cancer. Each year about 700,000 persons in the United States have a stroke, with about 80 percent of them being ischemic strokes.

Section 35.6

Neuregulin-1 Protects Neurons from Stroke Hours after the Event

"Opening the Window of Opportunity: Neuregulin-1 Protects Neurons from Stroke Hours after the Event" is from the National Institute of Neurological Disorders and Stroke (NINDS, www.ninds.nih.gov), part of the National Institutes of Health, March 8, 2006.

Stroke is the third leading cause of death in adults in the United States. Currently, the only approved drug treatment for acute stroke must be given within 3 hours from stroke onset. A recent study shows that a naturally occurring growth factor, called neuregulin-1, can protect nerve cells and decrease inflammation in an animal model of stroke when administered as long as 13 hours after the brain attack. This is the first study to show that neuregulin-1 can have a positive effect on the outcome after stroke in animals and could lead to new drug treatments for people.

"Even though you have cells dying immediately when there is a stroke, the cells continue to die for a time after the initial event. This is one of the reasons why it is so important to go immediately to the hospital once any sign of stroke is detected," says Byron Ford, Ph.D., of the Morehouse School of Medicine Neuroscience Institute in Atlanta. "The ability of neuregulin-1 to protect and prevent further neuronal damage could result in a better recovery." The study is published in the August 31, 2005 advance online publication of the *Journal of Cerebral Blood Flow & Metabolism* and was funded in part by the National Institute of Neurological Disorders and Stroke (NINDS).

There are two main types of stroke: hemorrhagic stroke, where a blood vessel ruptures, causing blood to leak into the brain, and ischemic stroke. With ischemic stroke, which accounts for 80 percent of the cases, a blood vessel that supplies blood to the brain gets clogged. Currently tPA (tissue Plasminogen Activator) is the only FDA approved treatment for stroke and is recommended for ischemic stroke treatment within 3 hours of the onset of symptoms. After 3 hours, the potential risk of hemorrhage or excessive bleeding outweighs the benefits of the drug treatment. Dr. Ford hypothesizes that the use of neuregulin-1 may offer an extended window of opportunity for therapeutic intervention after stroke.

In the Morehouse School of Medicine study, researchers blocked the middle cerebral artery in rats to interrupt the blood supply to the brain. Similar to stroke in humans, this deprivation of blood supply and oxygen caused brain cells to die within minutes and led to inflammation of tissue surrounding the site where the blood flow was obstructed. The scientists then examined the effects of administering neuregulin-1 to rats at different time intervals after the surgically induced stroke. Dr. Ford and his colleagues discovered that immediate administration of neuregulin-1 reduced cell death by 90 percent in the rats that were treated compared with rats that did not receive the compound. It also helped to prevent nerve cell loss after longer intervals.

"Neuregulin-1 protected neurons from damage even when administered as long as 13 1/2 hours after the stroke's onset. At that point it protected 60 percent of the neurons," says Dr. Ford. "Even two weeks after a single injection of neuregulin-1 we still saw no increase in the damage. The increased time period that neuregulin-1 is able to protect neurons after stroke would be a great benefit to stroke patients."

Neuregulin-1 acts by blocking delayed neuronal death and decreasing inflammatory responses. Normally, the brain doesn't make many receptors for neuregulin-1. However, after injury and inflammation, the number of receptors tends to increase. The scientists believe that this action helps to bind neuregulin-1 to the affected areas and helps to prevent further neuronal damage. The drug administration also translated to an improved clinical outcome in the model. The neuregulin-1 treated rats demonstrated significantly fewer neurological deficits when compared to animals that were untreated.

Previously, Dr. Ford had examined the protective effects of neuregulin-1 in vitro (in cells) and when administered before an induced stroke. However, this is the first study to demonstrate that the drug is an effective treatment when used after a stroke. The use of neuregulin-1 could have clinical benefits as both a pre- and poststroke treatment.

"Neuregulin-1 has the potential to be successful where others have not," says Dr. Ford. "Neuregulin-1 has the ability to not only protect neurons by blocking cell death but also by preventing inflammation." This contrasts with tPA which works by removing blood clots and does not protect neurons.

Although none of the doses resulted in obvious side effects in the rats, the laboratory will perform additional studies to determine if the drug is appropriate for clinical trials. Future studies will further examine how neuregulin-1 works from a molecular level. Given its ability to prevent inflammation, neuregulin-1 might also be a useful treatment for chronic inflammatory diseases such as arthritis, Dr. Ford says.

Xu Z, Croslan D, Harris A, Ford G, Ford B. "Extended therapeutic window and functional recovery after intraarterial administration of neuregulin-1 after focal ischemic stroke." *Journal of Cerebral Blood Flow and Metabolism,* advance online publication, August 31, 2005.

Section 35.7

Drug Prevents Brain Swelling after Stroke

From the National Institute of Neurological Disorders and
Stroke (NINDS, www.ninds.nih.gov), part of the National Institutes
of Health, June 14, 2006.

A drug long used to treat diabetes significantly reduces brain swelling, neuron loss, and death after stroke in rats, researchers have found. The finding may lead to improved ways of treating stroke and other disorders in humans.

The drug, called glibenclamide or glyburide, appears to work by blocking channels, or pore-like structures, that open in cell membranes when the brain is deprived of oxygen. The opening of these channels allows sodium ions and water to flow into the cells, causing them to swell (a condition called edema). The flow of sodium into cells also triggers a flood of sodium and water into surrounding tissues, which increases intracranial pressure and damages cells. Current treatments for brain edema are only moderately effective, and the swelling is believed to be responsible for much of the brain damage and death that occurs in people who have severe strokes.

The study was led by J. Marc Simard, M.D., Ph.D., of the University of Maryland at Baltimore School of Medicine. It was funded in part by the National Institute of Neurological Disorders and Stroke (NINDS) and appeared in the April 2006 issue of *Nature Medicine.*

Dr. Simard and his colleagues previously discovered a new type of ion channel, called an NCCa-ATP channel, in cells called astrocytes. These channels appeared to play a role in the cellular swelling that occurs after injury. Astrocytes normally act as support cells in the brain, but if the brain is damaged, they often swell and stop functioning correctly. They are then referred to as reactive astrocytes. Dr. Simard's group found that the number of NCCa-ATP ion channels increased dramatically in reactive astrocytes from brain regions that had been deprived of oxygen (a condition called hypoxia) due to insufficient blood flow. The opening of these channels is controlled by a protein called sulfonylurea receptor 1 (SUR1). The researchers wondered if the same ion channels might play a role in ischemic strokes, which are caused by a block of normal blood flow in the brain.

In the new study, Dr. Simard and his colleagues found that levels of SUR1 increased significantly in the core of the infarct, or damaged brain area, by 2 to 3 hours after a severe middle cerebral artery stroke. The levels of SUR1 remained high for several hours, then declined as cells began to die—about 8 hours after the stroke. In the area surrounding the core of the infarct (called the peri-infarct region), levels of SUR1 increased later but stayed elevated for much longer.

The investigators then gave continuous infusions of glibenclamide, which blocks SUR1, under the skin of rats that had experienced either severe middle cerebral artery occlusion (MCAO) strokes or less severe thromboembolic strokes. Similar groups of rats were treated with a saline solution for comparison. The researchers measured the amount of edema in the rats' brains as well as the extent of the brain damage after the strokes.

The overall effect of the glibenclamide was positive. Only 24 percent of rats given the glibenclamide treatment after severe MCAO strokes died, compared to 65 percent of rats that did not receive the treatment. The glibenclamide-treated rats had much less cerebral edema 8 hours after stroke. Brain-damaged regions were much smaller in rats treated with glibenclamide than in those treated with saline after thromboembolic strokes.

The researchers found evidence that poststroke changes in tiny blood vessels (capillaries) led to a breakdown of the blood-brain barrier. This, along with an increase in SUR1 and in the acidity of areas surrounding the original brain lesion, allowed glibenclamide to selectively target the damaged areas of the brain.

"An interesting observation in this study is that the NCCa-ATP channel, which was originally found in astrocytes, is also found in endothelial cells and neurons," says Tom Jacobs, Ph.D., NINDS program director for stroke and cerebrovascular biology. "Treatment that targets this channel on different cell types affected by stroke offers a promising new way to treat edema."

While a number of treatments have been devised to try to limit brain damage after stroke, many of them have side effects that have prevented widespread use. In contrast, glibenclamide has been used safely to treat type 2 diabetes for decades, and it has few side effects other than an increased risk of low blood sugar (hypoglycemia), Dr. Simard says. However, the drug is currently available only in pill form, and people who have had a stroke or other trauma are often unable to swallow pills. Also, a continuous infusion would be needed in order to block the NCCa-ATP channels while their numbers increase in damaged regions after a stroke. A version of glibenclamide that can be administered intravenously is now being developed. This type of delivery will allow researchers to test the drug in humans following strokes or other types of trauma.

The researchers are now looking retrospectively at records of people who have had strokes while they were taking a drug similar to glibenclamide in order to determine if they developed less brain damage than people who did not take then drug. They also are investigating whether glibenclamide can prevent the weakening of capillaries that makes it dangerous to give the drug tPA (tissue plasminogen activator) to stroke patients beyond the first 3 hours following a stroke, and whether the drug can prevent hemorrhage after spinal cord injury.

1. Simard JM, Chen M, Tarasov KV, Bhatta S, Ivanova S, Melnitchenko L, Tsymbalyuk N, Wed GA, Gerzanich V. "Newly expressed SUR1-regulated NCCa-ATP channel mediates cerebral edema after ischemic stroke." *Nature Medicine,* April 2006, Vol. 12, No. 3, pp. 433–440.

Chapter 36

Stents

Chapter Contents

Section 36.1

All about Stents

From "Stents," by the National Heart, Lung, and Blood Institute
(NHLBI, www.nhlbi.nih.gov), part of the National Institutes of Health,
May 2007.

What Is a Stent?

A stent is a small mesh tube that's used to treat narrowed or weakened arteries in the body.

You may have a stent placed in an artery as part of a procedure called angioplasty. Angioplasty can restore blood flow through narrowed or blocked arteries. Stents help prevent arteries from becoming narrowed or blocked again in the months or years after treatment with angioplasty. You may also have a stent placed in a weakened artery to improve blood flow and to help prevent the artery from bursting.

Stents are usually made of metal mesh, but sometimes they're made of fabric. Fabric stents, also called stent grafts, are used in larger arteries. Some stents are coated with medicines that are slowly and continuously released into the artery. These medicines help prevent the artery from becoming blocked again.

How Are Stents Used?

Stents for Arteries in the Heart

With age and some health conditions, the inside openings of the coronary arteries (arteries of the heart) tend to narrow due to deposits of a fatty substance called plaque. High cholesterol, diabetes, and smoking can cause the arteries to narrow. This narrowing of the coronary arteries can cause angina (chest pain) or lead to heart attack.

During angioplasty, doctors use an expanding balloon inside the artery to compress the plaque and widen the passageway. The result is improved blood flow to the heart and a decreased chance of heart attack.

Unless an artery is too small, doctors usually place a stent in the treated portion of the artery during angioplasty. The stent supports the inner artery wall and reduces the chance of the artery closing up again. A stent also can keep an artery open that was torn or injured during angioplasty.

When stents are placed in coronary arteries, there's a 1 in 5 chance that the arteries will close in the first 6 months after angioplasty. When stents aren't used, the risk of the arteries closing can be twice as high.

Stents for the Carotid Arteries in the Neck

Both the right and left sides of your neck have blood vessels called carotid arteries. These arteries carry blood from the heart to the brain. Carotid arteries can become narrowed by plaque. These plaque deposits limit blood flow to the brain and increase your risk for stroke. Your chance of developing plaque in your carotid arteries increases with age, and may increase if you smoke.

A new procedure uses stents to help keep the carotid arteries fully open after they're widened with angioplasty. Not all hospitals offer this procedure. How effective it is long term is still not known. The National Institute of Neurological Disorders and Stroke supports clinical studies to explore the risks and benefits of angioplasty and stenting of carotid arteries.

Stents for Other Arteries

The arteries in the kidneys also can become narrowed. This reduces blood flow to the kidneys, which can affect their ability to control blood pressure. This can cause severe high blood pressure.

The arteries in the arms and legs also can narrow with plaque over time. This narrowing can cause pain and cramping in the affected limbs. If the narrowing is severe, it can completely cut off the blood flow to a limb, which could require surgical treatment.

To relieve these problems, doctors may perform angioplasty on the narrowed kidney, arm, or leg arteries. This procedure often is followed by placing a stent in the treated artery. The stent helps keep the artery fully open.

Stents for the Aorta in the Abdomen or Chest

The major artery coming out of the heart and supplying blood to the body is called the aorta. The aorta travels through the chest and then down into the abdomen. Over time, some areas of the walls of the aorta can become weak. These weakened areas can cause a bulge in the artery called an aneurysm.

An aorta with an aneurysm can burst, leading to potentially deadly internal bleeding. When aneurysms occur, they're usually in the part of the aorta in the abdomen. To help avoid a burst, doctors place a fabric stent in the weakened area of the abdominal aorta. The stent creates a stronger inner lining for the artery.

Aneurysms also can develop in the part of the aorta in the chest. These aneurysms also can be treated with stents. But this new use of stents is not offered by all hospitals, and how effective it is long term is still not known.

Stents to Close off Aortic Tears

Another problem that can develop in the aorta is a tear in the inside wall. Blood can be forced into this tear, causing it to widen and eventually block blood flow through the artery or burst. When this occurs, it's usually in the part of the aorta that's in the chest.

Fabric stents are being developed and used experimentally to prevent aortic dissection by stopping blood from flowing into the tear. Tears in the aorta reduce blood flow to the tissues the aorta serves. A fabric stent placed within the torn area of the artery can help restore normal blood flow and reduce the risk of a burst aorta. Stents to treat aortic tears are still being researched. Only a few hospitals offer this procedure.

How Are Stents Placed?

To place a stent, your doctor will make a small opening in a blood vessel in your groin (upper thigh), arm, or neck. Through this opening, your doctor will thread a flexible, plastic tube (catheter) with a deflated balloon on the end. A stent may be placed around the deflated balloon. The tip of the catheter is threaded up to the narrowed artery section or to the aneurysm or aortic tear site. Special x-ray "movies" are taken of the tube as it is threaded up into your blood vessel. These movies help your doctor position the catheter.

For Arteries Narrowed by Plaque

Once the tube is in the area of the artery that needs treatment:

- Your doctor uses a special dye to help see narrowed areas of the blood vessel.

- Your doctor inflates the balloon. It pushes against the plaque and compresses it against the artery wall. The fully extended balloon also expands the surrounding stent, pushing it into place in the artery.

- The balloon is deflated and taken out along with the catheter. The stent remains in your artery. Cells in your artery eventually grow to cover the mesh of the stent and create an inner layer that resembles what is normally seen inside a blood vessel.

A very narrow artery, or one that is difficult to reach with the catheter, may require more steps to place a stent. This type of artery usually is first expanded by inflating a small balloon. The balloon is then removed and replaced by another larger balloon with the collapsed stent around it. At this point, your doctor can follow the standard practice of compressing the plaque and placing the stent.

When angioplasty and stent placement are performed on carotid arteries, a special filter device is used. The filter helps keep blood clots and loose pieces of plaque from passing into the bloodstream and brain during the procedure.

For Aortic Aneurysms

Placing a stent to treat an aneurysm in an artery is slightly different than treating an artery narrowed by plaque. The stent used to treat an aneurysm is made out of pleated fabric, often with one or more tiny hooks.

Once the catheter is positioned at the aneurysm site, the stent is threaded through the tube to the area that needs treatment. Then, your doctor places a balloon inside the stent. The balloon is inflated to expand the stent and have it fit tight against the artery wall. The hooks on the stent latch on to the artery wall to anchor the stent. Your doctor then removes the balloon and catheter, leaving the fabric stent behind.

The stent creates a new inner lining for that portion of the artery. Cells in the artery eventually grow to cover the fabric and create an inner layer that resembles what's normally seen inside a blood vessel.

What to Expect before a Stent Procedure

Most stent procedures require an overnight stay in the hospital and someone to take you home. Discuss with your doctor:

- when to stop eating and drinking before coming to the hospital;

- what medicines you should or shouldn't take on the day of the procedure; and

- when to come to the hospital and where to go.

You also should let your doctor know if you have diabetes, kidney disease, or other conditions that may require taking extra steps during or after the procedure to avoid complications.

What to Expect during a Stent Procedure

For Arteries Narrowed by Plaque

This procedure usually takes a few hours.

Before the procedure starts, you will get medicine to help you relax. You will be on your back and awake during the procedure so you can follow the doctor's instructions. The area where the catheter is inserted will be numbed and you won't feel the doctor threading the catheter, balloon, or stent inside the artery. You may feel some pain when the balloon is expanded to push the stent into place.

For Aortic Aneurysms

This procedure takes a few hours. It usually requires a 2- to 3-day stay in the hospital.

Before the procedure, you will be given medicine to help you relax. If a stent is placed in the abdominal portion of the aorta, your doctor may give you a regional anesthetic. This will make you numb from the area of the stent placement down, but it will allow you to be awake during the procedure. If a stent is placed in the chest portion of the aorta, usually a general anesthetic will be used, which will make you sleep through the procedure.

Once you're numbed or asleep, your doctor will make a small cut in your groin (upper thigh). The doctor will insert a catheter into the blood vessel through this cut. Sometimes, two cuts (one above each leg) are needed to place fabric stents that come in two parts. You will not feel the doctor threading the catheter, balloon, or stent into the artery.

What to Expect after a Stent Procedure

Recovery

After either type of stent procedure (for arteries narrowed by plaque or aortic aneurysm), once the stent has been placed and the balloon and catheter have been removed, the tube insertion site will be bandaged. A small sandbag or other type of weight may be put on top of the bandage to apply pressure to help prevent bleeding. You will recover in a special care area where your movement will be limited.

While you're in recovery, a nurse will check your heart rate and blood pressure regularly. The nurse also will see if there's any bleeding from the insertion site. Eventually, a small bruise and sometimes a small, hard "knot" will appear at the insertion site. This area may feel sore or tender for about a week.

You should let your doctor know if:

- you have a constant or large amount of bleeding at the site that can't be stopped with a small bandage; or

- you have any unusual pain, swelling, redness, or other signs of infection at or near the insertion site.

Common Precautions after a Stent Procedure

After a stent procedure, your doctor may have you take blood-thinning or anticlotting medicines for at least a few months. These medicines help prevent the development of blood clots in the stent. If your stent is coated with medicine, your doctor may advise you to take aspirin and an anticlotting medicine for months to years to lower the risk of blood clots.

You should avoid vigorous exercise and heavy lifting for a short time after the procedure. Your doctor will discuss with you when you can resume normal activities.

If you have a metal stent placed, you shouldn't have a magnetic resonance imaging (MRI) test within the first couple of months after the procedure. Metal detectors used in airports and other screening areas don't affect stents.

If you have an aortic fabric stent, your doctor will probably recommend that you have followup imaging tests (for example, x-ray) within the first year of having the procedure, and yearly imaging tests after that.

What Are the Risks of Having a Stent?

Risks Related to Angioplasty

Any medical procedure has risks, but major complications from angioplasty are rare. The most common risks from angioplasty include:

- bleeding from the site where the catheter was inserted into the skin;

- damage to the blood vessel from the catheter;

- infection; and

- allergic reaction to the dye used during the procedure.

Another common problem after angioplasty is too much tissue growth within the treated portion of the artery. This can cause the artery to narrow or close again, which is called restenosis. This problem is often avoided with the use of newer stents coated with medicines that help prevent too much tissue growth. Treating the tissue around the stent with radiation also can prevent tissue growth. For this procedure, the doctor puts a wire through a catheter to where the stent is placed. The wire releases radiation and stops cells around the stent from growing and blocking the artery.

Risks Related to Stent

About 1 to 2 percent of people with a stented artery develop a blood clot at the stent site. Blood clots can cause heart attacks, strokes, or other serious problems. The risk of blood clots is greatest during the first few months after the stent is placed in the artery. Your doctor will probably have you take blood-thinning or anticlotting medicines for at least a few months after having a stent procedure to prevent blood clots.

Stents coated with medicine (drug-releasing stents), which are often used to keep clogged heart arteries open, may increase your risk for potentially dangerous blood clots. But an expert Food and Drug Administration panel found no conclusive evidence that these stents increase the chances of having a heart attack or dying, if used as recommended. Patients with drug-releasing stents are usually advised to take aspirin and an anticlotting drug, such as clopidogrel, for months to years to lower the risk of blood clots.

Risks Related to Aortic Stents in the Abdomen

Whenever an aneurysm in the abdomen region of the aorta is repaired with either surgery or with a fabric stent, a few rare but serious complications can occur, including:

- a burst artery (aneurysm rupture);

- blocked blood flow to the stomach or lower body; and

- paralysis in the legs due to interruption of blood flow to the spinal cord. This is an especially rare complication.

Another possible complication is the fabric stent moving further down the aorta. This sometimes happens years after the stent is first placed. Such stent movement may require a doctor to place another fabric stent in the area of the aneurysm.

Section 36.2

Stenting Techniques and Outcomes Vary

A major study released in the March 2007 *New England Journal of Medicine* found that using stents (metal-mesh tubes) with heart angioplasty generally provides no more lasting benefit than using drugs alone to keep blood flowing properly and to treat angina or stable coronary artery disease.

The research looked at 2,287 non-emergency heart patients in the United States and Canada and was historic in that it called into question the widespread elective use of stents in treating heart conditions. But the conclusions should not be applied to measure the benefit of stenting in other parts of the body, says a Medical College of Wisconsin expert in strokes and new brain stenting procedures.

"When we talk about the brain and the heart, we need to keep in mind that we're talking about two very different organs," said Osama O. (Sam) Zaidat, M.D., MSc, Medical College Associate Professor of Neurology and Neurosurgery and Director of the MCW Neuro-Interventional Program. "They respond differently to different approaches and different medications.

"We have to be very careful when drawing any conclusion from the recently published heart study results. This study might only apply to the blocked arteries in the heart and in the same inclusion criteria applied in the study. We need additional future study to confirm these findings. I also would rather see the same results come out from further investigations. Generalizing the results from one study is not the right thing to do and clinical judgment remains the best approach.

"When it comes to brain stents, we need similar studies to show that the newly and specifically-designed cranial Wingspan stent is better than medical therapy, or vice versa." Dr. Zaidat is a principle investigator in studies to determine the safety and effectiveness of the Wingspan stent designed to help prevent subsequent strokes in ischemic stroke victims.

Heart Stent Findings "Astonishing"

Wide media attention greeted the heart stent study report, and several renowned heart specialists described the findings as "surprising" and even "astonishing." The patients studied were not emergency heart attack patients, but those with chest pain (angina) and coronary artery disease that was considered stable, with at least a 70% blockage of an artery.

Every patient in the study received aggressive treatment through what is known as "optimal medical therapy," which case-by-case may have included one or more of: blood thinners such as aspirin, cholesterol-lowering drugs, drugs such as nitroglycerin to relieve angina, and blood-pressure-lowering drugs.

About half of the heart patients also had stents placed to prop open narrowed arteries. In very general terms, after about five years' worth of follow-up was analyzed, the study revealed that the longer-term risks of heart attack, hospitalization for certain heart problems, stroke and death were not reduced by angioplasty with stenting compared with drug therapy alone.

This study added to the continuing debate over the use of elective angioplasty in general, in which a balloon is inserted and then blown up to widen the artery, not just the fairly recent development of also leaving a permanent stent in place to keep an artery open. In some news reports, Mayo Clinic cardiologist and American Heart Association president Raymond Gibbons went so far as to say that hundreds of thousands of elective angioplasties in the United States are not needed.

Other experts called for more considered analysis of when angioplasty or medical therapy, or a combination of the two, is most appropriate. An invasive procedure to treat a narrowed artery is not the only alternative, they said, when drugs can accomplish the same goals. Some also noted that the United States health care reimbursement system tends to pay more willingly for surgical procedures than for drug therapy that requires long-term maintenance and monitoring.

Heart and Brain: Different Tissues, Different Responses

While thinning the blood and addressing other heart conditions with drugs may prove equally beneficial and less costly than stenting in the heart, that simply may not be true for stenting to treat circulatory problems in the legs or prevent strokes in the brain, said Dr. Zaidat.

For example, the next phase of research into the new Wingspan brain stent will study longer-term outcomes from brain stenting as compared to using optimal medical therapy alone.

Dr. Zaidat stressed that thinning the blood with aspirin or other drugs to deal with narrowed arteries is not the same thing as using "clot-busters" (thrombolytic drugs) to literally break up acute blockages. However, he said, stenting may prove to be of benefit in the brain for both narrowed arteries and arteries that are acutely blocked by clots.

"Brain stenting with the Wingspan stent is for prevention of subsequent catastrophic stroke," said Dr. Zaidat. "Future studies may show that we can use stents to break up clots instead of trying to take them out. We may learn that stents show promise in treating acute blockage instead of using the thrombolytics. I have in fact treated three patients with this new stent for acute blockage, and they did very well, better than with thrombolytics.

"No matter what the brain stent will be used for, data from heart or leg artery studies cannot be applied to the brain and vice versa, because each tissue has a different response. That's one aspect of the dilemma we faced with brain stenting; we need more study to say whether the brain acts differently or not. And we're using a stent that is different from the heart stent from a safety perspective. The composition of arteries at different organ locations (brain, heart, leg, kidney) and the tissue surrounding specific organ arteries are also different and may react differently to placing different types of stents.

"The risk of stroke is different from the risk of heart attack from a blocked artery. The percentage of subsequent stroke when you have a brain artery blocked more than 70% is very high, about 35%. These are totally different creatures. You cannot say, because the stent use in a different body area is shown to be controversial in a single study, that one would recommend that people should be taking aspirin instead of undergoing angioplasty.

"Each specific scenario requires its own study to show whether the stent is better or the pills are better, and nothing supersedes clinical judgment by an experienced cardiologist for the heart and an experienced neurologist for the brain."

Section 36.3

Brain-Specific Stent Shows Promise in Preventing Strokes

A new stent designed for placement deep inside the narrow arteries of the brain has proved safe in holding blocked blood vessels open and reducing stroke survivors' risk of having another stroke, according to a study presented by Osama O. (Sam) Zaidat, M.D., MSc, Medical College of Wisconsin Associate Professor of Neurology and Neurosurgery and Director of the MCW Neuro-Interventional Program.

Like stents commonly used to treat clogged arteries in the heart and leg, the "Wingspan" stent is a tiny tube used to prop open the area of blockage. But this stent is even thinner and far more flexible than the others, made of a metal alloy mesh with enough "give" to navigate the tricky fragility of brain arteries.

"When we used this newly-designed brain stent across the country in 16 major U.S. institutions, we had a very good safety profile," said Dr. Zaidat. "That's the key finding of our study. Prior to this stent, the safety and complication rate using stents in the brain was not very good and were not very acceptable to patients or referring physicians. When we placed a stent that was not specifically designed for the brain we had to deal with a lot of technical and procedure-related issues, which have been associated in the past with a high morbidity."

The Wingspan stent is used to treat patients who have had ischemic strokes, the kind of stroke caused by a clot or other blockage in a brain

344

artery that inhibits blood flow. Ischemic strokes are the most common type of stroke, leaving tens of thousands of patients in the U.S. with brain damage—or killing them—each year.

Reducing Complications and Risk

Dr. Zaidat presented the Wingspan study findings at the 2007 International Stroke Conference. The study was completed in November 2006 using data from the first year after FDA approval of the stent. Before the new stent was developed, said Dr. Zaidat, attempts to deploy stents in the brain did not show good results in great part because the relatively cumbersome stents made for other parts of the body could not be accurately positioned in the brain.

Using a technique similar to other stenting procedures but refined to accommodate the physical characteristics and location of brain arteries, the Wingspan stent is "packaged/housed" within a tiny and flexible long brain catheter. The catheter is maneuvered to just the right point past the blockage, where it is pulled back to unsheathe and open the stent to be deployed. The blocked area is usually pre-dilated (angioplasty) with small, specifically-designed brain balloon.

"This study shows that the newly-designed "Wingspan" stent can be placed safely with a procedure risk (for complication) of less than five percent," said Dr. Zaidat. "The 161 patients enrolled had a success rate with this stent of 95.4%, which is quite an increase in the safety as compared to the old technique and the old devices that we were using before. The risk of complication using stents that are not specifically designed for the brain can be as high as 50%."

"And, a patient with a stroke related to a blocked or narrowed artery inside the head had a very high risk of subsequent strokes despite the use of the best medical therapy available at this point (such as aspirin and blood-thinning drugs). So if you give a patient with a blocked artery in the head the best medical therapy that's out there, and they have more than 70% blockage, the risk of subsequent stroke can be up to 35% over a two-year period."

Stroke, Brain Bleed, and Death

Finding ways to reduce the risk of subsequent stroke is the overall goal of the research, said Dr. Zaidat. In general terms, he said, it can be expected that 18% of ischemic stroke patients who receive only traditional drug therapy will experience another stroke or brain bleed or death within three months. According to data from the safety trials of the Wingspan stent, that number was just 12% for patients with the stent in place.

The new brain stenting technique is mostly performed by neuro-interventionalists (who are already fellowship-trained specialists in catheterizing and performing procedures on brain arteries) who must perform two such procedures under supervision before they are allowed to "go solo," said Dr. Zaidat. He is one of the proctors who travel the country training and assisting other neuro-interventionalists in use of the Wingspan device.

The next phase of study will specifically compare outcomes from brain stenting to those from optimal drug therapy in a major research effort led by academic and university centers across United States. Dr. Zaidat said he expects the need for 600 to 900 patients enrolled through about 40 medical centers nationwide to complete the future study.

"For example, and we certainly don't know this to be true yet, if this stent is proven in future studies to have a 15% risk of subsequent stroke within two years, that would be a dramatic improvement from the 35% risk with optimal medications," said Dr. Zaidat. "The risk with this disease is quite high, so it's clear that we need to do something besides the current medical therapy to try and bring that risk down."

Section 36.4

Stent-Assisted Coiling Procedure Can Prevent Aneurysm Rupture

"New Stent-Assisted Coiling Procedure Means Some Patients with Wide Neck Aneurysms May Avoid Brain Surgery," January 21, 2003, reprinted with permission from the University of Maryland Medical Center (www.umm.edu). The text that follows this document under the heading *"Health Reference Series* Medical Advisor's Notes and Updates" was provided to Omnigraphics, Inc. by David A. Cooke, M.D., February 25, 2008. Dr. Cooke is not affiliated with the University of Maryland Medical Center.

Doctors at the University of Maryland Medical Center are among the first in the country to perform a new procedure involving a stent, combined with coiling, to treat brain aneurysms. The treatment provides a non-surgical option for patients with "wide neck" aneurysms, who make up about 25 percent of the people with brain aneurysms. Those are weak spots in a blood vessel that balloon out and can rupture. When an aneurysm ruptures, it causes bleeding in the brain and a significant risk of death. With "wide neck" aneurysms, the bulge in the vessel has a wide opening where it attaches to the artery.

In recent years, doctors have been able to repair "narrow neck" aneurysms by inserting coils through a small catheter passed up through blood vessels in the brain. They fill the aneurysm with tiny, spring-like coils, redirecting the blood flow away from the weakened vessel wall. But before the new stenting procedure was developed, that therapy could not be offered to people with "wide neck" aneurysms because the coils would not stay in place with the wider opening.

"A stent is a very small, metal scaffold with lots of holes in it," says Gregg Zoarski, M.D., director of Neuroradiology at the University of Maryland Medical Center and associate professor of Diagnostic Radiology at the University of Maryland School of Medicine. "The stent provides a framework, bridging the wider neck, so we can insert the coils and keep them from falling out. Then the body's own natural healing abilities take over; blood clots on the coils, sealing off the weakened area, preventing a rupture."

One of Dr. Zoarski's first aneurysm patients treated with the stent-assisted coiling is 41-year-old Gerry Neal of Rosedale, Maryland. When she had an unusual pain on the right side of her head in August, she blamed it on the summer heat. The pain stretched from the back of her head to her temple and lasted for only a few seconds. When it happened several more times, Ms. Neal decided to see her doctor. An MRI [magnetic resonance imaging test] showed the problem: a large aneurysm in her brain.

At that time, because her aneurysm had a wide neck, Ms. Neal was not a candidate for coiling. Previously, patients with a wide neck aneurysm would need brain surgery with a procedure called surgical clipping. It involves drilling into the skull and placing a clip over the neck of the aneurysm, effectively cutting it off from the circulatory system. Recovery time for this procedure is much longer compared to coiling.

"With coiling, patients usually spend about two nights in the hospital and can typically get back to work in about a week," says Dr. Zoarski. "On the other hand, surgical clipping involves five to seven nights in the hospital, and patients are out of work for six to twelve weeks." But not all aneurysms can be clipped. In fact, doctors first tried clipping to fix Ms. Neal's aneurysm, but its location low on the skull base caused concerns during surgery. "Surgery wasn't easy," Ms. Neal says. "My head was shaved for the surgery, and afterward it swelled." She still has a scar on her head.

With the new stent-assisted coiling procedure, doctors do not need to enter the brain through the skull; instead, they enter the body through an artery in the groin. Using advanced computer x-ray scanners, skilled radiologists guide a microcatheter (less than one millimeter in diameter) through the blood vessels to the site of the aneurysm in the brain. They then deploy the stent that spans the neck of the aneurysm and conforms to the shape of the artery. Small gaps in the stent allow doctors to feed the tiny platinum coils into the bulge of the aneurysm. The number of coils needed depends on the size of the aneurysm. The coils themselves are only a few millimeters wide.

The stent prevents the coils from falling out of the aneurysm. "If they fell into the blood vessel, they could block the carotid artery or a smaller branch and cause a stroke," warns Dr. Zoarski. "Placing the stent across the neck of the aneurysm increases the safety of the procedure and helps us to fill the aneurysm completely with coils."

If left untreated, an aneurysm can rupture causing a subarachnoid hemorrhage. It's a dangerous condition that affects about 30,000 people every year in the United States. In up to half of these cases, this type of hemorrhage can be fatal; patients who do survive often face severe disabilities. An estimated five million Americans have some sort of cerebral aneurysm, and up to one quarter of those may have a wide neck.

Many patients may feel like they have a time bomb in their heads, fearing the aneurysm could burst at any time. Ms. Neal admits she had a tough time in the beginning and cried when she learned her diagnosis. "My family was upset, thinking I was going to die," she says. But she kept a positive attitude. "I resolved to get through it. I resolved to smile and laugh more."

Now, after the stent-assisted coiling procedure at the University of Maryland Medical Center on December 20th, Ms. Neal is doing well. She went back to work about a week after the procedure. "People are amazed to see me back at work so soon," she says. "My daughter is relieved that I'm going to be okay; my son says he knew it all the time."

Health Reference Series *Medical Advisor's Notes and Updates*

The combination stent-coiling technique described above has spread considerably since this article's original introduction. However, management of these wide-necked aneurysms remains difficult as stent use can introduce its own risks. Decisions still need to be made on a case-by-case basis, depending upon the features of the aneurysms and the experience of the treating physicians.

Chapter 37

Carotid Endarterectomy Performed to Prevent Stroke

What is a carotid endarterectomy?

A carotid endarterectomy is a surgical procedure in which a doctor removes fatty deposits blocking one of the two carotid arteries, the main supply of blood for the brain. Carotid artery problems become more common as people age. The disease process that causes the buildup of fat and other material inside the artery walls is called atherosclerosis, popularly known as "hardening of the arteries."

The fatty deposit is called plaque; the narrowing of the artery is called stenosis. The degree of stenosis is usually expressed as a percentage of the normal diameter of the opening.

Why is surgery performed?

Carotid endarterectomy is performed to prevent stroke. Two large clinical trials supported by the National Institute of Neurological Disorders and Stroke (NINDS) have identified specific individuals for whom the surgery is beneficial when performed by surgeons and in institutions that can match the standards set in those studies. The surgery has been found highly beneficial for persons who have already had a stroke or experienced the symptoms of a stroke and have a severe stenosis of 70 to 99 percent. In this group, surgery reduces the

"Questions and Answers about Carotid Endarterectomy" is from the National Institute of Neurological Disorders and Stroke (NINDS, www.ninds.nih.gov), part of the National Institutes of Health, October 18, 2004.

estimated 2-year risk of stroke or death by more than 80 percent, from greater than 1 in 4 to less than 1 in 10.

For patients who have already had transient or mild stroke symptoms due to moderate carotid stenosis (50 to 69 percent), surgery reduces the 5-year risk of stroke or death by 6.5 percent. The failure rate for ipsilateral stroke or death for the medical group is 22.2 percent, and for the surgery group is 15.7 percent from greater than 1 in 4 to less than 1 in 7. Individuals who have already had stroke symptoms, and who have carotid stenosis greater than 50 percent, may wish to consider surgery to prevent future stroke. With the completion of the NASCET [North American Symptomatic Carotid Endarterectomy] trial, patients with moderate (50 to 69 percent) stenosis will be better able to make more informed decisions.

In another trial, the procedure has also been found highly beneficial for persons who are symptom-free but have a carotid stenosis of 60 to 99 percent. In this group, the surgery reduces the estimated 5-year risk of stroke by more than one-half, from about 1 in 10 to less than 1 in 20.

What is a stroke?

A stroke occurs when blood flow is cut off from part of the brain. In the same way that a person suffering a loss of blood to the heart can be said to be having a "heart attack," a person with a loss of blood to the brain can be said to be having a "brain attack." There are two kinds of stroke, hemorrhagic and ischemic. Hemorrhagic strokes are caused by bleeding within the brain. Ischemic strokes, which are far more common, are caused by a blockage of blood flow in an artery in the head or neck leading to the brain. Some ischemic strokes are due to stenosis, or narrowing of arteries due to the buildup of plaque, fatty deposits and blood clots along the artery wall. A vascular disease that can cause stenosis is atherosclerosis, in which deposits of plaque build up along the inner wall of large- and medium-sized arteries, decreasing blood flow. Atherosclerosis in the carotid arteries, two large arteries in the neck that carry blood to the brain, is a major risk factor for ischemic stroke.

What are the symptoms of a stroke?

Symptoms of stroke include:

- sudden numbness, weakness, or paralysis of face, arm or leg, especially on one side of the body;

- sudden confusion, trouble talking or understanding speech;

- sudden trouble seeing in one or both eyes;

- sudden trouble walking, loss of balance, or coordination; and

- sudden severe headache with no known cause (often described as the worst headache in a person's life).

Symptoms may last a few moments and then disappear. When they disappear within 24 hours or less, they are called transient ischemic attacks (TIA).

How important is a blockage as a cause of stroke?

A blockage of a blood vessel is the most frequent cause of stroke and is responsible for about 80 percent of the approximately 700,000 strokes in the United States each year. With nearly 150,000 stroke deaths each year, stroke ranks as the third leading killer in the United States after heart disease and cancer. Stroke is the leading cause of adult disability in the United States with 2 million of the 3 million Americans who have survived a stroke sustaining some permanent disability. The overall cost of stroke to the nation is $40 billion a year.

How many carotid endarterectomies are performed each year?

In 1995, the most recent year for which statistics are available from the National Hospital Discharge Survey, there were about 132,000 carotid endarterectomies performed in the United States. The procedure was first described in the mid-1950s. It began to be used increasingly as a stroke prevention measure in the 1960s and 1970s. Its use peaked in the mid-1980s when more than 100,000 operations were performed each year. At that time, several authorities began to question the trend and the risk-benefit ratio for some groups, and the use of the procedure dropped precipitously. The NINDS-supported NASCET and the NINDS-supported Asymptomatic Carotid Atherosclerosis Study (ACAS) were launched in the mid-1980s to identify the specific groups of people with carotid artery disease who would clearly benefit from the procedure.

What are the risk factors and how risky is the surgery?

Important risk factors in addition to the degree of stenosis include: gender, diabetes, the type of stroke symptoms, and blockage of the carotid artery on the opposite side. Without other complicating illnesses, age alone is not a worrisome risk factor. Risk factors can affect patients in two ways. They can, particularly in combination, greatly increase a person's risk of having a stroke. In addition, these risk factors can increase the likelihood of surgical complications.

How is carotid artery disease diagnosed?

In some cases, the disease can be detected during a normal checkup by a physician. In other cases further testing is needed. Some of the tests a physician can use or order include ultrasound imaging, arteriography, and magnetic resonance angiography (MRA). Frequently these procedures are carried out in a stepwise fashion: from a doctor's evaluation of signs and symptoms to ultrasound, MRA, and arteriography for increasingly difficult cases.

History and physical exam. A doctor will ask about symptoms of a stroke such as numbness or muscle weakness, speech or vision difficulties, or lightheadedness. Using a stethoscope, a doctor may hear a rushing sound, called a bruit, in the carotid artery. Unfortunately, dangerous levels of disease sometimes fail to make a sound, and some blockages with a low risk can make the same sound.

Ultrasound imaging. This is a painless, noninvasive test in which sound waves above the range of human hearing are sent into the neck. Echoes bounce off the moving blood and the tissue in the artery and can be formed into an image. Ultrasound is fast, risk-free, relatively inexpensive, and painless compared to MRA and arteriography.

Arteriography. This can be used to confirm the findings of ultrasound imaging which can be uncertain in some cases. Arteriography is an x-ray of the carotid artery taken when a special dye is injected into the artery. A burning sensation may be felt when the dye is injected. An arteriogram is more expensive and carries its own small risk of causing a stroke.

Magnetic Resonance Angiography (MRA). This is a new imaging technique that avoids most of the risks associated with arteriography. An MRA is a type of image that uses magnetism instead of x-rays to create an image of the carotid arteries.

What is best medical therapy for stroke prevention?

The mainstay of stroke prevention is risk factor management: smoking cessation, treatment of high blood pressure, and control of blood sugar levels among persons with diabetes. Additionally, physicians may prescribe aspirin, warfarin, or ticlopidine for some individuals.

Chapter 38

Angioplasty

Coronary angioplasty is a medical procedure in which a balloon is used to open a blockage in a coronary (heart) artery narrowed by atherosclerosis. This procedure improves blood flow to the heart.

Atherosclerosis is a condition in which a material called plaque builds up on the inner walls of the arteries. This can happen in any artery, including the coronary arteries, which carry oxygen-rich blood to your heart. When atherosclerosis affects the coronary arteries, the condition is called coronary artery disease (CAD).

Angioplasty is a common medical procedure. It may be used to:

- improve symptoms of CAD, such as angina and shortness of breath.

- reduce damage to the heart muscle from a heart attack. A heart attack occurs when blood flow through a coronary artery is completely blocked. Angioplasty is used during a heart attack to open the blockage and restore blood flow through the artery.

- reduce the risk of death in some patients.

Angioplasty is done on more than 1 million people a year in the United States. Serious complications don't occur often, but can happen no matter how careful your doctor is, or how well he or she does the procedure.

From "Coronary Angioplasty," by the National Heart, Lung, and Blood Institute (NHLBI, www.nhlbi.nih.gov), part of the National Institutes of Health, July 2007.

Research on angioplasty is ongoing to make it safer and more effective, to prevent treated arteries from closing again, and to make the procedure an option for more people.

Other Names for Coronary Angioplasty

- Percutaneous coronary intervention (PCI)
- Percutaneous intervention
- Percutaneous transluminal angioplasty
- Percutaneous transluminal coronary angioplasty (PTCA)
- Balloon angioplasty
- Coronary artery angioplasty

Who Needs Coronary Angioplasty?

Coronary angioplasty is used to restore blood flow to the heart when the coronary arteries have become narrowed or blocked due to coronary artery disease (CAD).

When medicines and lifestyle changes, such as following a healthy diet, quitting smoking, and getting more physical activity, don't improve your CAD symptoms, your doctor will talk to you about other treatment options. These options include angioplasty and coronary artery bypass grafting (CABG), a type of open-heart surgery.

Your doctor will take into account a number of factors when recommending the best procedure for you. These factors include how severe your blockages are, where they're located, and other diseases you may have.

Angioplasty is often used when there is less severe narrowing or blockage in your arteries, and when the blockage can be reached during the procedure.

CABG might be chosen if you have severe heart disease, multiple arteries that are blocked, or if you have diabetes or heart failure.

Compared with CABG, some advantages of angioplasty are that it:

- has fewer risks than CABG;
- isn't surgery, so it won't require a large cut;
- is done with medicines that numb you and help you relax;
- unlike CABG, you won't be put to sleep for a short time;
- has a shorter recovery time.

Angioplasty also is used as an emergency procedure during a heart attack. As plaque builds up in the coronary arteries, it can burst, causing a blood clot to form on its surface. If the clot becomes large enough, it can mostly or completely block blood flow to part of the heart muscle.

Quickly opening a blockage lessens the damage to the heart during a heart attack and restores blood flow to the heart muscle. Angioplasty can quickly open the artery and is the best approach during a heart attack.

A disadvantage of angioplasty as compared with CABG is that the artery may narrow again over time. The chance of this happening is lower when stents are used, especially medicine-coated stents. However, these stents aren't without risk. In some cases, blood clots can form in the medicine-coated stents and cause a heart attack.

Your doctor will discuss with you the treatment options and which procedure is best for you.

How Is Coronary Angioplasty Done?

Before coronary angioplasty is done, your doctor will need to know whether your coronary arteries are blocked. If one or more of your arteries are blocked, your doctor will need to know where and how severe the blockages are.

To find out, your doctor will do an angiogram and take an x-ray picture of your arteries. During an angiogram, a small tube called a catheter with a balloon at the end is put into a large blood vessel in the groin (upper thigh) or arm. The catheter is then threaded to the coronary arteries. A small amount of dye is injected into the coronary arteries and an x-ray picture is taken.

This picture will show any blockages, how many, and where they're located. Once your doctor has this information, the angioplasty can proceed. Your doctor will blow up (inflate) the balloon in the blockage and push the plaque outward against the artery wall. This opens the artery more and improves blood flow.

A small mesh tube called a stent is usually placed in the newly widened part of the artery. The stent holds up the artery and lowers the risk of the artery renarrowing. Stents are made of metal mesh and look like small springs.

Some stents, called drug-eluting stents, are coated with medicines that are slowly and continuously released into the artery. These medicines help prevent the artery from becoming blocked again from scar tissue that grows around the stent.

In some cases, plaque is removed during angioplasty. In a procedure called atherectomy, a catheter with a rotating shaver on its tip is inserted into the artery to cut away plaque. Lasers also are used to dissolve or break up the plaque. These procedures are now rarely done because angioplasty gives better results for most patients.

What to Expect before Coronary Angioplasty

Meeting with Your Doctor

A cardiologist (a doctor who treats people with heart conditions) performs coronary angioplasty at a hospital. If your angioplasty isn't done as emergency treatment, you'll meet with your cardiologist before the procedure. Your doctor will go over your medical history (including the medicines you take), do a physical exam, and talk about the procedure with you. Your doctor also will order some routine tests, including:

- blood tests;
- an EKG (electrocardiogram); and
- a chest x-ray.

When the procedure is scheduled, you will be advised:

- when to begin fasting (not eating or drinking) before the procedure. Often you have to stop eating or drinking by midnight the night before the procedure.
- what medicines you should and shouldn't take on the day of the angioplasty.
- when to arrive at the hospital and where to go.

Even though angioplasty takes 1 to 2 hours, you will likely need to stay in the hospital overnight. In some cases, you will need to stay in the hospital longer. Your doctor may advise you not to drive for a certain amount of time after the procedure, so you may have to arrange for a ride home.

What to Expect during Coronary Angioplasty

Coronary angioplasty is performed in a special part of the hospital called the cardiac catheterization laboratory. The "cath lab" has special video screens and x-ray machines. Your doctor uses this equipment to see enlarged pictures of the blocked areas in your coronary arteries.

Preparation

In the cath lab, you will lie on a table. An intravenous (IV) line will be placed in your arm to give you fluids and medicines. The medicines will relax you and prevent blood clots from forming. These medicines may make you feel sleepy or as though you're floating or numb.

To prepare for the procedure:

- the area where the catheter will be inserted, usually the arm or groin (upper thigh), will be shaved; and

- the shaved area will be cleaned to make it germ free and then numbed. The numbing medicine may sting as it's going in.

Steps in Angioplasty

When you're comfortable, the doctor will begin the procedure. You will be awake but sleepy.

A small cut is made in your arm or groin into which a tube called a sheath is put. The doctor then threads a very thin guide wire through the artery in your arm or groin toward the area of the coronary artery that's blocked.

Your doctor puts a long, thin, flexible tube called a catheter through the sheath and slides it over the guide wire and up to the heart. Your doctor moves the catheter into the coronary artery to the blockage. He or she takes out the guide wire once the catheter is in the right spot.

A small amount of dye may be injected through the catheter into the bloodstream to help show the blockage on x-ray. This x-ray picture of the heart is called an angiogram.

Next, your doctor slides a tube with a small deflated balloon inside it through the catheter and into the coronary artery where the blockage is.

When the tube reaches the blockage, the balloon is inflated. The balloon pushes the plaque against the wall of the artery and widens it. This helps to increase the flow of blood to the heart.

The balloon is then deflated. Sometimes the balloon is inflated and deflated more than once to widen the artery. Afterward, the balloon and tube are removed.

In some cases, plaque is removed during angioplasty. A catheter with a rotating shaver on its tip is inserted into the artery to cut away hard plaque. Lasers also may be used to dissolve or break up the plaque.

If your doctor needs to put a stent (small mesh tube) in your artery, another tube with a balloon will be threaded through your artery. A stent is wrapped around the balloon. Your doctor will inflate the balloon, which will cause the stent to expand against the wall of the artery. The balloon is then deflated and pulled out of the artery with the tube. The stent stays in the artery.

After the angioplasty is done, your doctor pulls back the catheter and removes it and the sheath. The hole in the artery is either sealed with a special device, or pressure is put on it until the blood vessel seals.

During angioplasty, strong antiplatelet medicines are given through the IV to prevent blood clots from forming in the artery or on the stent. These medicines help thin your blood. They're usually started just before the angioplasty and may continue for 12–24 hours afterward.

What to Expect after Coronary Angioplasty

After coronary angioplasty, you will be moved to a special care unit, where you will stay for a few hours or overnight. While you recover in this area, you must lie still for a few hours to allow the blood vessels in your arm or groin (upper thigh) to seal completely.

While you recover, nurses will check your heart rate and blood pressure. They also will check your arm or groin for bleeding. After a few hours, you will be able to walk with help.

The place where the tube was inserted may feel sore or tender for about a week.

Going Home

Most people go home 1 to 2 days after the procedure. When your doctor thinks you're ready to leave the hospital, you will get instructions to follow at home, including:

- how much activity or exercise you can do.

- when you should follow up with your doctor.

- what medicines you should take.

- what you should look for daily when checking for signs of infection around the area where the tube was inserted. Signs of infection may include redness, swelling, or drainage.

- when you should call your doctor. For example, you may need to call if you have a fever or signs of infection, pain or bleeding where the catheter was inserted, or shortness of breath.

362

- when you should call 911 (for example, if you have any chest pain).

Your doctor will prescribe medicine to prevent blood clots from forming. Taking your medicine as directed is very important. If a stent was inserted, the medicine reduces the risk that blood clots will form in the stent. Blood clots in the stent can block blood flow and cause a heart attack.

Recovery and Recuperation

Most people recover from angioplasty and return to work about 1 week after being sent home. Your doctor will want to check your progress after you leave the hospital. During the followup visit, your doctor will examine you, make changes to your medicines if needed, do any necessary tests, and check your overall recovery. Use this time to ask questions you may have about activities, medicines, or lifestyle changes, or to talk about any other issues that concern you.

Lifestyle Changes. Although angioplasty can reduce the symptoms of coronary artery disease (CAD), it isn't a cure for CAD or the risk factors that led to it. Making healthy lifestyle changes can help treat CAD and maintain the good results from angioplasty. Talk with your doctor about your risk factors for CAD and the lifestyle changes you'll need to make. For some people, these changes may be the only treatment needed.

- Follow a healthy diet to prevent or reduce high blood pressure and high blood cholesterol and to maintain a healthy weight.

- Quit smoking if you smoke.

- Be physically active.

- Lose weight if you're overweight or obese.

- Reduce stress.

- Take medicines as your doctor directs to lower high blood pressure or high blood cholesterol.

Cardiac Rehabilitation. Your doctor may want you to take part in a cardiac rehabilitation (rehab) program. Cardiac rehab helps people with heart disease recover faster and return to work or daily activities.

Cardiac rehab includes supervised physical activity, education on heart-healthy living, and counseling to cut down on stress and help you return to an active life. Your doctor can tell you where to find a cardiac rehab program near your home.

What Are the Risks of Coronary Angioplasty?

Coronary angioplasty is a common medical procedure. Although angioplasty is normally safe, there is a small risk of serious complications, such as:

- bleeding from the blood vessel where the catheter was placed.
- damage to blood vessels from the catheter.
- an allergic reaction to the dye given during the angioplasty.
- an arrhythmia (irregular heartbeat).
- the need for emergency coronary artery bypass grafting during the procedure (2–4 percent of people). This may occur when an artery closes down, instead of opening up.
- damage to the kidneys caused by the dye used.
- heart attack (3–5 percent of people).
- stroke (less than 1 percent of people).

As with any procedure involving the heart, complications can sometimes, though rarely, cause death. Less than 2 percent of people die during angioplasty.

Sometimes chest pain can occur during angioplasty because the balloon briefly blocks off the blood supply to the heart.

The risk of complications is higher in:

- people aged 75 and older;
- people who have kidney disease or diabetes;
- women;
- people who have poor pumping function in their hearts; and
- people who have extensive heart disease and blockages.

Research on angioplasty is ongoing to make it safer and more effective, to prevent treated arteries from closing again, and to make the procedure an option for more people.

Complications from Stents

Restenosis. There is a chance that the artery will become narrowed or blocked again in time, often within 6 months of angioplasty. This is called restenosis.

When a stent isn't used, 4 out of 10 people have restenosis. When a nonmedicine-coated stent is used, 2 out of 10 people have restenosis.

The growth of scar tissue in and around the stent also can cause restenosis. Medicine-coated stents reduce the growth of scar tissue around the stent and lower the chance of restenosis. When medicine-coated stents are used, the chance of restenosis is lowered even more, to around 1 in 10 people.

Other treatments, such as radiation, can help prevent tissue growth within a stent. For this procedure, the doctor puts a wire through a catheter to where the stent is placed. The wire releases radiation to stop any tissue growth that may block the artery.

Blood Clots. Recent studies suggest that there is a higher risk of blood clots forming in medicine-coated stents compared to bare metal stents (nonmedicine-coated). The Food and Drug Administration (FDA) reports that medicine-coated stents usually don't cause complications due to blood clots when used as recommended.

When medicine-coated stents are used in people with advanced CAD, there is a higher risk of blood clots, heart attack, and death. The FDA is working with researchers to study medicine-coated stents, including their use in people with advanced CAD.

Taking medicine as prescribed by your doctor can lower the risk of blood clots. People with medicine-coated stents are usually advised to take an anticlotting drug, such as clopidogrel and aspirin, for months to years to lower the risk of blood clots.

As with all procedures, it's important to talk to your doctor about your treatment options, including the risks and benefits to you.

Chapter 39

Dealing with Recurrent Stroke

After stroke, survivors tend to focus on rehabilitation and recovery. But, preventing another (or recurring) stroke is also a key concern. Of the 750,000 Americans who have a stroke each year, 5 to 14 percent will have a second stroke within one year. Within five years, stroke will recur in 24 percent of women and 42 percent of men.

Table 39.1. Percentage of Recurrence after First Stroke

3% to 10%	30-Day
5% to 14%	1-Year
25% to 40%	5-Year

Stroke prevention is also crucial for those who have had transient ischemic attacks (TIAs) or mini-strokes. TIAs are brief episodes of stroke-like symptoms that last from a few minutes to 24 hours. TIAs usually don't cause permanent damage or disability. But, they can be a serious warning sign of an impending stroke. Up to one third of people who have a TIA are expected to have a stroke. Just like the first strokes, many recurrent strokes and TIAs can be prevented through lifestyle changes, surgery, medicine, or a mix of all three.

Your Lifestyle Choices

Everyone has some stroke risk. But, there are two types of stroke risk factors. One type you can't control. The other you can.

Stroke risk factors you can't change include:

- being over age 55;
- being a man;
- being African American;
- someone in your family has had a stroke; or
- having diabetes.

Having one or more of these factors doesn't mean you will have a stroke. By making simple lifestyle changes, you may be able to reduce the risk of a first or recurrent stroke.

These simple lifestyle changes can greatly reduce your chance of having a stroke:

- Control your blood pressure.
- Find out if you have atrial fibrillation (an irregular heartbeat which allows blood to pool in the heart and cause blood clots).
- Quit smoking.
- Limit alcohol.
- Monitor your cholesterol levels.
- Manage your diabetes.
- Exercise often.
- Eat foods low in sodium (salt) and fat.
- Monitor circulation problems with the help of your doctor.

Monitor Your Blood Pressure

High blood pressure is one of the most important and easily controlled stroke risk factors. So it's important to know your blood pressure range!

Blood pressure is given in two numbers, for example 120/80. The first number, the systolic blood pressure, is a measurement of the force your blood exerts on blood vessel walls as your heart pumps. The second, diastolic blood pressure, is the measurement of the force your blood exerts on blood vessel walls when your heart is at rest.

- For people over age 18, normal blood pressure is lower than 120/80. A blood pressure reading consistently 120/80 to 139/89 is pre-hypertension. If yours falls in this range, you are more likely to progress to high blood pressure. Also called hypertension, high blood pressure is a reading of 140/90 or higher.

- Have your blood pressure checked at least once each year— more often if you have high blood pressure, have had a heart attack or stroke, are diabetic, have kidney disease, have high cholesterol, or are overweight. If you are at risk for high blood pressure, ask your doctor how to manage it more aggressively.

Often blood pressure can be controlled through diet and exercise. Even light exercise—a brisk walk, bicycle ride, swim, or yard work— can make a difference. Adults should do some form of moderate physical activity for at least 30 minutes five or more days per week, according to the Centers for Disease Control and Prevention. Regular exercise may reduce your risk of stroke. Before you start an exercise program, check with your doctor.

Your Blood Pressure Is High

What do you do if you still have high blood pressure, even though you have made an effort to eat healthy foods and exercise? Then it's time to talk to your doctor.

A doctor can advise you about better lifestyle choices. Medicine may also be needed.

Many drugs can help treat high blood pressure. The most common are calcium channel blockers or ACE [angiotensin-converting enzyme]-inhibitors. You may have to try several different drugs before you find one that works for you. This is common. So, try not to be discouraged if it happens. Once you find a drug that works, take it as directed and exactly as prescribed, even when you feel fine.

Medicines

Medicine may help reduce stroke risk. In addition to those that treat high blood pressure, drugs are also available to control high cholesterol and treat heart disease. There are also drugs that can interfere with the blood's tendency to form potential stroke-causing blood clots.

Heart Disease

Many forms of heart disease can increase your stroke risk. One form—known as atrial fibrillation or AF—causes blood to form clots that can travel to the brain and cause a stroke. AF is an irregular heartbeat.

Warfarin (Coumadin®) and aspirin are often prescribed to treat AF. People taking warfarin should be monitored carefully by a doctor. Also, people taking this drug should limit foods rich in vitamin K, which in large quantities may offset the drug's effects. Examples of these foods include green leafy vegetables, alfalfa, egg yolks, soy bean oil, and fish livers.

High Cholesterol

High levels of cholesterol may also increase stroke risk by not letting blood move freely through the arteries. Cholesterol build-up can break off. This can cause a clot to form or a stroke to occur. A few drugs, such as statins, may help lower cholesterol. Some statins have helped reduce the risk of stroke or TIA in people who have had a heart attack. They have even helped some with average or only slightly high cholesterol.

Blood Clotting

There are also a few drugs that can prevent clots, helping reduce risk of a second stroke.

Aspirin is the least costly and longest lasting of these drugs. A newer, more effective option is a combination of aspirin and extended-release dipyridamole, called Aggrenox®. Or, your doctor might choose to treat you with Clopidogrel (Plavix®). Warfarin is often prescribed to prevent clots from forming in those with atrial fibrillation.

Surgical Options

For those whose first stroke was caused by a blockage in the carotid arteries (vessels that carry blood from the heart to the brain), surgery known as carotid endarterectomy may help reduce risk of another stroke.

During surgery, blockages and buildup in the arteries are removed to restore the free flow of blood. Your doctor is the best judge to decide if this is a good option for you.

Compliance Is Critical

The key to preventing recurrent stroke is simple: follow your doctor's suggestions about diet, exercise, and weight loss, and take any medicine as directed. Your doctor will decide what's best for you based on your general health and your medical history. By understanding the basis for these decisions, you'll be better able to follow the suggestions and make informed choices that will help reduce your risk of stroke.

Rehabilitation is a lifetime commitment and an important part of recovering from a stroke. Through rehabilitation, you relearn basic skills such as talking, eating, dressing, and walking. Rehabilitation can also improve your strength, flexibility, and endurance. The goal is to regain as much independence as possible.

Remember to ask your doctor, "Where am I on my stroke recovery journey?"

Chapter 40

Treating Stroke in Children

Chapter Contents

Section 40.1

Kids and Stroke

"Pediatric Stroke Center: Stroke Treatment," © 2006 Internet Stroke Center at Washington University in St. Louis. Reprinted with permission.

How Is Stroke Treated?

Unfortunately, stroke cannot be cured. The brain cannot heal itself the same way the rest of the body does. If a tiny part of the brain is injured by stroke, that tiny part of the brain will never "grow back" or be the same as it was before the stroke happened.

Fortunately, the brain has other ways of responding to an injury. If a small part of the brain is permanently injured and cannot do its job anymore, other parts of the brain often "pitch in" and take over the job the injured part of the brain used to do. Retraining parts of the brain to do different jobs is slow, difficult work. This is why, for many children with stroke, the most important part of their treatment is neurorehabilitation, where children work with doctors, nurses, and special therapists who are experts in helping children retrain their brains. Neurorehabilitation includes many different therapies, such as physical or speech therapy, that are selected to treat individual symptoms.

For example, a child who has trouble with words will probably spend a lot of time working with a speech therapist. A child who has a weak left hand may work with a physical therapist to strengthen the hand. An occupational therapist might help the child relearn how to do things with the hand that are important to daily life, like using a zipper or holding a cup. Often, children with weak hands and arms get constraint therapy, in which a large mitten is placed on the strong hand to help a child practice using the weak hand.

Neurorehabilitation is hard work for kids and parents, and there is no guarantee that a symptom will ever completely go away. However, the effort is worth it because most children can significantly improve their symptoms with the proper rehabilitative therapy.

Other treatment options are specific to the individual child. For example, a child who has seizures because of a stroke might need anti-seizure medication. Some kids might need to take blood-thinning medication. And if a child has a medical condition that caused a stroke, that medical condition should be treated as well. Your doctor will explain to you what treatments will work best for your child.

Section 40.2

Recognition and Treatment of Pediatric Stroke

Excerpted from "Recognition and Treatment of Stroke in Children," by the National Institute of Neurological Disorders and Stroke (NINDS, www. ninds.nih.gov), part of the National Institutes of Health, February 9, 2005.

Introduction

Despite growing appreciation by neurologists that cerebrovascular disorders occur more often in children than once suspected, the study of stroke in children and adolescents has remained largely descriptive. Child neurologists often encounter children with a cerebrovascular lesion, yet large scale clinical research is difficult because these disorders are less common than in adults and arise from diverse causes. Three fundamental problems hinder both clinical research and the routine clinical care of children with cerebrovascular disease:

- The infrequency of cerebrovascular disorders in children makes it difficult to organize multicenter controlled clinical trials of the sort done in adults in recent years. The relative rarity of stroke in children also contributes to the still remaining reluctance of some clinicians to consider the diagnosis in individual children.

- The causes of cerebrovascular disease in children are legion, and no one risk factor predominates. Thus, not only is stroke less common in children, but the diversity of risk factors creates a heterogeneous patient population which hinders clinical research.

- Despite improved diagnostic techniques which make rapid, noninvasive diagnosis of cerebrovascular disease possible, many

375

physicians still know very little about cerebrovascular disorders in children. This lack of awareness contributes to delayed diagnosis and in the near future will make it more difficult to use thrombolytic agents or other treatments which require early diagnosis and treatment.

Frequency of Pediatric Cerebrovascular Disease

Although cerebrovascular disorders occur less often in children than in adults, recognition of stroke in children has probably increased because of the widespread application of noninvasive diagnostic studies such as magnetic resonance imaging (MRI), magnetic resonance angiography (MRA), computed tomography (CT) and, in the neonate, cranial ultrasound studies. These studies allow confirmation of a diagnosis that in previous years would not have been suspected or at least not recognized as a vascular lesion. Also, the number of patients with cerebrovascular lesions from certain risk factors may have increased as more effective treatments for some causes of stroke have allowed patients to survive long enough to develop vascular complications. Patients with sickle cell disease or with leukemia, for example, now have a longer life expectancy, and during this time they may have a stroke.

Most of the pediatric cerebrovascular literature consists of single case reports or small groups of children with a common etiology. These reports offer some insight into the relative frequency of various causes of stroke and draw attention to individual risk factors, but their usefulness is otherwise limited. Larger series of children selected for a common anatomic lesion or a single cause offer additional insight into the unique features of cerebrovascular lesions in children, but patients collected from large medical centers may not be representative of all children with stroke. None of these studies can accurately judge the incidence of cerebrovascular disease in children.

Schoenberg and colleagues studied cerebrovascular disease in children of Rochester, Minnesota, from 1965 through 1974. Excluding strokes related to intracranial infection, trauma, or birth, they found three hemorrhagic strokes and one ischemic stroke in an average at risk population of 15,834, for an estimated average annual incidence rate of 1.89/100,000/year and 0.63/100,000/year for hemorrhagic and ischemic strokes respectively. Their overall average annual incidence rate for children through fourteen years of age was 2.52/100,000/year. In this population, hemorrhagic strokes occurred more often than ischemic strokes, while in the Mayo Clinic referral population, ischemic strokes were more common. The risk of childhood cerebrovascular disease in this study is about half the risk for neoplasms of the central nervous system of children, but neonates and children with traumatic lesions are excluded. Despite our impression that cerebrovascular disorders are recognized more often in children than in previous years, Broderick and colleagues found an incidence of 2.7 cases/100,000/year, similar to the figure reported by Schoenberg and colleagues. In the Canadian Pediatric Ischemic Stroke Registry incidence of arterial and venous occlusion is estimated to be 1.2/100,000 children/year.

The frequency of several individual risk factors for stroke in children is known, but in most instances, the occurrence of secondary cerebrovascular disease is so variable that it is difficult to assess the relative contribution of each risk factor to the problem of cerebrovascular disease as a whole. In one report which included both children and young adults, children were less likely than young adult stroke patients to have identifiable risk factors and more often fall victim to infectious or inflammatory disorders. The implication is that children may have additional, as yet unknown, risk factors.

Etiology of Stroke in Children

Probably the most fundamental difference between cerebrovascular diseases in children and adults is the wide array of risk factors seen in children versus adults. Congenital heart disease and sickle cell disease, for example, are common causes of stroke in children, while atherosclerosis is rare in children. No cause can be detected in about a fifth of the children with ischemic infarction, yet many of these children seem to do well. The recognized causes of cerebrovascular disorders in children are numerous, and the probability of identifying the cause depends on the thoroughness of the evaluation. A probable cause of cerebral infarction was identified in 184 of 228 (79%) children in the Canadian Pediatric Ischemic Stroke Registry. The source of an intracranial hemorrhage is even more likely to be found.

The most common cause of stroke in children is probably congenital or acquired heart disease. In the Canadian Pediatric Ischemic Stroke Registry, heart disease was found in 40 of 228 (19%) of the children with arterial thrombosis. Many of these children are already known to have heart disease prior to their stroke, but in other instances a less obvious cardiac lesion is discovered only after a stroke. Complex cardiac anomalies involving both the valves and chambers are collectively the biggest problem, but virtually any cardiac lesion can sometimes lead to a stroke. Of particular concern are cyanotic lesions with polycythemia, which increase the risk of both thrombosis and embolism.

Both the frequency and the cause of pediatric stroke may depend somewhat on both the geographic location and the specific hospital setting. The Canadian Pediatric Ischemic Stroke Registry, for example, lists only 5 children (2%) with cerebral infarction due to sickle cell anemia. A large metropolitan hospital in the United States might care for this many patients in a year, but early estimates that cerebral infarction occurred in 17% of people with sickle cell disease proved far higher than the 4–5% figure derived from more representative samples in Jamaica and in Africa.

Prehospital Emergency Care

Lack of general awareness of cerebrovascular disorders in children probably delays medical attention for children with cerebrovascular disorders. It is not unusual, for example, for children with a cerebral infarction to be brought to a physician several days after the onset of symptoms. In contrast, family members are usually well aware of the significance of an acute neurological impairment in older individuals, and these patients are typically seen by a physician earlier than children with a similar lesion.

Data from the Canadian Pediatric Ischemic Stroke Registry indicate that 48–72 hours often elapse between the onset of symptoms of arterial occlusion and a child's diagnosis. Venous occlusion was discovered a bit more quickly than arterial occlusion, at least in younger children, perhaps because of the common occurrence of epileptic seizures in children with venous thrombosis. This seems to be fairly typical of the pattern seen in the United States as well. The typical adult with a new onset neurological deficit from cerebrovascular disease undoubtedly sees a physician much sooner. It is likely that this delay in the diagnosis of children reflects a lack of awareness by both physicians and families that cerebrovascular disease occurs in children. To the extent that treatment might be improved by earlier evaluation and treatment, prompt recognition and treatment could improve management.

Treatment and Rehabilitation

No randomized controlled treatment trials have been completed in children with stroke; many of the procedures increasingly used in children with cerebrovascular disease have been adapted from studies in adults. Accumulating experience with antithrombotic and anticoagulant treatment in children suggests that these agents can be safely used in children, though their efficacy and proper dose still need to be established by controlled trials. Thrombolytic agents should be as effective in children as in adults, but the safety data are inadequate for children and the timing and dosage need to be determined for children and adolescents.

Chapter 41

Innovations in Treating Acute Stroke

Chapter Contents

Section 41.1

Removing Clots from Blocked Arteries: The MERCI Retriever

Excerpted from "Brain Attack—A Look at Stroke Prevention and Treatment," by Michelle Meadows, published in *FDA Consumer* magazine, by the U.S. Food and Drug Administration (FDA, www.fda.gov), March-April 2005.

In August 2004, the Food and Drug Administration cleared the first device to remove blood clots in the brain in people with ischemic stroke. The MERCI Retriever—Mechanical Embolus Removal for Cerebral Ischemia—is made by Concentric Medical Inc. of Mountain View, California.

"The device is a catheter with a coiled tip that grasps the clot and allows it to be removed by the physician," says Miriam Provost, deputy director of the FDA's Division of General, Restorative and Neurological Devices. "It may provide an option for some patients who aren't eligible for tPA [tissue plasminogen activator]."

The risks of the MERCI Retriever include bleeding and vessel punctures. The National Institute of Neurological Disorders and Stroke is funding a clinical trial that continues to study the device. The MERCI Retriever is intended for use by interventional radiologists, doctors who are specially trained to use imaging techniques to view the inside of the body while they guide small instruments through blood vessels to the site of the problem.

Section 41.2

The Hyperbaric Oxygen Therapy Debate

"Hyperbaric Oxygen Therapy Debate," *Stroke Smart* Magazine, January-February 2006. © National Stroke Association. Reprinted with permission.

When consumers began hearing about hyperbaric oxygen therapy as a treatment for stroke survivors as recently as 10 years ago, questions poured in to federal agencies on whether the alternative therapy helped the recovery process.

"People were asking a lot of questions so we decided to study it as a topic for one of our reports," said Susan Carson, senior research associate of the Oregon Evidence-Based Practice Center, which prepared a report for the federal Agency for Healthcare Research and Quality. Although the treatment is FDA-approved for conditions like deep-sea sickness seen in scuba divers and wound healing, it is not approved for stroke.

The center examined studies on hyperbaric oxygen therapy—a treatment in which patients inhale 100 percent oxygen while inside a special chamber that is pressurized to greater than 1 atmosphere (atm). Oxygen has weight and the air we breathe is made up of about 21% oxygen. One atm is the pressure caused by the air's weight (the atmosphere) at sea level. If the oxygen content of the air rises, it weighs more and exerts more pressure. Most hyperbaric oxygen chambers have a pressure from 1 to 3 atm because the amount of oxygen in the chamber is greater than in the air we breathe. The extra oxygen in the air has the potential to help heal tissues, like skin damaged by wounds or burns. For stroke, the idea is that increased oxygen in the body can help heal the damaged brain tissue.

Hyperbaric treatment sessions generally are 90 to 120 minutes, although duration and frequency were not standardized, according to Carson.

"In addition to looking at studies, we talked to patients and practitioners as part of our research," said Carson. "Some thought it was almost miraculous and others thought there was no benefit at all."

At the Brain Therapeutics Medical Clinic in Mission Viejo, California, David Steenblock, D.O., is a strong proponent of hyperbaric oxygen therapy and has combined it with physical therapy, biofeedback, vitamins, and more typical stroke treatments in treating 1,200 survivors.

"It's one more tool you can use in the recovery process," said Steenblock. "Strokes are caused by lack of oxygen to part of the brain. Hyperbaric oxygen therapy increases oxygen to the damaged cells." Steenblock said 90 to 95 percent of his patients had "significant improvement to one or more of their faculties (communication, thinking, or movement skills) damaged by stroke" after participating in the program, which includes a 60 daily treatments in a hyperbaric chamber at a cost of $6,000 to $9,000. Combined with physical therapy and other treatments, his program generally costs $20,000 to $23,000. The costs are not covered by insurance.

"I've seen patients come in [with] a wheelchair and walk out with a cane," said Steenblock. "They regain some independence and it eliminates the use and cost of a caregiver so why not give it a try. I wish I could tell you that 95 percent of the people see total improvement, but I can't. But your chances are much enhanced under this program."

When Carson and her team set out to study hyperbaric oxygen therapy for stroke, they found a handful of controlled studies, including just three she categorized as "fair quality studies." A controlled study uses two groups of patients that use different treatments (one a real treatment and the other a placebo/no treatment) so the effectiveness can be compared. In scientific terms, a controlled study carries more weight than an uncontrolled study, which looks at one treatment.

"Overall, our findings were that the best evidence shows no benefits from treatments. But, we couldn't conclude that we were sure there was no benefit because the studies were so small," she said.

She noted that the studies often weren't blind, meaning those in the study knew they were getting the treatment and not a placebo, which could have biased them. The type of patient who participated in the studies varied, too.

"Sometimes they were treated within 24 hours, sometimes three months later, so that also made it hard to make any kind of generalization," she said. Uncontrolled or observational studies were even more uncertain, she said, as they reported favorable and sometimes dramatic results, but failed to prove that these results were directly related to hyperbaric oxygen therapy.

"It would be very hard for a patient or a clinician to make a decision about this treatment and the best thing they can do is educate themselves and to look at the source of the information they find in trying to make a decision," said Carson.

For more information about hyperbaric oxygen therapy, visit the National Center for Complementary and Alternative Medicine at http://nccam.nih.gov or call 888-644-6226 (866-464-3615 for TTY users). The government's latest reports on hyperbaric oxygen treatment for stroke can be found at www.ahrq.gov or by calling 301-427-1364.

Section 41.3

Snake Venom Used to Treat Stroke Patients

"NJ doctors tap snake venom to treat stroke patients," by Angela Davis, *The Star-Ledger,* February 5, 2008. © 2008 *The Star-Ledger.* All rights reserved. Reprinted with permission.

The venom of the Malaysian pit viper is the potent ingredient found in an experimental drug called Viprinex now being tested at three New Jersey hospitals. When given intravenously, Viprinex has been shown to help dissolve clots that plug arteries and cut off oxygen and blood flow to the brain.

According to doctors, the major advantage of Viprinex, which also thins the blood, is that it may be effective as long as six hours after a stroke patient's symptoms begin. That would double the window of the only government-approved clot-busting therapy, called tPA, which must be given within three hours.

The fact that less than five percent of stroke victims get to a hospital in time has greatly limited the use of tPA, or tissue plasminogen activator. In addition, some doctors are hesitant to use the drug, which has been available since 1996, because it causes bleeding in the brain in about six percent of patients.

"What many investigators have been looking for is something that can dissolve clots with less risk of bleeding," said Martin Gizzi, the neurologist who heads the New Jersey Neuroscience Institute at JFK Medical Center in Edison, which is participating in a clinical trial of Viprinex.

Under the trial's guidelines, some patients will receive Viprinex, while others get a placebo. Doctors won't know who got the real thing until the research—which is being conducted at 200 sites worldwide—has

385

been completed in 2009. Patients are followed for 90 days after receiving the drug so their level of recovery can be assessed.

The drug is derived from the venom of the Malaysian pit viper, an aggressive snake that inhabits forest edges across much of Southeast Asia and grows to about three feet in length. The venom is frozen before being purified and converted to a drug product, explained Warren Wasiewski, the scientist overseeing the trial for Neurobiological Technologies Inc., the Edgewater drug company that makes the drug.

Section 41.4

Arthritis Drug Shows Promise for Reducing Brain Hemorrhage in Premature Babies

From the National Institute of Neurological Disorders and Stroke (NINDS, www.ninds.nih.gov), part of the National Institutes of Health, August 27, 2007.

A drug that is commonly used to reduce the pain of arthritis may eventually be used in pregnant women with preterm labor to lessen the risk of brain damage in very low birth weight babies, a study suggests.

Premature infants, especially those born before 32 weeks of gestation and weighing under 1,500 grams (about 3 pounds, 5 ounces), are at high risk of brain hemorrhages, or bleeding, that can lead to cerebral palsy, seizures, and other long-term problems. Brain hemorrhages affect about 12,000 premature infants each year in the United States. Most of these bleeds occur in a part of the brain called the germinal matrix, a structure near the brain ventricles where all the developing baby's brain cells originate. This structure normally disappears by 36 weeks of gestation.

In the new study, led by Dr. Praveen Ballabh at New York Medical College-Westchester Medical Center in Valhalla, New York, and Dr. Maiken Nedergaard at the University of Rochester Medical Center in New York, researchers traced the high risk of germinal matrix hemorrhage to newly formed blood vessels in that part of the brain.

Administering the drug celecoxib, which is commonly used to treat arthritis pain, reduced the proliferation of these blood vessels and substantially decreased the incidence of brain hemorrhage in an animal model. The study was funded in part by the National Institute of Neurological Disorders and Stroke (NINDS) and appears in the journal *Nature Medicine.*[1]

The germinal matrix produces new neurons and glial cells that then migrate to other parts of the brain. Maintaining this activity requires a large amount of blood and oxygen, so the germinal matrix grows many temporary blood vessels to support the neuron development, Dr. Ballabh explains. This process of forming new blood vessels, called angiogenesis, is triggered by proteins called vascular endothelial growth factor (VEGF) and angiopoietin-2 (ANGPT-2).

Unfortunately, newly developed blood vessels in the germinal matrix are very fragile. When a baby is born before the germinal matrix disappears, the premature infant's unstable medical condition can cause fluctuations in blood pressure, which in turn can rupture the fragile germinal matrix blood vessels. Some hemorrhages are very small and cause few problems, but others cause severe brain damage.

In the new study, Dr. Ballabh and his colleagues examined autopsied human brain tissue from fetuses, premature infants, and full-term babies. They found that, in fetuses and premature infants, VEGF and ANGPT-2 were more abundant in the germinal matrix than in the brain's cortex and white matter. The amount of blood vessel proliferation was also much greater in the germinal matrix than in other areas. The proliferation decreased soon after birth. The researchers suspect that the increased blood oxygen after babies began to breathe air reduced the level of VEGF, halting the development of new blood vessels.

Dr. Ballabh reasoned that reducing the amount of VEGF and ANGPT-2 in the brain just prior to birth might temporarily stop the development of new blood vessels in the germinal matrix and make the brain less likely to bleed. The researchers tested this idea by giving pregnant rabbits either of two inhibitors of angiogenesis, celecoxib or another drug called ZD6474, for several days prior to birth. Both drugs reduced the level of VEGF and decreased the incidence and severity of brain hemorrhage in premature rabbit pups.

While both drugs appeared to be safe in pregnant rabbits, most of the pups born after ZD6474 treatment died 3 to 4 days after birth, Dr. Ballabh says. In contrast, the celecoxib-treated pups remained apparently healthy. Celecoxib is sometimes used to suppress preterm labor in women, and it has few known adverse effects.

The researchers are now planning additional studies to examine the safety and effectiveness of celecoxib and ZD6474 in animal models. These studies will examine whether the drugs affect neuron development, lung function, and other characteristics in newborn animals. The investigators will also try to determine the best dose of the medication to prevent brain hemorrhage without causing adverse effects. The doses of medication used in the initial study were quite large, so it is unclear whether smaller doses would be effective. If all goes well, Dr. Ballabh hopes to eventually begin a clinical trial to determine if treating women in preterm labor with celecoxib or a similar drug can prevent brain damage in premature babies.

1. Ballabh P, Xu H, Hu F, Braun A, Smith K, Rivera A, Lou N, Ungvari Z, Goldman SA, Csiszar A, Nedergaard M. Angiogenic inhibition reduces germinal matrix hemorrhage. *Nature Medicine,* April 2007, vol. 13, no. 4, pp. 477–485.

Chapter 42

Gene Therapy for Cardiovascular Diseases and Stroke

Chapter Contents

Section 42.1

What Is Gene Therapy?

Excerpted from "Gene Therapy," by the U.S. Department of Energy
Office of Science (www.ornl.gov), Office of Biological and Environmental
Research, Human Genome Program, August 6, 2007.

What is gene therapy?

Genes, which are carried on chromosomes, are the basic physical and functional units of heredity. Genes are specific sequences of bases that encode instructions on how to make proteins. Although genes get a lot of attention, it's the proteins that perform most life functions and even make up the majority of cellular structures. When genes are altered so that the encoded proteins are unable to carry out their normal functions, genetic disorders can result.

Gene therapy is a technique for correcting defective genes responsible for disease development. Researchers may use one of several approaches for correcting faulty genes:

- A normal gene may be inserted into a nonspecific location within the genome to replace a nonfunctional gene. This approach is most common.

- An abnormal gene could be swapped for a normal gene through homologous recombination.

- The abnormal gene could be repaired through selective reverse mutation, which returns the gene to its normal function.

- The regulation (the degree to which a gene is turned on or off) of a particular gene could be altered.

How does gene therapy work?

In most gene therapy studies, a "normal" gene is inserted into the genome to replace an "abnormal," disease-causing gene. A carrier molecule called a vector must be used to deliver the therapeutic gene to the patient's target cells. Currently, the most common vector is a

390

virus that has been genetically altered to carry normal human DNA [deoxyribonucleic acid]. Viruses have evolved a way of encapsulating and delivering their genes to human cells in a pathogenic manner. Scientists have tried to take advantage of this capability and manipulate the virus genome to remove disease-causing genes and insert therapeutic genes.

Target cells such as the patient's liver or lung cells are infected with the viral vector. The vector then unloads its genetic material containing the therapeutic human gene into the target cell. The generation of a functional protein product from the therapeutic gene restores the target cell to a normal state.

Some of the different types of viruses used as gene therapy vectors:

- **Retroviruses**—A class of viruses that can create double-stranded DNA copies of their RNA [ribonucleic acid] genomes. These copies of its genome can be integrated into the chromosomes of host cells. Human immunodeficiency virus (HIV) is a retrovirus.

- **Adenoviruses**—A class of viruses with double-stranded DNA genomes that cause respiratory, intestinal, and eye infections in humans. The virus that causes the common cold is an adenovirus.

- **Adeno-associated viruses**—A class of small, single-stranded DNA viruses that can insert their genetic material at a specific site on chromosome 19.

- **Herpes simplex viruses**—A class of double-stranded DNA viruses that infect a particular cell type, neurons. Herpes simplex virus type 1 is a common human pathogen that causes cold sores.

Besides virus-mediated gene-delivery systems, there are several nonviral options for gene delivery. The simplest method is the direct introduction of therapeutic DNA into target cells. This approach is limited in its application because it can be used only with certain tissues and requires large amounts of DNA.

Another nonviral approach involves the creation of an artificial lipid sphere with an aqueous core. This liposome, which carries the therapeutic DNA, is capable of passing the DNA through the target cell's membrane.

Therapeutic DNA also can get inside target cells by chemically linking the DNA to a molecule that will bind to special cell receptors. Once bound to these receptors, the therapeutic DNA constructs are engulfed by the cell membrane and passed into the interior of the target cell. This delivery system tends to be less effective than other options.

Researchers also are experimenting with introducing a 47th (artificial human) chromosome into target cells. This chromosome would exist autonomously alongside the standard 46—not affecting their workings or causing any mutations. It would be a large vector capable of carrying substantial amounts of genetic code, and scientists anticipate that, because of its construction and autonomy, the body's immune systems would not attack it. A problem with this potential method is the difficulty in delivering such a large molecule to the nucleus of a target cell.

What is the current status of gene therapy research?

The Food and Drug Administration (FDA) has not yet approved any human gene therapy product for sale. Current gene therapy is experimental and has not proven very successful in clinical trials. Little progress has been made since the first gene therapy clinical trial began in 1990. In 1999, gene therapy suffered a major setback with the death of 18-year-old Jesse Gelsinger. Jesse was participating in a gene therapy trial for ornithine transcarboxylase deficiency (OTCD). He died from multiple organ failures 4 days after starting the treatment. His death is believed to have been triggered by a severe immune response to the adenovirus carrier.

Another major blow came in January 2003, when the FDA placed a temporary halt on all gene therapy trials using retroviral vectors in blood stem cells. FDA took this action after it learned that a second child treated in a French gene therapy trial had developed a leukemia-like condition. Both this child and another who had developed a similar condition in August 2002 had been successfully treated by gene therapy for X-linked severe combined immunodeficiency disease (X-SCID), also known as "bubble baby syndrome."

FDA's Biological Response Modifiers Advisory Committee (BRMAC) met at the end of February 2003 to discuss possible measures that could allow a number of retroviral gene therapy trials for treatment of life-threatening diseases to proceed with appropriate safeguards. In April of 2003 the FDA eased the ban on gene therapy trials using retroviral vectors in blood stem cells.

What factors have kept gene therapy from becoming an effective treatment for genetic disease?

- **Short-lived nature of gene therapy**—Before gene therapy can become a permanent cure for any condition, the therapeutic

DNA introduced into target cells must remain functional and the cells containing the therapeutic DNA must be long-lived and stable. Problems with integrating therapeutic DNA into the genome and the rapidly dividing nature of many cells prevent gene therapy from achieving any long-term benefits. Patients will have to undergo multiple rounds of gene therapy.

- **Immune response**—Anytime a foreign object is introduced into human tissues, the immune system is designed to attack the invader. The risk of stimulating the immune system in a way that reduces gene therapy effectiveness is always a potential risk. Furthermore, the immune system's enhanced response to invaders it has seen before makes it difficult for gene therapy to be repeated in patients.

- **Problems with viral vectors**—Viruses, while the carrier of choice in most gene therapy studies, the patient—toxicity, immune and inflammatory responses, and gene control and targeting issues. In addition, there is always the fear that the viral vector, once inside the patient, may recover its ability to cause disease.

- **Multigene disorders**—Conditions or disorders that arise from mutations in a single gene are the best candidates for gene therapy.

Unfortunately, some the most commonly occurring disorders, such as heart disease, high blood pressure, Alzheimer disease, arthritis, and diabetes, are caused by the combined effects of variations in many genes. Multigene or multifactorial disorders such as these would be especially difficult to treat effectively using gene therapy.

Section 42.2

Gene Therapy Could Prevent Stroke Damage

Reprinted with permission from "UI Study Identifies Damaging Mechanism in Transplants, Heart Attacks," University of Iowa News Services, March 2, 2004. © 2004 The University of Iowa. All rights reserved.

A University of Iowa [UI] study suggests that inhibiting a certain protein involved in inflammation might be of therapeutic benefit in organ transplantation, heart attacks, and possibly stroke. The study, led by John Engelhardt, Ph.D., UI professor and interim head of anatomy and cell biology, found that blocking the action of this protein can prevent the tissue damage caused by ischemia/reperfusion injury. The study is published in the March 1 [2004] issue of the *Journal of Clinical Investigation.*

Ischemia/reperfusion injury is a common, damaging component of organ transplantation, heart attack, and stroke and is a determinant of organ failure in all cases. In this type of injury, the organ is initially deprived of oxygen-carrying blood (ischemia). During reperfusion (the re-establishment of blood supply), toxins are briefly generated from the oxygen that lead to tissue damage and trigger a potentially detrimental inflammatory response.

Although inflammation is an important bodily response to environmental injuries including bacterial and viral infection as well as ischemia/reperfusion injury, too much inflammation can damage healthy tissue and cause problems.

"In this study we looked at a well-known 'master switch' type of protein called NF-kB that controls the expression of genes that regulate inflammatory responses," said Engelhardt, who also is professor of internal medicine in the UI Roy J. and Lucille A. Carver College of Medicine and director of the UI Center for Gene Therapy of Cystic Fibrosis and Other Genetic Diseases.

Engelhardt and his colleagues, including graduate student and lead author of the study, Chenguang Fan, compared the activation of NF-kB in response to bacterial infection and ischemia/ reperfusion injury. Historically, these two types of injury were thought to produce inflammation via the same cellular pathway. However, the UI researchers found that there are two distinct pathways for the two different types of injury.

"Important health implications have emerged from these studies, which may aid us in treating environmental injuries that have both ischemic and inflammatory components. We can now selectively remove, like a molecular surgeon, activation of one or both of these pathways using gene therapy approaches," Engelhardt said. "We found that selective inhibition of the pathway triggered by ischemia/reperfusion injury was better for the organ and better for the animal."

Activation of NF-kB is tightly controlled by so-called inhibitory proteins. Two of these inhibitory proteins, IkB alpha and IkB beta, keep NF-kB in an inactive state. However, injury leads to modification of the inhibitory proteins, causing them to release NF-kB. The activated master switch protein can then regulate expression of genes that mount a response to the injury.

The UI team used gene manipulation to replace IkB alpha with IkB beta in mice. Mice with only IkB beta protein respond to bacterial infection in the same way that normal mice do. However, these mice sustain less liver damage and were more likely to survive ischemic/reperfusion injury to that organ than mice with both inhibitory proteins.

The study found that the two inhibitory proteins function similarly in response to bacterial infection, but have different abilities to activate NF-kB after ischemia/reperfusion injury. Furthermore, the results suggest that inhibiting the IkB alpha pathway could prevent ischemic/reperfusion injury to transplanted organs and therefore improve the success of this procedure.

Similarly, Engelhardt speculated that blocking this pathway in patients at risk of a heart attack—a patient undergoing angioplasty, for example—potentially could benefit those patients in the event of a heart attack.

In addition to the animal experiments, the UI team also used gene therapy to manipulate the activation of NF-kB. These experiments helped reveal the different molecular pathways that activate NF-kB as a result of different types of injury.

"Gene therapy was a tool we used to address the mechanism of the disease process. But once you understand the process, those gene therapy tools become potential therapeutic tools," Engelhardt added. "This research has led to a better understanding of the disease process that occurs following ischemic/ reperfusion injury and a better understanding will allow us to potentially prevent or treat ischemic organ injury disorders."

In addition to Engelhardt and Fan, the research team also included Qiang Li, Yulong Zhang, Xiaoming Liu, D.V.M., Ph.D., Meihui Luo, Duane Abbott, and Weihong Zhou, M.D. The research was supported by grants from the National Institutes of Health.

Part Four

Stroke Complications

Chapter 43

Complications and Medical Problems Associated with Stroke

Stroke is a complicated medical condition which can affect each person differently. Some problems resulting from stroke can be very serious; others are more minor. Here is a list of common medical problems associated with stroke.

Heart/Cardiovascular Complications

- Congestive heart failure
- Atrial fibrillation
- Coronary artery disease
- Angina
- Hypertension
- Orthostatic hypotension

Signs

- Chest pain
- Sweating
- Nausea or vomiting
- Shortness of breath

- Jaw, neck, shoulder, or arm pain
- Dizziness; falling
- Restlessness or fatigue
- Rapid weight gain—two or three pounds within a day
- Swelling, especially in legs and feet
- Frequent coughing or urination at night

If these symptoms occur, call your doctor or 911 immediately.

Prevention

- Take medicines as instructed.
- Follow dietary guidelines as instructed.
- Exercise every day to prevent loss of muscle tone, strengthen the heart, and improve blood flow. Follow your home program but stop and call your doctor if you notice any of the warning signs.
- Follow your bowel program and do not push down when moving your bowels.

Seizures

Signs

- Sudden involuntary movements
- Staring
- Loss of control including bladder and bowel
- Teeth clenching
- Drooling
- Rigid posturing

If these symptoms occur, lie down on one side with a soft cushion under the head. Protect from sharp objects or corners. Call your doctor or 911 immediately.

Prevention

- Take medicines as instructed.

- If using antiseizure drugs, follow doctor's advice for regular blood checks.

Pneumonia

A disease of the lungs caused by infection

Signs

- Very fast or very slow breathing
- Shallow breaths
- Confusion or behavior changes
- Chills or fever
- Chest pains
- Problems swallowing
- Vomiting

If these symptoms occur, call your doctor or 911 immediately.

Prevention

- Use extra pillows to sleep with the head elevated. This helps make breathing easier.
- Drink plenty of fluids. This can help make coughing up secretions easier.
- Stay warm and comfortable as much as possible.
- Do breathing exercises as ordered by your doctor or therapist.
- Change position at least once every two hours when you are in bed.
- Take deep breaths, using muscles of the chest to strengthen them.

Pulmonary Embolism

A blood clot in the lungs

Signs

- Coughing or wheezing

- Shortness of breath
- Chest pain
- Blue color around the mouth
- Dizziness

If these symptoms occur, call your doctor or 911 immediately.

Prevention

- Keep as active as possible.
- Take all medicines as ordered by your doctor. Blood thinners are often used to prevent clots.
- Wear elastic stockings (TED hose) when sitting or standing to prevent swelling in the legs and feet.

Deep Vein Thrombosis

Swelling of a vein with a blood clot, usually in the calf or thigh

Signs

- Redness, swelling, or warmth in an area that is different when compared to the other leg.

If this occurs, check for fever. Stay in bed. Do not rub or exercise legs. Call doctor, home health nurse, or go to an emergency room immediately.

Prevention

- Stay active.
- Do exercises as instructed.
- Wear elastic stockings if prescribed.

Shoulder Problems

Signs

- Pain when resting and with movement.
- Limited movement of the shoulder.

If this occurs, contact your doctor or therapist. A sling or other device may be necessary.

Prevention

- Do exercises as instructed.
- Take ordered medicines to help with pain.

Shoulder Hand Syndrome

Signs

- Pain in the shoulder
- Limited movement
- Swelling or tenderness over the top of the hand

If these occur, contact your doctor or therapist.

Prevention

- Do exercises as instructed by the doctor or therapist.
- Take medicines as prescribed.
- Use heat and massage to help manage pain.
- Elevate hand on a pillow while in bed.
- Wear a compression glove on the swollen hand if prescribed.

Spasticity

Signs

- Pain in arms or legs
- Muscle spasms
- Muscle tightness

If these occur, talk to your doctor. Discuss whether spasticity is interfering with your recovery.

Prevention

- Do range of motion and stretching exercises as ordered by your doctor or therapist.

- Wear prescribed splints.
- Take medicines.

Swallowing Problems (Dysphagia)

Signs

- Food getting stuck on the weaker side of the mouth
- Coughing before, during, or after swallowing
- Food or fluid feeling stuck in the throat after swallowing
- Swallowing repeatedly

If this occurs, call your doctor or therapist. A swallowing test and special swallowing tips may be necessary.

Sleep Problems

Signs

- Early morning waking
- Getting up frequently in the night

If this occurs, talk to your doctor about sleep habits.

Prevention

- Avoid using bed for activities other than sleeping such as eating, watching TV, and talking on the phone.
- Limit fluid intake after 6:00 p.m.
- Empty bladder right before going to bed.
- If not getting enough sleep at night, try taking a scheduled nap.

Chapter 44

Pain after Stroke

A stroke can leave someone with various physical effects, such as weakness, paralysis, or changes in sensation. Unfortunately some people also experience pain after stroke. This text outlines some of the different causes of pain after stroke and the treatments that are available.

Stroke causes interruption and damage to the normal functioning of the brain, often resulting in weakness (hemiparesis) or paralysis (hemiplegia) on one side of the body. This can unfortunately lead to spasticity and other painful conditions.

As with many aspects of stroke, pain may have to be lived with for some time, but there are coping techniques that can be learned, and physiotherapy and other treatments are successful in many instances.

Frozen Shoulder (Adhesive Capsulitis)

This is not uncommon after a stroke and always occurs on the affected side, resulting in prolonged stiffness, loss of movement, and often severe pain. This can be avoided by:

- **Correct positioning and handling:** After the stroke, good movement and positioning, including shoulder care, are vital (see below).

- **Mobilizing the shoulder:** In the first stage of treatment, passive movement can be applied by the physiotherapist to counteract the paralysis and loss of coordination arising from the stroke and keep the shoulder joint mobile.

- **Avoiding overstrenuous arm movements:** If a particular activity makes the shoulder hurt, the individual should stop it immediately. Carrying on with it will not make the pain wear off and may make things worse.

Shoulder Care

Stroke people are vulnerable on their weak side—where the weight of the affected limb may cause tissue damage, which is then difficult to treat. Some people can feel a gap at the shoulder joint. This does not mean that the shoulder is dislocated, but it is a warning sign that the joint is not supported properly by the muscles. There is a risk that the soft tissue around the joint can become nipped between the bones, causing inflammation, pain, and damage, or "shoulder subluxation."

The affected arm initially needs to be placed on a pillow to provide support, as gravity alone can dislocate the joint. Stroke people should not be pulled, however gently, by the arm. A skilled physiotherapist will then work to restore normal movement and postural control.

Spasticity and Contractures after Stroke

Spasticity means stiffness, and results from the brain losing control of the muscles, allowing them to tighten or develop "increased muscle tone." From the beginning, people who need it should have help with the correct positioning of their limbs, which we now realize can help prevent spasticity developing.

Some degree of spasticity is found in almost every patient with hemiplegia. The tightness is always there, and although regular physiotherapy can help to partly release it, it means that movement still requires extra effort.

Some people who have had a stroke find they develop contractures in their affected limbs (where the muscles tighten up and can't be straightened out). This can make normal mobility impossible and cause painful muscular spasms. It can happen sometimes even if the person has had regular physiotherapy.

Once the muscles start tightening, it is difficult to get them to relax again and the doctors may want to consider using drugs or Botox to help reduce the pain and disability that can follow from what is termed high, or excessive, muscle tone.

Central Poststroke Pain

Approximately 5 percent of people who have a stroke will develop nerve pain from the stroke called central poststroke pain (CPSP). The pain is often described as an icy burning sensation. The onset of pain may occur at the time of the stroke but more often several months later.

The pain is felt in the part of the body affected by the stroke. In 20 percent of people, the pain gets better over a period of years. In 30 percent of these, there is a lessening of pain over the first year.

The precise cause of the pain is unknown. In some cases it is due to damage to the thalamus, the brain's "pain center." Because the brain is damaged, it feels pain when it should be feeling a sensation that is not painful.

Usual painkillers have little effect on this pain. Some medications originally developed for epilepsy and depression can have a positive effect. Referral to a pain clinic, relaxation, visualization techniques, meditation, aromatherapy, counseling, and hypnotherapy can also be helpful.

Transcutaneous Electrical Nerve Stimulation (TENS)

This alternative to drugs for pain management is widely used by hospitals and pain clinics throughout the United Kingdom. It is best for treating "localized" pain including arthritis, sciatica, lumbago, etc. There are no side effects and it can be used alongside any other medication without fear of interference. (People fitted with a cardiac pacemaker are advised not to use TENS unless under medical direction.)

The standard treatment time is around 40 minutes and this can provide several hours of significant or total relief from even chronic pain. Self adhesive pads (electrodes) are placed directly onto the skin around or adjacent to the area of pain. At the higher frequencies, it instigates "gateway control," which prevents the pain signals from moving along the nerve pathways. The lower frequencies help the body to release natural painkillers called endorphins.

Chapter 45

Stroke and Thinking Abilities

Stroke can cause physical problems. It can also affect cognition. Cognition refers to thinking abilities. It's how people use their brains to talk, read, write, learn, understand, reason, and remember. Losing skills in this area may affect how you manage everyday tasks, take part in rehabilitation, and live on your own after stroke.

Stroke and Thinking Abilities

Every stroke is unique. The effect the stroke has on your thinking abilities depends on where and how the stroke injured the brain, and your overall health.

Each side of the brain controls different things. So, a stroke on one side of the brain will cause different problems than a stroke on the other side.

Damage to one side of the brain can cause loss of language skills (talking, reading, writing, understanding what people say). It can also cause "verbal memory" loss or the ability to remember things having to do with words. Damage to the other side may cause attention, thinking, and behavior problems.

Stroke can also damage the front of the brain. In this case, you are more likely to lose your ability to control and organize thoughts and behavior. This makes it hard to think through the steps to complete a task. Front-brain strokes may not affect your ability to do or remember specific things.

Memory Loss

Memory loss after stroke is common, but not the same for everyone. There are many ways your memory can be affected by stroke.

- Verbal memory—memory of names, stories, and information having to do with words.

- Visual memory—memory of faces, shapes, routes, and things you see.

- If you have memory damage, you may have trouble learning new information or skills. Or you may be unable to remember and retrieve information.

- Stroke can cause vascular dementia (VaD), a greater decline in thinking abilities. Some experts believe that 10–20% of Americans over age 65 with dementia have VaD. This makes it second only to Alzheimer disease as a leading cause of dementia.

- Therapies or medicines almost never fully restore memory after stroke. But, many people do recover at least some memory spontaneously after stroke. Others improve through rehabilitation.

What may help:

- Try to form a routine—doing certain tasks at regular times during the day.

- Try not to tackle too many things at once. Break tasks down into steps.

- If something needs to be done, make a note of it or do it right away.

- Make a habit of always putting things away in the same place where they can be easily seen or found.

Aphasia

After a stroke, one of the most common thinking problems is trouble with communication. Aphasia is one of these problems. About one million people in the United States have aphasia. Most cases are the result of stroke.

Aphasia is a partial or total loss of ability to talk, understand what people say, read, or write. It may affect only one aspect of language. For example, you may be unable to remember the names of objects or put words together into sentences. More often, many aspects are affected at the same time.

There are several types of aphasia. They differ by where the brain is damaged.

- Global aphasia is the most severe form. People with global aphasia can speak few familiar words and barely understand what people say. They cannot read or write.

- Another form is Broca, or nonfluent, aphasia. People with this often omit certain kinds of words from sentences, speak slowly and with effort, and have a hard time with grammar. They mainly speak short statements of less than four words, like "walk dog."

- People with Wernicke, or fluent, aphasia talk easily. But they use the wrong sounds in words, say the wrong words, or even make up words.

You may recover from aphasia without treatment. Most, however, benefit from therapy by a speech and language therapist. The goal is to improve your ability to communicate with other people. This is done by helping you get back some of your language skills and learning new ways of getting your message across when needed.

Communication tips:

- Use props to make conversation easier (photos, maps).

- Draw or write things down on paper.

- Take your time. Make phone calls or try talking to people only when you have plenty of time.

- Show people what works best for you.

- Stay calm. Take one idea at a time.

- Create a communication book that includes words, pictures, and symbols that are helpful to you.

The internet can be used to talk to people via e-mail or to create a personal web page for yourself.

What Can Help

- Get information on stroke recovery from National Stroke Association. Visit www.stroke.org or call 800-STROKES (800-787-6537).

- Contact your local stroke association.

- Join a stroke support group. Other survivors will understand, validate your issues, and offer encouragement and ideas for dealing with memory loss.

Professionals Who Can Help

- Neuropsychologist—a doctor who can diagnose and treat changes in thinking, memory, and behavior after stroke. Ask your neurologist for a referral.

- Speech and language therapist—to find one in your area call the American Speech-Language-Hearing Association at 800-638-8255.

Rehabilitation is a lifetime commitment and an important part of recovering from a stroke. Through rehabilitation, you relearn basic skills such as talking, eating, dressing, and walking. Rehabilitation can also improve your strength, flexibility, and endurance. The goal is to regain as much independence as possible.

Remember to ask your doctor, "Where am I on my stroke recovery journey?"

Chapter 46

Impaired Cognition: Frequently Asked Questions

What is cognition?

Cognition is another word for thinking. Cognition is the process that is used to understand and interact with the world. Cognition is also used to describe how our brain functions to perceive and express our experiences.

What is meant by impaired cognition?

Impaired cognition means that the skills and abilities that a person had before their accident or medical problem now either are absent or have some defect in some important way. There are special names for some of these impairments; for example, an impairment in language skills that makes it hard for people to speak or understand speech is called aphasia.

How is cognition affected by brain injury?

Since a brain injury can affect any part of the brain, any of the thinking abilities the brain performs can be changed. Some of these abilities are attention, communication, visual perception (the ability to understand what we see), and memory. Very often, it is the parts

"Impaired Cognition: Frequently Asked Questions," by Robert J. Hartke, Ph.D. © 2008 Rehabilitation Institute of Chicago (www.lifecenter.ric.org). All rights reserved. Reprinted with permission.

413

of the brain located toward the front of the skull that are most severely damaged. People with damage in this area may have problems with attention and concentration, organization ability, and the ability to remember things that have happened since their injury. People with damage in the front of the brain may lose their awareness of what they are doing or how others see them. They may seem inconsiderate and selfish like they don't care how they make others feel. However, it is probably more accurate to say they are no longer aware of how they make other people feel.

How does brain injury affect the way you act and how you feel?

Sometimes brain injuries damage the part of the brain that controls emotions. As a result, people may become angry much more easily than before and their anger may be much more forceful. Often, people with this problem feel embarrassed after an angry outburst because they know their reaction was inappropriate. Other people may laugh or cry at inappropriate times because of the same problem. Doctors describe this lack of control of emotions by a number of terms including "emotional lability" or "affective dysregulation." People may also act before they think and may do and say things they would never have done or said before. Such behavior is sometimes described as "impulsivity" or "disinhibition."

How long does it take to recover from a brain injury?

Recovery time depends on how severe the injury was. If someone was unconscious for less than thirty minutes, they will usually recover within three months. If someone was unconscious for more than 24 hours, their recovery may take up to a year. Recovery is usually most rapid in the days and weeks immediately after an injury (improvements can often be noticed from one day to another). Recovery slows down after a while (improvements may not be noticeable unless a comparison is made with how the person was a month ago).

What does it mean to be recovered from a brain injury— what is the definition of recovery?

Rehabilitation helps people to recover but recovery may not mean being just like the person was before. One way to think of recovery is that the person with the injury (impairment) has acknowledged that there is a change, has learned techniques to do things differently or compensate for problems, and has decided to do as much in life as they can. It means enjoying life as much as possible and feeling good as a person while being aware of one's limitations. It means feeling valuable to others. It does not mean being exactly the same as "before the injury." Recovery is an ongoing process, and after all, everybody changes over time.

Will I recover all of my abilities after my brain injury?

It has always been very difficult to predict the amount of recovery some one has after brain injury. When someone has been hurt enough to be hospitalized and be unconscious for a long time, there are usually some lasting effects from the injury. But is it hard to predict how much they could interfere with your life. Depending upon how severe the injury is, the effects and changes to life can be permanent. In less severe cases, some functions may recover, while others remain weak, such as short-term memory. Either way, recovery can take a long time. At some point, it becomes hard to know if improvement comes from brain recovery or just learning to do things differently. Either way, improvement is possible and life goes on.

What kind of activities can I do in everyday life to help myself recover from brain injury?

It's most important not to sit and wait for recovery to come to you, but to work at it. That's why therapies are so important, even after leaving the hospital. Keeping to a routine and staying active during and after therapies have stopped helps a lot. Think of the brain as a muscle. It will weaken if it is not exercised. Aside from therapy assignments, look for ways to stimulate thinking. Games, puzzles, reading and performing everyday tasks that offer mental challenge can be useful. Remember to try to strike a balance and not do too little or too much. Don't hesitate to ask for help and advice to get this balance right.

What kind of activities could make recovery more difficult or interfere with recovery?

Try to balance the level of mental stimulation during recovery. Slow down and do only one thing at a time. Use of nonprescribed drugs, especially recreational drugs and alcohol, can interfere with recovery. Aside from the direct effects these chemicals can have on the brain, they can impair judgment and put a person at risk for further injury.

So be careful when using them, if at all, and consult with your doctor if you have questions about any particular substance. Of course, avoid risky activities (like extreme sports) that could cause another brain injury.

When will I be able to start doing the things that I used to do like work, driving, school?

Some of these things can be restarted as soon as a person becomes aware of their limitation, has mastered some techniques to make up for weaknesses, and has realistic goals. Doctors and therapists will have advice on these matters. Work and driving are very complex behaviors. Limitations that you do not yet fully understand may make it hard to be successful returning to work. Driving can be very dangerous if there are impairments that affect vision or speed or reflexes or problem solving. A special driving evaluation can be done for individuals with brain impairments. The goal should be to do things in a way that is safe and rewarding. This may require changes in the definition of acceptable behaviors. It is more important to go slow and be successful at "things that you used to do," than think that nothing has changed and do things that result in hurt feelings and failures.

What does the term "minimally conscious" mean?

People who are minimally conscious are more awake than someone in a deep coma, but they may actually have little awareness of their surroundings. They may even open their eyes and look around the room, but they may not respond to what they see or hear in the room.

What is the best way to talk to or help a person in this state?

Some people have suggested that it helps minimally conscious people to give them things to think about; for example, to bring in a lot of visitors, to talk to them a lot, to leave the TV on, to read to them, etc. None of these activities have been proven to help the person recover, but there are some stories that suggest it may be helpful to do certain simple activities. It may help for the minimally conscious person to start using their different senses again, so some people talk to them or play music for them. They hold their hand, or bring them sweet smelling flowers. Some have said that playing tape recorded messages from family or friends can be helpful. It is probably not helpful to expose them to complex stimuli they can no longer understand (e.g., playing books on tape, making them watch TV). When people are around minimally conscious patients, it is best to avoid speaking about them as if they are not there and cannot hear you.

How can I talk to my kids about brain injury?

Children need to know some basic things about brain impairment. You might tell them that people with brain impairments may act confused or have trouble remembering or talking about things. Remind your children that the brain impaired person is not "retarded," "stupid," or "child like" even if other adults use those labels. Ask your child what questions they have and if you do not have an answer for them, don't hesitate to ask for help to understand both the question and the appropriate response. Do not think that you have to be an expert in brain impairment. Ask staff and professionals you trust for help.

What are the ways that family members react to a person with a brain injury?

A brain injury can be scary and confusing. Sometimes someone with a brain injury is treated like a child or a baby by other family members. This is not a good response. Sometimes family members get angry at the person with the impairment because they think that they were somehow responsible for their problem. This is understandable under some circumstances, but usually not a helpful way to respond. Sometimes family members have different ideas about what is best for the individual and they disagree with each other. This usually makes everyone feel upset because everyone likes others to see things the same way they do. Brain impairments can make family members feel personally vulnerable, frustrated, and misunderstood. Like any other big family problem, it is not always possible to agree about what to do, but it is important that family members try to listen to different points of view and treat others with respect and kindness. Even under the best of conditions, there will be times when some family members will stay upset and distant and may even withdraw from family contact. With patience and time, they will hopefully come to a better understanding of the injury and re-establish contact.

What should I do if my brain injured family member has problems with anger and becomes violent?

Sometimes people have difficulty with emotional control after brain injury and this can include having a short temper. Family members need to learn different ways to respond to someone with a brain injury who is easily angered. The best way to deal with violence is to learn how to prevent it. Watch for patterns or triggers that set off the brain injured family member and avoid responses that will only make anger build. It is important to remain calm. It is usually not a good idea to argue logically when a brain injured person has become upset. Diversion or redirection in any form is often the best response. This takes away the irritation or trigger and allows the person time to calm down. Try not to physically restrict the person within limits and allow them to freely express themselves physically and verbally. If they become physically violent or threatening, direct appeals for calm can be tried, but may not have the desired effect. In extreme situations, where physical restraint seems necessary, it is always a good idea to have a phone available and numbers to call (such as the doctor or police) for quick, efficient use. Don't try to handle these situations alone. If anger control is a chronic problem, consult with your doctor about the possibility of using medication to help manage the behavior.

How should I respond when my loved one denies that s/he has an impairment?

One of the most difficult challenges facing family members can be helping a brain injured person fully realize the changes brought on by their accident. Denial or lack of awareness can be an actual part of the injury effects and not just a lack of information or an emotional defense. It is important to realize that sometimes a brain injury survivor is never capable of fully understanding their impairments. In this case, it is not a good idea to logically argue or explain their impairment to them, especially during times of conflict. It may be best to provide a simple, short reason why they are restricted (e.g., it's from the accident; your doctor has said so) and leave it at that. Sometimes, over a long period of time and experiences, the survivor may come to learn that the injury has put limits on them that they must live with.

Additional Resources

American Stroke Association, a division of the American Heart Association. National Center, 7272 Greenville Avenue, Dallas, Texas 75231, 800-242-8721.

Brain Injury Association of America, Inc., 8201 Greensburro, Suite 611, McLane, Virginia 22102, 703-761-0750.

Crimmins, C.E. *Where is the Mango Princess?* Knopf, 2000.

Gronwall, DMA, Wrightson, P, and Waddell, P. *Head Injury: The Facts: A guide for families and care-givers.* Oxford Press, 1999.

National Stroke Association, 9707 Easter Lane Building B, Centennial, Colorado 80112, 800-787-6537.

Osborn, Claudia Over My Head: *A doctor's own story of head injury from the inside looking out.* Kansas City: Andrews McMeel Publishing, 1998.

Stoler, D and Hill, BA. *Coping with Mild Traumatic Brain Injury.* Avery Press, 1998.

Chapter 47

Vascular (Multi-Infarct) Dementia

Introduction

Serious forgetfulness, mood swings, and other behavioral changes are not a normal part of aging. They may be caused by poor diet, lack of sleep, or too many medicines, for example. Feelings of loneliness, boredom, or depression also can cause forgetfulness. These problems are serious and should be treated. Often they can be reversed.

Sometimes, however, mental changes are caused by diseases that permanently damage brain cells. The term dementia describes a medical condition that is caused by changes in the normal activity of very sensitive brain cells. These changes in the way the brain works can affect memory, speech, and the ability to carry out daily activities.

Alzheimer disease is the most common cause of dementia in older people. The second most common cause of dementia in older adults is vascular dementia, which affects the blood vessels in the brain. Alzheimer disease (AD) affects approximately 4 million people in the United States. Abnormal proteins collect in the brain and appear to cause loss of nerve cells in the areas vital to memory and thinking.

Alzheimer disease develops slowly. At first, people with AD may have trouble remembering recent events, or the names of familiar people or things. Skills are lost continuously and gradually, though

Excerpted from "Multi-Infarct Dementia Fact Sheet," by the National Institute on Aging (NIA, www.nia.nih.gov), part of the National Institutes of Health, August 30, 2006. NIH Publication No. 02-3433.

some people decline faster than others. As the disease goes on, symptoms become more easily noticed and serious enough to cause people with AD or their family members to seek medical help.

Multi-infarct dementia is the most common form of vascular dementia, and accounts for 10–20% of all cases of progressive, or gradually worsening, dementia. It usually affects people between the ages of 60–75, and is more likely to occur in men than women.

Multi-infarct dementia is caused by a series of strokes that disrupt blood flow and damage or destroy brain tissue. A stroke occurs when blood cannot get to part of the brain. Strokes can be caused when a blood clot or fatty deposit (called plaque) blocks the vessels that supply blood to the brain. A stroke also can happen when a blood vessel in the brain bursts.

Some of the main causes of strokes are:

- untreated high blood pressure (hypertension);
- diabetes;
- high cholesterol; and
- heart disease.

Of these, the most important risk factor for multi-infarct dementia is high blood pressure.

Because strokes occur suddenly, loss of thinking and remembering skills—the symptoms of dementia—also occurs quickly and often in a step-wise pattern. People with multi-infarct dementia may even appear to improve for short periods of time, then decline again after having more strokes.

Symptoms

Sudden onset of any of the following symptoms may be a sign of multi-infarct dementia:

- confusion and problems with recent memory
- wandering or getting lost in familiar places
- moving with rapid, shuffling steps
- loss of bladder or bowel control
- laughing or crying inappropriately
- difficulty following instructions
- problems handling money

422

Multi-infarct dementia is often the result of a series of small strokes. Some of these small strokes produce no obvious symptoms and are noticed only on brain imaging studies, so they are sometimes called "silent strokes." A person may have several small strokes before noticing serious changes in memory or other signs of multi-infarct dementia.

Transient ischemic attacks, or TIAs, are caused by a temporary blockage of blood flow. Symptoms of TIAs are similar to symptoms of stroke and include mild weakness in an arm or leg, slurred speech, and dizziness. Symptoms generally do not last for more than 20 minutes. A recent history of TIAs greatly increases a person's chance of suffering permanent brain damage from a stroke. Prompt medical attention is required to determine what may be causing the blockage in blood flow and to start proper treatment (such as aspirin or warfarin).

If you believe someone is having a stroke—if a person experiences sudden weakness or numbness on one or both sides of the body, or difficulty speaking, seeing, or walking—call 911 immediately. If the physician believes the symptoms are caused by a blocked blood vessel, treatment with a "clot buster," such as tPA (tissue plasminogen activator), within 3 hours can reopen the vessel and may reduce the severity of the stroke.

Diagnosis

People who show signs of dementia and who have a history of strokes should be evaluated for possible multi-infarct dementia. The doctor usually will ask the patient and the family about the person's diet, medications, sleep patterns, personal habits, past strokes, and other risk factors (such as high blood pressure, diabetes, high cholesterol, and heart disease). The doctor also may ask about recent illnesses or stressful events, like the death of someone close or problems at home or work, which may account for the symptoms. To look for signs of stroke, the doctor will check for weakness or numbness in the arms and legs, difficulty with speech, or dizziness. To check for other health problems that could cause symptoms of dementia, the doctor may order office or laboratory tests. These tests may include a blood pressure reading, an electroencephalogram (EEG), a test of thyroid function, or blood tests.

The doctor also may ask for x-rays or special tests such as a computerized tomography (CT) scan or a magnetic resonance imaging (MRI) scan. Both CT scans and MRI scans take pictures of sections of the brain. The pictures are displayed on a computer screen to allow the doctor to see inside the brain and check for signs of stroke, tumors, or other sources of brain injury. Specialists called radiologists and neurologists interpret these scans. In addition, the doctor may send the patient to a psychologist or psychiatrist to assess reasoning, learning ability, memory, and attention span.

Sometimes multi-infarct dementia is difficult to distinguish from AD because their symptoms can be very similar. It is possible for a person to have both diseases, making it hard for the doctor to diagnose either.

Treatment

While no treatment can reverse brain damage that has already been caused by a stroke, treatment to prevent further strokes is very important. For example, high blood pressure, the primary risk factor for multi-infarct dementia, and diabetes are treatable. To prevent more strokes, doctors may prescribe medicines to control high blood pressure, high cholesterol, heart disease, and diabetes. They will counsel patients about good health habits such as exercising, avoiding smoking and drinking alcohol, and eating a low-fat diet.

To reduce symptoms of dementia, doctors may change or stop medications that can cause confusion, such as sedatives, antihistamines, strong painkillers, and other medications. Some patients also may have to be treated for additional medical conditions that can increase confusion, such as heart failure, thyroid disorders, anemia, or infections.

Doctors sometimes prescribe aspirin, warfarin, or other drugs to prevent clots from forming in small blood vessels. Medications also can be prescribed to relieve restlessness or depression or to help patients sleep better.

To improve blood flow or remove blockages in blood vessels, doctors may recommend surgical procedures, such as carotid endarterectomy, angioplasty, or stenting. Studies are under way to see how well these treatments work for patients with multi-infarct dementia. Scientists are also studying drugs that can improve blood flow to the brain, such as antiplatelet and anticoagulant medications; drugs to treat symptoms of dementia, including Alzheimer disease medications; as well as drugs to reduce the risk of TIAs and stroke, such as cholesterol-lowering statins and blood pressure medications.

Helping Someone with Multi-Infarct Dementia

Family members and friends can help someone with multi-infarct dementia cope with mental and physical problems. They can encourage individuals to maintain their daily routines and regular social and physical activities. By talking with them about events and daily experiences, family members can help their loved ones use their mental abilities as much as possible. Some families find it helpful to use reminders such as lists, alarm clocks, and calendars to help the patient remember important times and dates.

A person with multi-infarct dementia should see their primary care doctor regularly. Health problems such as high blood pressure, diabetes, high cholesterol, and heart disease should be carefully monitored. If a person has additional medical conditions, such as depression, mental health experts may be consulted as well.

Help for home caregivers is available from a variety of sources, including nurses, family doctors, social workers, and physical and occupational therapists. Home health care and respite or neighborhood day care services can provide much-needed relief to caregivers. Support groups offer emotional support for family members caring for a person with dementia. A state or local health department, a local hospital, or the patient's doctor may be able to provide telephone numbers for such services.

Chapter 48

Communication Problems after Stroke

Communication problems are one of the most common effects of stroke. Losing the ability to speak or understand is frightening and frustrating, and it happens to about a third of people who have had a stroke. This text explains the different types of communication problems that can arise after a stroke and offers some practical tips to aid communication.

Communication problems after a stroke often result from damage to the parts of the brain responsible for language, but the ability to control the muscles involved in speech may also be affected. The specific problems experienced by any one individual will depend on the extent of the damage and which area of the brain has been affected.

For most people, the area of the brain mainly responsible for aspects of language is located in the left hemisphere (side). This means that damage in this region can affect the ability to speak, understand, read, and write. However, damage to the right side may still make communication difficult because it may limit someone's ability to control crucial movements, affect memory, and make coherent organization of language difficult.

Defining the Problem

There are many different ways in which the ability to communicate may be affected but, generally, the problems are related either to speaking, or understanding what other people are saying. Short-term memory lapses and difficulty in concentrating can make communication even more problematic for some.

Dysphasia

One of the most difficult and common situations is when someone suddenly cannot speak at all after a stroke or what they say does not make sense to you. This is called dysphasia. Dysphasia (sometimes called aphasia) does not damage intelligence, but does affect how someone can use language. Speaking, understanding what is said, reading, and writing are all communication skills, and can all be changed by a stroke.

It can be frustrating for the stroke person as they may believe that they are speaking normally but that other people cannot understand them. Often this arises because the words that come out are not the ones they want to say, or because their sentences are fractured and missing crucial words. The stroke person may be unaware of this. Some people use words with related meanings to the one they want—food instead of drink, for example—while others mix the sounds up in words.

Dysarthria

Someone who has problems forming the right words because of muscle weakness in the mouth has dysarthria. Dysarthria may also affect breath control and the ability to make sounds, so that speech may sound flat, slurred, nasal, or have a jerky rhythm.

Dyspraxia

An inability to control and coordinate the movements that are needed to talk normally is called dyspraxia. A person with dyspraxia may be unable to speak clearly and, in severe cases, to make deliberate sounds at all. It is different from dysarthria because it is not caused by muscle weakness, and is often seen and treated as part of dysphasia. Dyspraxia can affect sequencing and the ability to coordinate other actions as well as speech, and so may be dealt with by a number of health care professionals.

What Help Is Available?

Anyone with communication difficulties after a stroke should be referred to a speech and language therapist. This can be done by the medical team if they are in hospital or by the doctor if they are at home.

Initially, the therapist will assess the person's strengths and needs in terms of communication and their speech and language skills. Dealing with the problem may involve other people, including health professionals and family and friends, who may be offered advice on how to help the stroke person to communicate.

Different approaches to treatment are needed, depending on whether the person has dysphasia or dysarthria, although some people have both after a stroke. The therapist will also use various methods to try to establish the precise nature of the difficulties, for example by using pictures.

Every person who has a stroke is different, and the amount of recovery someone will make is very difficult to predict. Unfortunately some people will have long-term communication difficulties and may need to find alternative ways of communicating, such as using signs or gestures or a communication chart.

How Can I Help?

There are a number of ways that family and friends can help someone with their communication, but do ask if your help is needed before giving it.

- Establish communication by finding out whether someone can use yes or no (or a signal such as thumbs up/thumbs down) accurately. If they can do this most of the time, then you can ask questions to which the answer is yes or no, to narrow down what they want to say.

- Don't rush the conversation. Give the person time to take in what you say and to respond, and don't interrupt them. It is better to assume someone can hear and understand what you say, even if they are not responding much.

- Adjust your communication to the right level. Speak in a normal tone of voice and try to use sentences that are short and to the point. You may need to speak slightly slower than usual. For example, instead of saying, "Your wife called and she will be here tomorrow to pick you up and take you home," say, "Your wife called." (pause) "She will be here tomorrow." (pause) "You can go home then."

- Use visual aids to reinforce your verbal message, such as facial expressions, gestures, writing, drawing, or even a Word and Picture chart.

- Stand or sit where you can be seen and heard clearly—poor lighting or distractions do not help.

Top Tips for Helping Someone with Aphasia

- Remember that spoken words are not the only way to communicate. Help the person to develop skills in as many ways as possible, perhaps making pictures or using gestures and mime.

- Don't give up. If you can't work out or guess what someone is trying to say, suggest you take a break and come back to it later. Don't forget to!

- Don't pretend to understand. If you're having difficulty understanding someone, be honest and tell them: "I'm sorry, I don't understand—let's try again."

- Be positive and encouraging and remind them of any progress they have made.

- Make a record. Write down what works best for you both when communicating because a person with dysphasia might forget the different ways available to him/her. Make a list and refer to it when communication breaks down.

- Try writing down key words. Drawings and pictures can also help.

- Remember the person has not become less intelligent, so treat them as an adult. You may need to remind less tactful friends and relatives of this.

- Communication is not about perfect grammar and proper sentences, so don't feel you must always correct "mistakes."

- Don't visit in a large group. It is much easier for someone to concentrate if it is just you and them. Background noise and distractions do not help.

- Keep visits short, or take a break during a visit. Someone with dysphasia will get tired easily and will not respond well when they are tired.

- What is right for one person may be wrong for another, and you will need to respect the individual's inclinations and interests just as you did before the stroke.

- Do not get discouraged if you have a day when communication seems completely impossible. The effort can leave all involved feeling tired and frustrated.

Recovery Need Not Stop after Speech Therapy

Stopping therapy does not mean that there will be no future progress. Self-confidence and skills can be increased by practicing speech naturally in different settings over time. Try and identify places where the person can practice and develop, and find interests and pursuits that can be enjoyed socially.

They might consider joining a group set up to support people after stroke (stroke club), a communication (or dysphasia) support group (run by The Stroke Association or Speakability in the United Kingdom [UK]) or a local adult education class (some colleges run courses in communication skills, reading, and writing).

It is not unusual for someone with dysphasia to be depressed and frustrated, and they may need some form of counseling to try and express their feelings about the changes in their life after stroke.

What Can Be Done at Home?

There are many activities, which can be done at home to build communication skills and boost confidence. Having friends' and family input can really make a difference, as they know the person best, and may share their interests. The younger ones will enjoy the opportunity to join in some games to help re-establish memory and communication, so enlist as much help as possible.

Sometimes it helps to plan a certain time or times to do communication tasks. These are most successful if they are kept short (less than 30 minutes) and planned around times when the person is rested. If you hit a block, stop for the day or change activities.

The following is a list of ideas for tasks and activities that a friend or family member might initiate with the person affected by dysphasia, or which might be practiced at a communication or dysphasia support group.

- Find and use gestures for common action words (for example, eating, drinking, writing, sleeping, shopping, etc.).

- Gather a box of common objects. Make actions around them. For example: "point to the one you clean your teeth with," "pick up the cup."

- Draw pictures of common objects. Say and write their names. Use simple word-search puzzle books.

- Cut headlines and pictures with captions out of newspapers and tell a story about each one. Make a news scrapbook and include whole articles when you are able to read more easily.

- Make a book of family photos, pictures of friends and places visited, and encourage the person to talk about them.

- Print the names of common objects and rooms at home on cards. Encourage the person to read the cards and locate the item or place.

- Play card games such as Beat Your Neighbor or Pontoon to practice numbers.

- Make a chart of daily chores around the house, perhaps with actual photographs of the person doing them.

- Adapt a favorite, simple recipe using pictures and/or drawings for the ingredients and measurements.

- Use maps of the town you live in, the UK, and the world. Put them in a book and refer to the maps when talking about various locations.

- Practice writing activities daily, such as copying letters or words, and pick words at random for the person to write down. Encourage the person to write short letters, cards, and thank you notes.

- Keep a large monthly calendar in view for birthdays and anniversaries. Encourage the person to enter all appointments and events or write an item of interest for each day.

- Make a journal and include something to mark each day, written or drawn, and items such as a photo, article, invitation, or keepsake.

- Limit the amount of TV they watch and seek out interaction with other people to restore the art of communicating.

Chapter 49

Involuntary Emotional Expression Disorder in Stroke Survivors

What Is IEED?

Involuntary emotional expression disorder (IEED) is a medical condition that causes sudden and unpredictable episodes of crying, laughing, or other emotional displays. IEED is also called Pseudobulbar Affect, Emotional Lability, or emotional incontinence.

If you have this problem, a diagnosis of IEED can come as a relief. The diagnosis can help explain why you may find yourself crying hard when you don't feel sad, why you may laugh at a sad story, or why you get angry over things that didn't used to make you mad.

IEED may occur when disease or injury damages the area of the brain that controls normal expression of emotion. This damage can disrupt brain signaling causing a "short circuit," triggering episodes of emotional outbursts. The emotions you display may be out of proportion to the situation. Or, they may be out of context. For example, you may laugh at a funeral or other solemn occasion.

If you have IEED, the inappropriateness, intensity, and suddenness of the outbursts can make you feel as if you have lost control over your life. The disconnect between your internal emotions and external expressions can be frustrating—both for you and your loved ones.

Understanding the condition can be a big step to reclaiming your confidence and improving your relationships and quality of life.

Who Gets IEED?

IEED is triggered by damage to an area of the brain, sometimes from stroke. It is thought to impact more than 1 million Americans who may also suffer from stroke, traumatic brain injury, or neurologic diseases such as multiple sclerosis, amyotrophic lateral sclerosis (ALS, Lou Gehrig Disease), Parkinson disease, and dementias including Alzheimer disease.

Do I Have IEED?

Only a doctor can diagnose IEED. But you can look for signs. First of all, do you suffer from Alzheimer, Parkinson, ALS, or MS [multiple sclerosis] or have you had a stroke or traumatic brain injury?

If yes, then ask yourself the following:

- Do you cry easily?

- Do you find that even when you try to control your crying you can't?

- Do you laugh at inappropriate times?

- Do you have emotional outbursts that are inappropriate to the situation?

If you answered yes to one or more of these questions, ask your doctor about IEED.

Why Is IEED So Distressing?

IEED can be emotionally painful for both those that have it and their loved ones. One of the hardest things for people with IEED is a feeling of loss of control. IEED-related episodes can happen without warning in social and professional situations. This can fuel feelings of embarrassment and anxiety. Many people don't go out in public for fear of crying or laughing inappropriately. Some start missing days of work, stop eating in restaurants, and/or avoid family gatherings. This can lead to feelings of isolation. Also, many people with IEED are frustrated that they can't seem to manage something as basic as their own emotions.

How Can I Manage It?

The first step to treating IEED is to get an accurate diagnosis. Then ask your doctor about ways to manage IEED.

Try not to be embarrassed when you talk to your doctor. Your doctor probably has not seen your episodes, so be as specific as possible when describing your emotions.

Remember that IEED is a distinct neurologic disorder and should be diagnosed and treated separately from stroke. While there is some promising research, there is no medical treatment for IEED approved by the U.S. Food and Drug Administration.

Because people with IEED may cry a lot, they may be diagnosed with depression. But, IEED is not depression. IEED episodes are often sudden, unpredictable, and may be contrary to the person's actual mood. Since it is often confused with depression, many people with IEED are prescribed anti-depressant drugs by their doctors.

Stroke survivors may see their IEED symptoms lessen over time as the brain heals.

You are not alone—you can connect with other people who have similar conditions. Support groups can be very helpful. Your physician may be able to provide you with a list of support/patient organizations.

Handling Social Situations with IEED

Be open and honest about this condition with your family, friends and co-workers. This will help them to better understand your emotional episodes. Warn people that you cannot always control your emotions. Explain that the emotions you show on the outside do not always reflect how you feel on the inside.

When you meet new people, inform them of your IEED as soon as you feel comfortable with them. Give them an idea of what happens when you have an episode.

At times, you may want to politely excuse yourself from the social situation if you feel an episode coming on. For example, if you feel an episode coming on while you are at work or dinner with friends, excuse yourself until the episode passes.

Coping with IEED

Learning about IEED and accepting that it is a distinct neurologic condition may help.

Try these things to cope with an episode of IEED:

- Be open about the problem; that way, people are not surprised or confused when you have an episode.

- When you feel an episode coming on, try to distract yourself by counting the number of objects on a shelf or by thinking about something unrelated.

- Take a slow deep breath and continue doing this until you're in control.

- Relax your forehead, shoulders, and other muscle groups that tense up during an emotional episode.

Chapter 50

Spasticity Often Seen in Association with Stroke

What Is Spasticity?

Spasticity is a term used to describe abnormal involuntary tightening of muscles that either occurs spontaneously or when the body is stimulated in certain ways (for example, when a joint is moved). Spasticity may be seen in association with rapid repetitive muscle spasms, called clonus. These muscles spasms are often found at the ankle.

What Causes Spasticity?

Spasticity is a nerve and muscle condition that occurs after an injury to the brain or the spinal cord. Nerve cells below the level of the injury become disconnected from the brain. These nerves are then in a "turned on" state, constantly sending a chemical signal to the muscle, causing it to tighten. Spasticity is often not seen immediately after an injury, but may become gradually worse weeks to months following the event. Conditions that commonly lead to spasticity include strokes, cerebral palsy, spinal cord injuries, traumatic brain injuries, and multiple sclerosis.

What Makes Spasticity Worse?

- Rapidly moving a joint

- Sensory stimulation (such as pressure or touch)

- Medical problems such as pain or skin breakdown

- Infections of the bladder or kidney

- Constipation

- Restrictive or tight clothing

- Certain body positions, e.g., sitting, lying in bed, walking, or other activities

- Fatigue

- Certain times of the day or night

All these factors should be considered and checked if someone experiences a sudden increase in their spasticity.

What Are the Consequences of Spasticity?

Spasticity may be mild and cause only slight muscle stiffness. As it becomes more severe, the stiffness may lead to muscle, tendon, and joint shortening, called contracture. The tightening may also be painful. Involuntary tightening can be reduced with medicines; however, a fixed contracture, which occurs when the muscle and the other structures become permanently short, will not be helped by the anti-spasticity medicine. This can only be treated by stretching, splinting, serial casting (progressive casts that gradually stretch out the muscle), or surgery.

Spasticity and contractures may impact a person's ability to do the daily activities such as dressing, eating, toileting, and grooming. Severe tightness in the armpit, groin, or hand can cause problems for hygiene and can lead to skin breakdown. In the upper body or leg, spasticity can affect sitting, transfers, and walking. Sometimes spasticity is helpful. For example, some people are able to trigger a spasm to help roll over, or leg tightness can help someone stand when his or her leg muscles are weak. These aspects of spasticity need to be considered when spasticity is treated.

What Treatments Are Available to Treat Spasticity?

Spasticity does not always need to be treated. It is best to consult with a medical professional who is familiar with spasticity and its treatment. There are different types of treatments available.

- Stretching is an important part of any program to help prevent contracture development.

- Splinting can be used in addition to stretching to help maintain joint position.

- Medications that relax the muscles may also be tried. These can be given orally, injected into muscles, or into the space around the spine that contains the spinal fluid. Some patients with severe spasticity may need to be on multiple medicines, or may need to use oral medicines in combination with muscle or nerve injections, called chemodenervation.

With severe spasticity, a treatment team may be needed to assess the best methods of intervention. This team can include rehabilitation professionals and physicians including a physical therapist, occupational therapist, speech therapist, rehabilitation engineer, nurse, and physiatrist (rehabilitation doctor). A neurosurgeon or an orthopedic surgeon may be involved, particularly if surgery is anticipated. Some centers have spasticity clinics where patients may be seen by these multiple professionals for an assessment.

References

- www.WeMove.org

- *Muscle and Nerve,* Supplement 6/1997: Spasticity: Etiology, Evaluation, Management, and the Role of Botulinum Toxin Type A.

Chapter 51

Balance Problems after Stroke

Stroke can cause many different physical effects such as weakness or paralysis, and can also cause problems with balance. This can cause feelings of dizziness, unsteadiness, or nausea, and people can lose confidence in moving and walking around. This information explains how balance is controlled, how it can be affected by stroke, and what can be done to help.

Balance problems can make you feel dizzy or unsteady, which can increase the chance of suffering from a fall. Falls and fall-related injuries are among the most common complications after a stroke but the majority of falls, although distressing, are not very serious.

What Is Balance?

Balance means the ability to hold your body up and to change its position while doing other activities. Balance is important because it is involved in day-to-day activities, such as getting up from a chair, walking, and bending over to pick up something.

How Is Balance Controlled?

Balance is very complex and is controlled by a number of different systems in the body.

- **Eyes:** In order to have a good sense of balance, we need to be able to see where we are in relation to the world around us.

- **Sensors in joints, tendons, and muscles:** The brain needs to know how the feet and legs are positioned in relation to the ground, and how the head is positioned in relation to the chest and shoulders. This information is detected by the sensors, which are located in your muscles, tendons, and joints.

- **Cognition:** The ability of the brain to understand where the body is and to provide a mental "map" of surroundings and plan movements.

- **Muscle strength and joint flexibility:** The muscles and joints must be able to carry out the "orders" from the brain.

- **Ears:** Balance organs within the ears inform the brain about the movements and position of your head. The balance organs are located in the inner ear, which is called the "labyrinth."

Why Can a Stroke Cause Balance Problems?

A stroke can cause problems with balance due to:

- injury to one of the systems that control balance and movement;
- injury to the nerves that send messages to the brain;
- injury to the balance centers of the brain itself; and
- paralysis and weakness on one side of the body, which can make stroke sufferers unsteady on their feet.

Can Balance Problems after a Stroke Be Improved?

Balance problems often improve naturally as the brain slowly repairs itself in the weeks after a stroke. Recovery is helped by trying as far as possible to keep moving. Many people who have had a stroke regain their balance within three months.

However, everyone is different and there is no fixed time that it will take to get better. The problems caused by the stroke may mean that you are not able to move around a lot and this can affect how long it takes for balance problems to improve. For some people, balance problems will never completely go away.

Balance Retraining Exercises

Balance retraining exercises may help people who have had a stroke improve their balance. Because there are several possible causes of balance problems after stroke, different types of exercises will be appropriate for different people.

A physiotherapist can help you to work out which movements you need to practice and therefore which exercises are most suitable for you. The most common exercises will be simple tasks practicing everyday movements in an environment in which you feel safe. At first these will be practiced with the therapists and then either on your own or with a nurse or relative.

- If your balance has been badly affected, it may be that the first thing to tackle is sitting balance—practicing reaching and dressing without toppling over.

- Next would be "transfers"—moving from bed to chair, or chair to toilet. The therapist may provide grab rails to help you.

- For most people, the majority of the work will be practicing sitting to standing and walking around the room/ward. A walking aid may help you.

You may feel uncomfortable or scared about some of the exercises that you need to carry out. It is often the fear of falling that stops people from practicing their exercises.

However, challenging your brain is an important part of your rehabilitation and you will need to do the exercises for several weeks before you see real progress. Don't be disheartened if you fall a few times—if you practice when somebody else is around, they can help you.

Tips to Avoid a Fall

The following tips may help to prevent you from suffering a fall:

- Be careful of rugs, carpets, uneven floors, and loose steps which could make a person trip.

- Be aware of cupboards or shelves that are too high or too low to reach easily, which could cause you to overbalance.

- Footwear—don't wear baggy slippers!

- Dim lighting in rooms and hallways increases the risk of falling—leave a light on at night if you need to use the toilet.

- Check that any walking aid (especially the rubber tip at the bottom) is safe and use it.

- Wear your hearing aid.

- Ask an occupational therapist to check if you need any aids or adaptations (such as grab rails or raised toilet seats).

Chapter 52

Swallowing Problems after Stroke

The ability to swallow is a complex activity involving the coordination of many nerves and muscles that can be damaged by a stroke. Nearly half of people who have had a stroke will initially experience difficulty swallowing. This is called dysphagia. This information explains how this can be a serious problem and outlines the skilled help needed to manage it.

What Are the Signs?

The signs of swallowing problems include a drooping mouth, gurgling or slurred speech, coughing or choking, and feelings of discomfort in the throat. Most people recover their swallow within a matter of weeks. Some will take longer, and for a small proportion of people, the ability to swallow does not return.

What Are the Hazards?

Without treatment, people with dysphagia are vulnerable to dehydration and undernutrition. There is also a risk that food may "go down the wrong way," getting into the windpipe (trachea) and so into the lungs. This is called aspiration. This can cause infection and, in serious cases, can lead to a chest infection or to pneumonia. It may cause the stroke person to choke and cough, or there may be no obvious signs of it happening.

What Are the Immediate Tests and Treatment?

Where the person is conscious and able to sit up, a nurse will give a simple test for signs of swallowing problems using a small amount of water on a teaspoon. If the person manages to swallow this safely without coughing or choking, it will be repeated, before they are given a small glass of water.

If the problem persists, a speech and language therapist will carry out a full assessment. This may involve a test called a video-fluoroscopy where the person swallows a small amount of fluid containing barium. The precise area of the swallowing problem is then highlighted on a video x-ray machine. If there are serious difficulties, the person will be kept 'nil by mouth,' that is, without food or liquid. Their fluid levels will be maintained using a drip into a vein, and a dietitian will advise on any nutritional supplements required.

It is important when receiving 'nil by mouth' that the person's mouth does not become dry or sore and is kept clean, fresh, and free from infection. Dried saliva and mucus from the nose and chest can lead to discomfort and bad breath. A visiting relative can assist by moistening the dry mouth with wet swabs provided by nursing staff, regularly brushing the teeth, cleaning dentures, and using salve to moisturize the lips.

Is There Any Therapy to Speed up the Recovery of Swallowing?

By about two weeks after a stroke, over two thirds of people with swallowing difficulties will be swallowing safely again. A speech and language therapist may recommend exercises to help coordinate the swallowing muscles and restimulate the nerves that trigger the swallowing reflex. They will try ways of compensating for individual difficulties and they will suggest techniques to help food go down more easily.

How Is Food Reintroduced?

As swallowing is being recovered, food and fluid consistencies are altered to suit individual needs, and a speech therapist or dietitian will advise on what is appropriate. Drinks and foods can be thickened using commercial thickeners, which make thin liquids and puréed foods safer and easier to swallow. Some pre-thickened juices and milk drinks are now available on prescription. Thickeners can also be used as soaking solutions to make cakes, sandwiches, and biscuits a safe consistency to swallow.

Puréed fruit or yogurt may be given, while skimmed-milk powder, boneless fish, or mashed potatoes or other starchy vegetables can be used to thicken soup.

When someone has not eaten for a while, their appetite often needs to be encouraged with smaller meals at more frequent intervals. Nutritional supplement drinks may be used to increase calorie intake. A dietitian will advise on individual food requirements. Physical disability may make it difficult for the person to feed him or herself, and they may need special cutlery. It may be helpful for a relative to visit around mealtimes so that they can offer encouragement and assistance. However, it is important that any other visitors are kept to a minimum during meals as it is easier to chew and swallow properly in a calm and quiet environment.

Some Tips for Safe Swallowing

- Eat in a quiet, relaxed environment.

- Sit upright while eating and stay upright for 30 minutes after eating.

- Take only one teaspoonful at a time, ensuring that the food has been swallowed before the next spoonful.

- Close your lips around the spoon.

- Do not mix food and drink in the same mouthful.

- Ask your doctor if your medicines can be prescribed in liquid or syrup form.

What Is the Longer-Term Treatment?

If swallowing difficulties persist, tube feeding will be required to remove the risk of food or fluid entering the lungs.

A nasogastric tube (NG) is a narrow tube that is inserted through the nose into the back of the throat and down into the stomach. The tube is secured to the nose with medical tape. A liquid diet is then dripped slowly into the tube. Some people find this slightly uncomfortable and there is a risk of it being inadvertently pulled out.

If swallowing problems continue and artificial feeding is necessary for longer than a few weeks, a gastrostomy tube (or PEG) may be recommended. A local anesthetic will be used while the PEG (a flexible, fine, hollow tube) is inserted directly into the stomach through the abdominal wall. It is held in place by a flat plastic disk. The PEG is less likely to irritate or to fall out than a nasogastric tube and is hidden under clothing.

Before leaving hospital, the stroke person and their carer need to be taught how to care for the skin around the tube and how to recognize any sign that the area may be infected. If the tube blocks, or there is infection, then the doctor or community nurse will be able to help. A dietitian will offer advice about the types of liquid food that can be taken.

The ability to eat and drink safely and with enjoyment is a major part of life. Swallowing problems have a huge impact on someone who has had a stroke and their family. It is important to manage any difficulties with support and help from local health professionals.

Chapter 53

Bladder and Bowel Function after Stroke

Incontinence after a stroke—problems with bladder and/or bowel control—is very common. Though this can be extremely distressing, many of these problems will resolve over time. This text explains the common continence problems that can happen, and the treatments available.

Incontinence means the loss of control of the bladder or bowel. It is extremely common after a stroke. It is estimated that about half of all people admitted to hospital after a stroke will have some problem with bowel or bladder control. About 15 percent of people who have had a stroke will have ongoing continence problems a year after their stroke.

Common Problems

There are many different types of continence problems that can occur as a result of stroke. These include:

- Frequency—Needing to pass urine very often.

- Urge incontinence—When someone suddenly feels an urgent, uncontrollable need to go to the toilet. Often this does not give the person enough time to go to the toilet, so they may wet or soil themselves.

- Nocturnal incontinence—Wetting the bed while asleep.

- Functional incontinence—Due to the physical effects of a stroke, someone may not be able to get to the toilet in time, or may have difficulty unfastening their clothes in time to use the toilet.

- Reflex incontinence—This is also called neurogenic incontinence and means passing urine without realizing you have done so. This happens when the part of the brain controlling the bladder is affected by the stroke. For most people this lasts only a few months and improves as recovery happens in the brain.

- Overflow incontinence—This is where the bladder leaks due to being too full. This can be due to a loss of feeling in the bladder, or a difficulty in emptying the bladder completely.

- Fecal incontinence—Problems controlling bowel movements. This can be caused by not being able to get to the toilet in time, damage to the part of the brain controlling the bowel, or by overflow leakage of feces due to constipation.

- Constipation—People who are less mobile are more prone to constipation. This can be caused by nerve damage, the effects of lying for long periods in a hospital bed, and/or by not eating or drinking as much as usual. It can also make bladder-emptying problems worse when hard stools press on the bladder.

Why Problems Develop

There are several different reasons why continence problems can develop following a stroke. For example if the person is not fully aware of their surroundings, they may be unaware of the need to use the toilet and may wet or soil themselves without realizing or noticing.

The stroke may have damaged the part of the brain that controls the bladder and/or the bowel. It is possible that they may be able to relearn the skills of bladder and/or bowel control.

Continence difficulties may also occur if someone has difficulty walking or moving around, or they need help getting to the toilet—they may not be able to get there in time. The same is true if someone also has communication problems as they may not be able to tell anyone when they need to go to the toilet.

Professional Help

An assessment by a doctor or nurse is essential in finding the nature and cause of a person's continence problems and in devising an effective treatment program. One of a number of tests may be performed, ranging from a simple physical examination to x-rays of the bladder or bowel, or specialist investigations to determine exactly how the bladder is working.

A referral may be made to a local continence advisor or specialist, such as a urologist, gastroenterologist, gynecologist, or geriatrician. Nurses, including district nurses, practice nurses, community nurses, and health visitors, are also experienced in dealing with continence problems.

Continence advisors are specialist nurses who are trained to help with continence problems. They can develop a plan specially tailored for the individual's circumstances. Physiotherapists can provide training and exercises to improve walking and transferring from a bed or chair to a commode or toilet. Occupational therapists can help if the home needs to be adapted or equipment is needed to make it easier to use the toilet. Social workers can help with financial issues, such as a grant to adapt the bathroom or to build a new one, and can also arrange for a variety of support services, such as walking aids or wheelchairs.

Treatment

Once the underlying cause of the continence problem has been determined, suitable treatment will be offered. This may include:

- Bladder training which reduces urgency and frequency by gradually retraining the bladder to be less active and to hold more urine. If the stroke has damaged the bladder control center in the brain, the bladder can become overactive and start to release urine without warning. Bladder training teaches you how to "hold on."

- Pelvic floor exercises help strengthen muscles so that they provide support. This will help improve bladder control and improve or stop leakage of urine.

- Medication can help reduce urine production, and decrease urgency and frequency. There are also drugs for bowel incontinence; these help decrease movement in the bowel or make the sphincter muscle tighter to avoid leakage.

- In severe cases of incontinence a catheter may be used. This involves using a tube to drain urine from the bladder. If the bladder is not emptying completely, catheterization may need to be done several times a day (intermittent catheterization) to reduce the risk of developing a urinary tract infection. If this cannot be carried out for physical or social reasons, a permanent catheter, in which the bag is attached to the leg and worn under clothing, may be necessary.

Continence products, such as pads, pants, liners, and bed covers, are available to help people manage issues with continence. They are available in a variety of sizes and shapes; some are disposable and some are washable. For men a drainage appliance may be suitable. Talk to the continence advisor about which would be the most suitable.

Some continence products are available from the NHS [National Health Service] free of charge, although every area has its own criteria for who is eligible. Products can also be purchased from some pharmacies and by mail order.

Helping Yourself

- Drink plenty of fluids—try to have 6.8 glasses of fluid each day. Try to cut down on drinks which contain caffeine such as tea, coffee, and cola, and alcoholic drinks as they can irritate the bladder.

- Eat a balanced diet with plenty of fruit and vegetables which contain valuable fiber which helps bowel movements.

- Keep as active as you are able to.

- Try to use the toilet as soon as you need to, and empty your bladder fully. This can help to avoid infections.

Chapter 54

Sleep Disorders after Stroke

Getting a good night's sleep is an important part of stroke recovery. And yet, sleep problems are common among stroke survivors. When these sleep problems go on for a long time, they are considered sleep disorders. Having a sleep disorder can be frustrating. It can make you tired and irritable. It can affect your health and quality of life. It can also pose serious dangers by increasing your risk for another stroke. The good news is that there are things you can do to get a good night's sleep again. Your sleepless nights are numbered.

Sleep Disorders Caused by Breathing Problems

About two-thirds (2/3) of stroke survivors have sleep-disordered breathing (SDB). This type of sleep disorder is caused by abnormal breathing patterns. With SDB, your sleep is interrupted several times throughout the night. So, during the day you may be really sleepy or have trouble thinking or solving problems. SDB also poses dangerous health risks because it can increase blood pressure, heart stress, and blood clotting.

There are several types of SDB. The most common is obstructive sleep apnea (OSA). With OSA, you may stop breathing for 10 seconds or more, many times during the night. You usually won't have breathing problems during the day when you are awake.

Symptoms

There are several telltale signs that you have sleep-disordered breathing. Some are seen at night and others during the day.

Symptoms you might see at night include:

- loud snoring

- waking up frequently during the night, gasping for breath

- increased sweating

- shortness of breath

- insomnia, or being unable to fall asleep or remain asleep throughout the night

Sleeping problems at night can cause problems the next day, including:

- excessive daytime sleepiness

- memory or attention problems

- headaches

- fatigue (low energy level)

- irritability

- depression or extreme sadness

Diagnosing a Sleep Disorder

Most often, your bed partner is the first to notice the symptoms. Or you may notice them yourself. Either way, you should talk to your doctor if you think you may have a sleeping disorder. To officially diagnose the problem, your doctor may arrange a sleep test called a polysomnogram (PSG). This painless, all-night test will study your sleep patterns. It is typically done in a special sleep center.

Treating Your Sleep Disorder

Treatments vary, depending on whether your case is mild or more serious.

- You may be able to improve mild cases by losing weight, staying away from alcohol, and avoiding sleep medicines.

- For mild to moderate cases, your doctor may prescribe a special dental appliance. Worn at night while you sleep (like a retainer), this tool can open up your airways and improve your breathing.

- In some cases, the problem is caused by your sleeping position and can be treated by keeping you from turning onto your back at night. This can be done by sewing an object such as a tennis ball to your pajamas, making it uncomfortable for you to turn over.

- The most successful treatment is usually continuous positive airway pressure (CPAP), a form of breathing assistance during sleep. CPAP uses air pressure to open up your airways. The CPAP machine is a little larger than an average toaster. It blows heated, humidified air through a short tube to a mask that you wear. The mask must fit snugly to prevent air from leaking. The CPAP machine is portable and can be taken on trips. People using CPAP report having higher energy levels, better thinking abilities, and improved well being during the day. They also say they are less sleepy.

- Severe cases may require surgery.

Other Sleep Disorders

There are a few other sleep disorders commonly seen in stroke survivors.

- About 20-40% of survivors have "circadian disturbances" or sleep-wake cycle disorders (SWDs). With this sleep problem, your sleep schedule is no longer determined by day and night. Bright light therapy may help you get your sleep-wake schedule back on track.

- Another frequent sleeping problem after stroke is insomnia, or trouble falling asleep or staying asleep throughout the night. Treating this often complex problem may involve behavioral or medical intervention.

Professionals Who Can Help

- A doctor or sleep medicine specialist
- Health psychologist or behavioral sleep medicine specialist
- Certified sleep center

Rehabilitation is a lifetime commitment and an important part of recovering from a stroke. Through rehabilitation, you relearn basic skills such as talking, eating, dressing, and walking. Rehabilitation can also improve your strength, flexibility, and endurance. The goal is to regain as much independence as possible.

Remember to ask your doctor, "Where am I on my stroke recovery journey?"

Part Five

Life after Stroke: Rehabilitation and Daily Living Concerns

Chapter 55

Facts about Poststroke Rehabilitation

In the United States more than 700,000 people suffer a stroke each year, and approximately two thirds of these individuals survive and require rehabilitation. The goals of rehabilitation are to help survivors become as independent as possible and to attain the best possible quality of life. Even though rehabilitation does not "cure" stroke in that it does not reverse brain damage, rehabilitation can substantially help people achieve the best possible long-term outcome.

What Is Poststroke Rehabilitation?

Rehabilitation helps stroke survivors relearn skills that are lost when part of the brain is damaged. For example, these skills can include coordinating leg movements in order to walk or carrying out the steps involved in any complex activity. Rehabilitation also teaches survivors new ways of performing tasks to circumvent or compensate for any residual disabilities. Patients may need to learn how to bathe and dress using only one hand, or how to communicate effectively when their ability to use language has been compromised. There is a strong consensus among rehabilitation experts that the most important element in any rehabilitation program is carefully directed, well-focused, repetitive practice—the same kind of practice used by all people when they learn a new skill, such as playing the piano or pitching a baseball.

"Post-Stroke Rehabilitation Fact Sheet," is from the National Institute of Neurological Disorders and Stroke (NINDS, www.ninds.nih.gov), part of the National Institutes of Health, NIH Publication No. 02-4846, October 19, 2007.

Rehabilitative therapy begins in the acute-care hospital after the patient's medical condition has been stabilized, often within 24 to 48 hours after the stroke. The first steps involve promoting independent movement because many patients are paralyzed or seriously weakened. Patients are prompted to change positions frequently while lying in bed and to engage in passive or active range-of-motion exercises to strengthen their stroke-impaired limbs. ("Passive" range-of-motion exercises are those in which the therapist actively helps the patient move a limb repeatedly, whereas "active" exercises are performed by the patient with no physical assistance from the therapist.) Patients progress from sitting up and transferring between the bed and a chair to standing, bearing their own weight, and walking, with or without assistance. Rehabilitation nurses and therapists help patients perform progressively more complex and demanding tasks, such as bathing, dressing, and using a toilet, and they encourage patients to begin using their stroke-impaired limbs while engaging in those tasks. Beginning to reacquire the ability to carry out these basic activities of daily living represents the first stage in a stroke survivor's return to functional independence.

For some stroke survivors, rehabilitation will be an ongoing process to maintain and refine skills and could involve working with specialists for months or years after the stroke.

What Disabilities Can Result from a Stroke?

The types and degrees of disability that follow a stroke depend upon which area of the brain is damaged. Generally, stroke can cause five types of disabilities: paralysis or problems controlling movement; sensory disturbances including pain; problems using or understanding language; problems with thinking and memory; and emotional disturbances.

Paralysis or Problems Controlling Movement (Motor Control)

Paralysis is one of the most common disabilities resulting from stroke. The paralysis is usually on the side of the body opposite the side of the brain damaged by stroke, and may affect the face, an arm, a leg, or the entire side of the body. This one-sided paralysis is called hemiplegia (one-sided weakness is called hemiparesis). Stroke patients with hemiparesis or hemiplegia may have difficulty with everyday activities such as walking or grasping objects. Some stroke patients have problems with swallowing, called dysphagia, due to damage to the part of the brain that controls the muscles for swallowing. Damage to a lower part of the brain, the cerebellum, can affect the body's ability to coordinate movement, a disability called ataxia, leading to problems with body posture, walking, and balance.

Sensory Disturbances Including Pain

Stroke patients may lose the ability to feel touch, pain, temperature, or position. Sensory deficits may also hinder the ability to recognize objects that patients are holding and can even be severe enough to cause loss of recognition of one's own limb. Some stroke patients experience pain, numbness or odd sensations of tingling or prickling in paralyzed or weakened limbs, a condition known as paresthesia.

Stroke survivors frequently have a variety of chronic pain syndromes resulting from stroke-induced damage to the nervous system (neuropathic pain). Patients who have a seriously weakened or paralyzed arm commonly experience moderate to severe pain that radiates outward from the shoulder. Most often, the pain results from a joint becoming immobilized due to lack of movement and the tendons and ligaments around the joint become fixed in one position. This is commonly called a "frozen" joint; "passive" movement at the joint in a paralyzed limb is essential to prevent painful "freezing" and to allow easy movement if and when voluntary motor strength returns. In some stroke patients, pathways for sensation in the brain are damaged, causing the transmission of false signals that result in the sensation of pain in a limb or side of the body that has the sensory deficit. The most common of these pain syndromes is called "thalamic pain syndrome," which can be difficult to treat even with medications.

The loss of urinary continence is fairly common immediately after a stroke and often results from a combination of sensory and motor deficits. Stroke survivors may lose the ability to sense the need to urinate or the ability to control muscles of the bladder. Some may lack enough mobility to reach a toilet in time. Loss of bowel control or constipation may also occur. Permanent incontinence after a stroke is uncommon. But even a temporary loss of bowel or bladder control can be emotionally difficult for stroke survivors.

Problems Using or Understanding Language (Aphasia)

At least one fourth of all stroke survivors experience language impairments, involving the ability to speak, write, and understand spoken and written language. A stroke-induced injury to any of the brain's language-control centers can severely impair verbal communication.

Damage to a language center located on the dominant side of the brain, known as Broca's area, causes expressive aphasia. People with this type of aphasia have difficulty conveying their thoughts through words or writing. They lose the ability to speak the words they are thinking and to put words together in coherent, grammatically correct sentences. In contrast, damage to a language center located in a rear portion of the brain, called Wernicke's area, results in receptive aphasia. People with this condition have difficulty understanding spoken or written language and often have incoherent speech. Although they can form grammatically correct sentences, their utterances are often devoid of meaning. The most severe form of aphasia, global aphasia, is caused by extensive damage to several areas involved in language function. People with global aphasia lose nearly all their linguistic abilities; they can neither understand language nor use it to convey thought. A less severe form of aphasia, called anomic or amnesic aphasia, occurs when there is only a minimal amount of brain damage; its effects are often quite subtle. People with anomic aphasia may simply selectively forget interrelated groups of words, such as the names of people or particular kinds of objects.

Problems with Thinking and Memory

Stroke can cause damage to parts of the brain responsible for memory, learning, and awareness. Stroke survivors may have dramatically shortened attention spans or may experience deficits in short-term memory. Individuals also may lose their ability to make plans, comprehend meaning, learn new tasks, or engage in other complex mental activities. Two fairly common deficits resulting from stroke are anosognosia, an inability to acknowledge the reality of the physical impairments resulting from stroke, and neglect, the loss of the ability to respond to objects or sensory stimuli located on one side of the body, usually the stroke-impaired side. Stroke survivors who develop apraxia lose their ability to plan the steps involved in a complex task and to carry the steps out in the proper sequence. Stroke survivors with apraxia may also have problems following a set of instructions. Apraxia appears to be caused by a disruption of the subtle connections that exist between thought and action.

Emotional Disturbances

Many people who survive a stroke feel fear, anxiety, frustration, anger, sadness, and a sense of grief for their physical and mental losses. These feelings are a natural response to the psychological trauma of stroke. Some emotional disturbances and personality changes are caused by the physical effects of brain damage. Clinical depression, which is a sense of hopelessness that disrupts an individual's ability to function, appears to be the emotional disorder most commonly experienced by stroke survivors. Signs of clinical depression include sleep disturbances, a radical change in eating patterns that may lead to sudden weight loss or gain, lethargy, social withdrawal, irritability, fatigue, self-loathing, and suicidal thoughts. Poststroke depression can be treated with antidepressant medications and psychological counseling.

What Medical Professionals Specialize in Poststroke Rehabilitation?

Poststroke rehabilitation involves physicians; rehabilitation nurses; physical, occupational, recreational, speech-language, and vocational therapists; and mental health professionals.

Physicians

Physicians have the primary responsibility for managing and coordinating the long-term care of stroke survivors, including recommending which rehabilitation programs will best address individual needs. Physicians are also responsible for caring for the stroke survivor's general health and providing guidance aimed at preventing a second stroke, such as controlling high blood pressure or diabetes and eliminating risk factors such as cigarette smoking, excessive weight, a high-cholesterol diet, and high alcohol consumption.

Neurologists usually lead acute-care stroke teams and direct patient care during hospitalization. They sometimes remain in charge of long-term rehabilitation. However, physicians trained in other specialties often assume responsibility after the acute stage has passed, including physiatrists, who specialize in physical medicine and rehabilitation.

Rehabilitation Nurses

Nurses specializing in rehabilitation help survivors relearn how to carry out the basic activities of daily living. They also educate survivors about routine health care, such as how to follow a medication schedule, how to care for the skin, how to manage transfers between a bed and a wheelchair, and special needs for people with diabetes. Rehabilitation nurses also work with survivors to reduce risk factors that may lead to a second stroke, and provide training for caregivers.

Nurses are closely involved in helping stroke survivors manage personal care issues, such as bathing and controlling incontinence. Most stroke survivors regain their ability to maintain continence, often with the help of strategies learned during rehabilitation. These strategies include strengthening pelvic muscles through special exercises and following a timed voiding schedule. If problems with incontinence continue, nurses can help caregivers learn to insert and manage catheters and to take special hygienic measures to prevent other incontinence-related health problems from developing.

Physical Therapists

Physical therapists specialize in treating disabilities related to motor and sensory impairments. They are trained in all aspects of anatomy and physiology related to normal function, with an emphasis on movement. They assess the stroke survivor's strength, endurance, range of motion, gait abnormalities, and sensory deficits to design individualized rehabilitation programs aimed at regaining control over motor functions.

Physical therapists help survivors regain the use of stroke-impaired limbs, teach compensatory strategies to reduce the effect of remaining deficits, and establish ongoing exercise programs to help people retain their newly learned skills. Disabled people tend to avoid using impaired limbs, a behavior called learned non-use. However, the repetitive use of impaired limbs encourages brain plasticity and helps reduce disabilities.

Strategies used by physical therapists to encourage the use of impaired limbs include selective sensory stimulation such as tapping or stroking, active and passive range-of-motion exercises, and temporary restraint of healthy limbs while practicing motor tasks. Some physical therapists may use a new technology, transcutaneous electrical nerve stimulation (TENS), that encourages brain reorganization and recovery of function. TENS involves using a small probe that generates an electrical current to stimulate nerve activity in stroke-impaired limbs.

In general, physical therapy emphasizes practicing isolated movements, repeatedly changing from one kind of movement to another, and rehearsing complex movements that require a great deal of coordination and balance, such as walking up or down stairs or moving safely between obstacles. People too weak to bear their own weight can still practice repetitive movements during hydrotherapy (in which water provides sensory stimulation as well as weight support) or while being partially supported by a harness. A recent trend in physical therapy emphasizes the effectiveness of engaging in goal-directed activities, such as playing games, to promote coordination. Physical therapists frequently employ selective sensory stimulation to encourage use of impaired limbs and to help survivors with neglect regain awareness of stimuli on the neglected side of the body.

Occupational and Recreational Therapists

Like physical therapists, occupational therapists are concerned with improving motor and sensory abilities. They help survivors relearn skills needed for performing self-directed activities and occupations— such as personal grooming, preparing meals, and housecleaning. Therapists can teach some survivors how to adapt to driving and provide on-road training. They often teach people to divide a complex activity into its component parts, practice each part, and then perform the whole sequence of actions. This strategy can improve coordination and may help people with apraxia relearn how to carry out planned actions.

Occupational therapists also teach people how to develop compensatory strategies and how to change elements of their environment that limit activities of daily living. For example, people with the use of only one hand can substitute Velcro closures for buttons on clothing. Occupational therapists also help people make changes in their homes to increase safety, remove barriers, and facilitate physical functioning, such as installing grab bars in bathrooms.

Recreational therapists help people with a variety of disabilities to develop and use their leisure time to enhance their health, independence, and quality of life.

Speech-Language Pathologists

Speech-language pathologists help stroke survivors with aphasia relearn how to use language or develop alternative means of communication. They also help people improve their ability to swallow, and they work with patients to develop problem-solving and social skills needed to cope with the aftereffects of a stroke.

Many specialized therapeutic techniques have been developed to assist people with aphasia. Some forms of short-term therapy can improve comprehension rapidly. Intensive exercises such as repeating the therapist's words, practicing following directions, and doing reading or writing exercises form the cornerstone of language rehabilitation. Conversational coaching and rehearsal, as well as the development of prompts or cues to help people remember specific words, are sometimes

465

beneficial. Speech-language pathologists also help stroke survivors develop strategies for circumventing language disabilities. These strategies can include the use of symbol boards or sign language. Recent advances in computer technology have spurred the development of new types of equipment to enhance communication.

Speech-language pathologists use noninvasive imaging techniques to study swallowing patterns of stroke survivors and identify the exact source of their impairment. Difficulties with swallowing have many possible causes, including a delayed swallowing reflex, an inability to manipulate food with the tongue, or an inability to detect food remaining lodged in the cheeks after swallowing. When the cause has been pinpointed, speech-language pathologists work with the individual to devise strategies to overcome or minimize the deficit. Sometimes, simply changing body position and improving posture during eating can bring about improvement. The texture of foods can be modified to make swallowing easier; for example, thin liquids, which often cause choking, can be thickened. Changing eating habits by taking small bites and chewing slowly can also help alleviate dysphagia.

Vocational Therapists

Approximately one fourth of all strokes occur in people between the ages of 45 and 65. For most people in this age group, returning to work is a major concern. Vocational therapists perform many of the same functions that ordinary career counselors do. They can help people with residual disabilities identify vocational strengths and develop resumes that highlight those strengths. They also can help identify potential employers, assist in specific job searches, and provide referrals to stroke vocational rehabilitation agencies.

Most important, vocational therapists educate disabled individuals about their rights and protections as defined by the Americans with Disabilities Act of 1990. This law requires employers to make "reasonable accommodations" for disabled employees. Vocational therapists frequently act as mediators between employers and employees to negotiate the provision of reasonable accommodations in the workplace.

Where Can a Stroke Patient Get Rehabilitation?

Rehabilitation should begin as soon as a stroke patient is stable, often within 24 to 48 hours after a stroke. This first stage of rehabilitation usually occurs within an acute-care hospital. At the time of discharge from the hospital, the stroke patient and family coordinate with hospital social workers to locate a suitable living arrangement. Many stroke survivors return home, but some move into some type of medical facility.

Inpatient Rehabilitation Units

Inpatient facilities may be freestanding or part of larger hospital complexes. Patients stay in the facility, usually for 2 to 3 weeks, and engage in a coordinated, intensive program of rehabilitation. Such programs often involve at least 3 hours of active therapy a day, 5 or 6 days a week. Inpatient facilities offer a comprehensive range of medical services, including full-time physician supervision and access to the full range of therapists specializing in poststroke rehabilitation.

Outpatient Units

Outpatient facilities are often part of a larger hospital complex and provide access to physicians and the full range of therapists specializing in stroke rehabilitation. Patients typically spend several hours, often 3 days each week, at the facility taking part in coordinated therapy sessions and return home at night. Comprehensive outpatient facilities frequently offer treatment programs as intense as those of inpatient facilities, but they also can offer less demanding regimens, depending on the patient's physical capacity.

Nursing Facilities

Rehabilitative services available at nursing facilities are more variable than are those at inpatient and outpatient units. Skilled nursing facilities usually place a greater emphasis on rehabilitation, whereas traditional nursing homes emphasize residential care. In addition, fewer hours of therapy are offered compared to outpatient and inpatient rehabilitation units.

Home-Based Rehabilitation Programs

Home rehabilitation allows for great flexibility so that patients can tailor their program of rehabilitation and follow individual schedules. Stroke survivors may participate in an intensive level of therapy several hours per week or follow a less demanding regimen. These arrangements are often best suited for people who lack transportation or require treatment by only one type of rehabilitation therapist. Patients

467

dependent on Medicare coverage for their rehabilitation must meet Medicare's "homebound" requirements to qualify for such services; at this time lack of transportation is not a valid reason for home therapy. The major disadvantage of home-based rehabilitation programs is the lack of specialized equipment. However, undergoing treatment at home gives people the advantage of practicing skills and developing compensatory strategies in the context of their own living environment.

What Research Is Being Done?

The National Institute of Neurological Disorders and Stroke (NINDS), a component of the Federal Government's National Institutes of Health (NIH), has primary responsibility for sponsoring research on disorders of the brain and nervous system, including the acute phase of stroke and the restoration of function after stroke. The NINDS also supports research on ways to enhance repair and regeneration of the central nervous system. Scientists funded by the NINDS are studying how the brain responds to experience or adapts to injury by reorganizing its functions (plasticity) by using noninvasive imaging technologies to map patterns of biological activity inside the brain. Other NINDS-sponsored scientists are looking at brain reorganization after stroke and determining whether specific rehabilitative techniques, such as constraint-induced movement therapy and transcranial magnetic stimulation, can stimulate brain plasticity, thereby improving motor function and decreasing disability. Other scientists are experimenting with implantation of neural stem cells, to see if these cells may be able to replace the cells that died as a result of a stroke.

Chapter 56

Innovations in
Stroke Rehabilitation

Chapter Contents

Section 56.1

New Approaches in Stroke Rehab

"Rat Race Rehabilitation" by Bob Stott, *Therapy Times,*
October 22, 2007. © 2007 *Therapy Times.* Reprinted with permission.

According to the American Heart Association, stroke is the third highest killer and leading cause of long-term disability in the United States, with 700,000 people suffering a new or recurrent stroke each year. In light of these statistics and with a baby boomer population entering their golden age, stroke rehabilitation is pushing its way to the forefront of the therapy industry.

Strokes can attack almost without warning. A previously undetected blood clot or burst blood vessel can suddenly turn disastrous, blocking circulation to large portions of the brain, depriving the tissue of necessary oxygen and glucose. Once blockage occurs, some brain cells can die within minutes, while others may take several hours to die, depending on the severity of the stroke. As a result, stroke victims can often lose a range of physical and mental functions, and most motor-function disabilities can become permanent.

And They're Off . . .

Due to the small window of opportunity available for stroke patients to recover normal function, stroke rehabilitation needs to start as soon as possible, and may last for several months. While some patients have been known to continue to recover function years after the occurrence of a stroke, most significant return of function is seen within the first weeks of therapy. According to the Copenhagen Stroke Study, no significant functional recovery was seen in stroke patients later than 24 weeks poststroke; a time estimate many clinicians and health insurers use as a limit for therapy services. In light of these estimates, stroke patients are inclined to take on as much therapy as possible before time runs out on their prospects of recovery.

"Among [stroke victims] who survive, only 10 percent recover completely and many of the remaining survivors need rehabilitation because of resulting impairments," write J. Xie, M.D., Ph.D., and colleagues from the Division for Heart Disease and Stroke Prevention, National Center for Chronic Disease Prevention and Health Promotion, U.S. Centers for Disease Control and Prevention (CDC). "Long-term disability not only affects functional status and social roles among stroke survivors, but also results in substantial costs; the combined direct and indirect costs of stroke are projected to be $62.7 billion in the United States in 2007."

However, as the general populace is becoming better informed about the repercussions of stroke and its therapies, there is a growing trend of active patient involvement with their therapy. Also, as a wide range of alternative therapies are better publicized than in prior years, informed patients are able to discuss the course of their own therapy with their physicians. As a result, new avenues of communication allow patients to have some degree of influence over their own rehabilitation.

Cross-Rehabilitation Takes the Lead

While physical and occupational therapies tend to be the focus for most rat racers struggling through stroke rehabilitation, developing technologies are now allowing for separate therapies to overlap in more concise coordinated treatments. With the introduction of several of these new treatments, therapists have the chance to extend the window of recovery for stroke patients, as well as augmenting the patient's range of function.

Providing a meeting point between the three focal stroke therapies (physical, occupational, speech), a new technology program called the Interactive Metronome® has become prevalent for usage in stroke patients suffering from multiple function loss. Developed by Interactive Metronome Inc., the Metronome combines the standard musical metronome—a device that produces a regulated audible pulse, used to establish a steady beat, or tempo—with a computer program that measures, assesses, and improves a patient's foundational skills for learning and development. The program's auditory guide tones direct a patient to match a series of hand and foot exercises in sync to the metronome beat.

As result of these neurosensory and neuromotor exercises, the patient is strengthening areas of their brain that foster increased attention span, motor control/coordination, language processing, and reading and mathematics skills.

Another recent introduction to the rehabilitation field is haptics, a virtual reality technology that allows users to see and feel daily tasks

471

in a computer-generated environment. Haptics programs are custom-designed to target and improve specific skills, such as grasping, squeezing, and rotating the wrist, measuring the physical force used for a patient to do each task. This combination of physical and mental exercise presents therapists with a wider range of exercises to view patient recovery. Virtual tasks, such as pouring milk or cracking an egg into a pan, can be modified to fit each patient's level of level of impairment, while immediate feedback enables therapists to adjust programs according to patient recovery progress.

"Designing one [haptics program] is very much like creating an aircraft simulator to test and train pilots," says Albert Rizzo, Ph.D., a research scientist at the University of Southern California Institute for Creative Technologies, Los Angeles. "But now we've created simulations that can assess and rehabilitate a stroke patient under a range of stimulus conditions. These are conditions that aren't easily deliverable or controllable in the real world."

An additional breakthrough in stroke rehabilitation studies comes with the advent of cortical stimulation; the process of electrically arousing the cerebral cortex, the outermost layer of the brain. Cortical stimulation operates on the working theory that the precise delivery of low-level electricity via an implanted system can help the brain form alternate pathways to regain function lost after a stroke.

"The old thinking is that the brain [poststroke] is not retrainable," says Mark Huang, M.D., who is leading a Northstar Neuroscience Inc. study at the Rehabilitation Institute of Chicago. But, the new thinking, he says, is that the brain can be retrained. "Brain mapping trials have shown that, after brain trauma, other areas of the brain can take over function of the impaired area. Using cortical stimulation, areas of the brain that represent motor control are altered so the patient has better control of the impaired limbs."

In the continuing Northstar study, surgeons place a small stimulating electrode—approximately the size of a postage stamp—on the protective membrane of the cortex over the particular areas where brain function is affected by the stroke. Similar in design to an artificial pacemaker, the electrode connects to a wire running under the skin to the collarbone where it hooks up to an implanted pulse generator.

The cortical stimulant is only used during periods when the patient is attempting physical activity, and the procedure is intended to coincide with other forms of therapy for greatest results in recovery. Once therapy sessions have concluded, the electrode and generator are removed.

472

"The theory based on the model studies is that if therapists apply electrical stimulation, they enhance the ability of the brain to recover beyond the limits of traditional rehab therapies," says Huang. The focus of the study is that the treatment is not growing new brain cells, but there is unproven potential that cortical stimulation is capable of growing new connections between brain cells.

While stroke patients continue to push themselves to recovery, researchers and therapists are likewise pushing the folds of accepted medicine outward by investigating alternate therapies and experimental procedures. In the hectic rat race to overcome the debilitating effects of stroke, every individual victory contributes to the improvement of recovery therapy.

Bob Stott is a staff writer for *Therapy Times*.

Section 56.2

Repetitive Transcranial Magnetic Stimulation May Offer Promise for Stroke Patients

"Ask the Experts: Can repetitive transcranial magnetic stimulation (rTMS) be used to treat stroke victims or those with head injuries?" by Sarah Lisanby, M.D., Chief, Brain Stimulation and Therapeutic Modulation Division © 2006 Columbia University Medical Center Department of Psychiatry. Reprinted with permission.

Can repetitive transcranial magnetic stimulation (rTMS) be used to treat stroke victims or those with head injuries? Specifically, can motor control and reflexes, as well as memory and speech be improved through rTMS?

Repetitive transcranial magnetic stimulation (rTMS) refers to the use of magnetic fields to stimulate the brain. The magnetic fields induce small electrical currents in the brain, which can activate circuits in the brain. Repeatedly activating functional networks in the brain can alter the functioning of those networks in ways that might be therapeutic. The therapeutic potential of rTMS is under study.

rTMS is under study for the treatment of a range of psychiatric and neurological disorders, including depression, schizophrenia, anxiety disorders, Parkinson's disease, and stroke, just to name a few. rTMS is not presently approved by the Food and Drug Administration (FDA), therefore rTMS is considered experimental.

Several studies have examined the potential use of rTMS for neurorehabilitation following stroke. One theory behind using rTMS following stroke is that rTMS might be able to activate circuits damaged by the stroke to strengthen their connections. In these studies, rTMS is typically given at or near the site of the stroke. Physical therapy, an important aspect of neurological recovery following stroke, relies on the person's ability to voluntarily move the muscles affected by the stroke, to strengthen the damaged circuits. rTMS is being studied in this context to see if directly activating these circuits could be effective. Some studies have combined rTMS with physical training, and demonstrated that pre-treatment with rTMS enhanced the degree to which the person's movement improved during the physical training. Other studies have used different forms of rTMS, such as Paired Associative Stimulation (PAS) where rTMS is paired with electrical stimulation of the affected muscle), and theta burst stimulation (TBS) where bursts of high frequency rTMS are repeated at 5 per second.

An alternative theory behind the use of rTMS following stroke is that the brain's response to the stroke may trigger changes in brain function that are maladaptive. In these studies, rTMS is typically given to the hemisphere (side of the brain) opposite to the side of the stroke. For example, the theory suggests that a stroke in the left hemisphere may trigger an increase in activity in the opposite hemisphere, and that this abnormal hyperexcitability in the right hemisphere interferes with normal functioning. rTMS is then given to the right hemisphere in an attempt to dampen or block the development of this abnormal hyperexcitability. This approach has been studied in the treatment of aphasia (language impairment from stroke).

Finally, rTMS has been studied in the treatment of poststroke depression. In addition to motor function and speech, mood can also be affected by stroke. There are forms of depression that are thought to result from stroke, either large strokes, or multiple small strokes that may be "clinically silent." This is commonly called "vascular depression" because it is a depression that has its origins in vascular disease. Studies have examined whether rTMS could be useful in treating vascular depression, with encouraging results.

Research with rTMS in stroke is at the early stages. The research has been very promising, but is not yet at the stage that rTMS could be recommended as a routine clinical treatment. Several research studies are available that use rTMS following stroke. If you are interested in these studies, it is important to discuss the risks, benefits, and alternatives with your doctor. rTMS carries a risk of seizure, which could be higher in persons with neurological damage such as stroke.

For more information, see:

1. Castel-Lacanal E, Gerdelat-Mas A, Marque P, Loubinoux I, Simonetta-Moreau M. Induction of cortical plastic changes in wrist muscles by paired associative stimulation in healthy subjects and post-stroke patients. *Exp Brain Res.* 2007 Jun;180(1): 113–22.

2. Kim YH, You SH, Ko MH, Park JW, Lee KH, Jang SH, Yoo WK, Hallett M. Repetitive transcranial magnetic stimulation-induced corticomotor excitability and associated motor skill acquisition in chronic stroke. *Stroke.* 2006 Jun;37(6):1471–6.

3. Talelli P, Greenwood RJ, Rothwell JC. Exploring Theta Burst Stimulation as an intervention to improve motor recovery in chronic stroke. *Clin Neurophysiol.* 2007 Feb;118(2):333–42.

4. Webster BR, Celnik PA, Cohen LG. Noninvasive brain stimulation in stroke rehabilitation. *NeuroRx.* 2006 Oct;3(4):474–81.

Section 56.3

TROY: A Newly Identified Stop Signal in the Pathway for Nerve Regeneration

From the National Institute of Neurological Disorders
and Stroke (NINDS, www.ninds.nih.gov), part of the National
Institutes of Health, March 5, 2005.

One of the major puzzles in neuroscience is how to get nerves in the brain and spinal cord to regrow after injury. A new study has identified a protein, TROY, that inhibits nerve cell repair and plays a role in preventing nerve regeneration. This finding is an important step in developing new methods for treatment of spinal cord injury, stroke, and degenerative nerve disorders such as multiple sclerosis (MS).

Most of the cells in the human body have the ability to repair themselves after injury. However, neurons in the central nervous system (CNS) are unable to regenerate their injured axons. One of the major obstacles to regeneration in the adult CNS is the presence of inhibitory molecules that are associated with myelin, a fatty coating that forms a sheath around nerve cells. Research in recent years has focused on identifying the chain of events that prevents regeneration.

Part of the inhibitory or "braking" machinery that stops nerve regeneration is Nogo, a protein normally found in myelin. Studies have suggested that a necessary partner or coreceptor to Nogo is a protein called p75, which is common in the developing nervous system but decreases during adulthood. However, while most neurons in the central nervous system do not have p75, these neurons still demonstrate myelin inhibition and cannot repair themselves. In the new study, Dr. Zhigang He and colleagues from the Children's Hospital of Harvard Medical School in Boston asked, "Why do neurons without p75 still fail to regenerate after injury?" Their findings appear in the February 3, 2005, issue of *Neuron*. This research was funded in part by the National Institute of Neurological Disorders and Stroke (NINDS).

"We hypothesized that either these neurons without p75 have a completely different mechanism to prevent regeneration, or that a different version of the protein exists," says Dr. He. "This investigation led us to the newly identified TROY protein, a member of the same receptor family as p75. While TROY has a similar action to the p75 protein, it is widely expressed throughout the CNS. TROY also has a well researched biochemical pathway that could help us to possibly target new strategies for clinical therapy."

This study is the first to show that TROY is a critical player in blocking nerve regeneration. Although the research does not eliminate the possibility that other molecules are also involved in regeneration, the study helps scientists to understand how myelin inhibition may be regulated. The finding that more than one protein may be involved in myelin inhibition adds a new level of complexity to designing therapeutic strategies for treating CNS injury.

"Designing a therapeutic strategy to block myelin inhibition would be an efficient way to promote regeneration. This research may provide important insights into development of future treatment for spinal cord injuries," says Dr. He.

Researchers caution that any strategy to alter the inhibitor proteins would need to be carefully designed. Since both p75 and TROY are expressed in many types of cells in the CNS and are also involved in inflammatory responses, simply blocking these proteins could lead to many undesirable side effects.

The discovery of the TROY protein enhances understanding of nerve injury and provides a piece in the puzzle of CNS nerve regeneration. Investigators hope this information will point to ways to stimulate nerve repair in the brain, which is vital for restoring functions in persons with MS, spinal cord injury, stroke, and other CNS injury conditions.

Reference: Park JB, Yiu G, Kaneko S, Wang J, Chang J, He Z. "A TNF receptor family member, TROY, is a coreceptor with Nogo receptor in mediating the inhibitory activity of myelin inhibitors." *Neuron,* February 3, 2005, Vol.45, pp. 345–351.

Chapter 57

Choosing Stroke Rehabilitation Services

Rehabilitation, often referred to as rehab, is an important part of stroke recovery. Through rehab, you:

- Relearn basic skills such as talking, eating, dressing, and walking.
- Increase your strength, flexibility, and endurance.
- Regain as much independence as possible.

You and your loved ones want the best rehab program possible. But, it is important to remember that all stroke survivors are not the same. Not only do they have different brain injuries and disabilities, but also different interests, lifestyles, and priorities. What is best for you may not be the best for someone else.

So, how do you choose the best rehab program for you?

Use this guide to learn more about stroke rehab programs and to help you find a good fit. After reading this guide, you will be able to:

- Tell the difference between one stroke rehab setting and another.
- Identify who's who on the stroke rehab team.
- Understand "discharge planning" and what it can include.

- Determine if a rehab program meets current rehabilitation industry standards.

- Set apart an excellent program from a good to average program.

- Figure out if a rehab program meets your personal needs.

Understanding Stroke Rehabilitation Programs

Most stroke survivors will receive treatment in a stroke rehab program. There are several types of rehab programs for stroke survivors. These programs differ from each other in three ways:

- type and range of services provided

- frequency of services

- setting (where the treatment occurs)

Stroke Rehab Settings

Stroke rehab programs can be found in many different settings. Your doctors will usually suggest the most rigorous program you can handle. They will decide what you can handle based on your age, overall health, and degree of disability.

Some stroke rehab programs are inpatient programs and others are outpatient programs. An inpatient program will assign you a room to live in while you are being treated. An outpatient program will provide treatment to you but not admit you to stay overnight.

Stroke Rehabilitation Team

To help you meet your stroke recovery goals, your rehab program will be planned by a team of professionals. This team may include some of the following:

- **Physiatrist:** Specializes in rehabilitation following injuries, accidents, or illness

- **Neurologist:** Specializes in the prevention, diagnosis, and treatment of stroke and other diseases of the brain and spinal cord

- **Rehabilitation Nurse:** Specializes in helping people with disabilities; helps survivors manage health problems that affect stroke (diabetes, high blood pressure) and adjust to life after stroke

Table 57.1. Comparing Stroke Rehab Settings

Programs	Services	Setting	Frequency	Likely Candidates
Acute care (inpatient) and rehab hospitals	24-hour medical care and a full range of rehab services	Hospital or special rehab unit of a hospital	Several hours each day (most demanding)	Survivors who have many medical issues and may develop problems without continued medical treatment
Sub-acute facilities	Provide daily nursing care and a fairly wide range of rehab services	Rehab center, rehab unit of a hospital, skilled nursing facility (short-term nursing care) or skilled nursing home (long-term), skilled nursing unit in a hospital	Less demanding than acute programs, but continue for longer periods of time	Survivors who have serious disabilities but are unable to handle the demands of acute programs
Long-term care facilities	One or more treatment areas	Nursing home, skilled nursing facility	2–3 days per week	Survivors who have their medical problems under control but still need 24-hour nursing care
Outpatient facilities	One or more treatment areas	Doctor's office, outpatient center of a hospital, other outpatient centers	2–3 days per week	Survivors who have their medical problems under control enough to live in their own homes and can travel to get their treatment
Home health agencies	Specific rehab services in one or more treatment areas	In the home	As needed	Survivors who live at home but are unable to travel to get their treatment

481

- **Physical Therapist (PT):** Helps stroke survivors with problems in moving and balance; suggests exercises to strengthen muscles for walking, standing, and other activities

- **Occupational Therapist (OT):** Helps stroke survivors learn strategies to manage daily activities such as eating, bathing, dressing, writing, or cooking

- **Speech-Language Pathologists (SLP):** Helps stroke survivors re-learn language skills (talking, reading, and writing); shares strategies to help with swallowing problems

- **Dietitian:** Teaches survivors about healthy eating and special diets (low salt, low fat, low calorie)

- **Social Worker:** Helps survivors make decisions about rehab programs, living arrangements, insurance, and support services in the home

- **Neuropsychologist:** Diagnoses and treats survivors who may be facing changes in thinking, memory, and behavior after stroke

- **Case Manager:** Helps survivors facilitate follow-up to acute care, coordinate care from multiple providers, and link to local services

- **Recreation Therapist:** Helps stroke survivors learn strategies to improve the thinking and movement skills needed to join in recreational activities

Discharge Planning

Discharge planning is the process of preparing you to live independently in the home. The purpose is to help maintain the benefits of rehabilitation after you have been released from the program. It begins early during rehabilitation and involves you, your family and the stroke rehab team. You should be discharged from rehab soon after your goals have been reached.

Discharge planning can include:

- Making sure you have a safe place to live after discharge.

- Deciding what care, assistance, or special equipment you will need.

- Arranging for more rehab services or for other services in the home.

- Choosing the health care provider who will monitor your health and medical needs.

- Determining the caregivers who will provide daily care, supervision, and assistance at home.

- Determining which community services may be helpful now or after some time. Examples include meal delivery, volunteer rides to the rehab center, visitor programs, and caregiver relief programs.

Finding the Right Fit

Standards of Excellence—CARF and JCAHO

Many industries have a formal system of recognizing organizations that meet standards of excellence in their field. This is called accreditation or certification. For hospitals and rehabilitation centers, the Commission on Accreditation of Healthcare Organizations (CARF) and the Joint Commission on Accreditation of Healthcare Organizations (JCAHO) set these standards. Medicare also certifies rehab programs and centers that meet minimum health and safety standards.

Some examples of requirements for CARF accreditation include:

- A medical director and doctors who are board certified in rehab-related specialties such as physiatry or neurology.

- A team approach for patient care.

- Regular rehab team meetings to evaluate each patient's progress.

- Involvement of family members in the program.

- Regular family meetings to keep them up-to-date with the progress of their loved ones.

- Patient and family education.

- Patient and family support.

- Defined process for handling emergencies.

- Ongoing assessment of each patient's progress in terms of abilities and level of independence in activities of daily living (such as dressing and walking).

You may want to ask rehabilitation centers to explain how they handle some of these areas.

Narrowing down Your Options

An excellent stroke rehab program should also meet standards of excellence not required for CARF or Medicare certification. This can set apart an excellent program from a good to average program. Use the following checklist to help you find the excellent program that you deserve.

After you narrow down your list of programs that meet current rehabilitation standards, you can focus on finding a nearby program that meets your personal needs. The second checklist can help you determine if a rehab program meets your needs.

Checklist: Finding an Excellent Program

Questions to Ask

- Has the program been in operation at least one year?

- Does the program have a formal system for evaluating the progress made by its patients and the overall outcomes of the stroke rehab program?

- Does the program have any partners that offer rehab services at other levels of care that I may eventually need (day treatment, outpatient treatment, or home care)?

- Does the program provide a wide range of therapy services? (physical therapy, occupational therapy, speech therapy)

- Does the program have on staff a full-time physiatrist or another doctor who is experienced in stroke and rehab medicine?

- Is medical care available at the rehab center if I need it?

- Can my doctor visit me at the rehab center? (Does he/she have visiting privileges?)

- Does the program have a stroke support group for survivors and their families? If not, can they refer me to a local group?

- Does the program use outside groups (such as consumer advocacy groups) to get ideas for serving disabled people?

- Does the program conduct home visits before checking people out of the center and releasing them to their homes?

- Are staff members required to keep up with new information about stroke and rehabilitation? How do they do so?

Checklist: Meeting Personal Needs

Treatments and Services

- Does the facility offer the rehab treatments that I need?
- Am I eligible for those treatments?
- How can these treatments help me?
- Will there be bilingual staff members if I need them?
- Will there be sign language interpreters if I need them?
- Will medical information be explained in simple terms?
- Is help available with discharge? How does it work?
- What percent of people will return home after discharge?
- What percent of people will be placed in nursing homes?

Location

- Is it convenient to me?
- Is it close to public transportation?
- Is it convenient to family and friends?

Hours

- Are the days and times convenient for me?
- What are the visiting hours?
- Are the visiting hours convenient for family and friends?
- Are the visiting hours long enough for a good quality visit?

Cost and Insurance

- What is the estimated cost of my treatment?
- Will my insurance plan or government funding (Medicare, Medicaid, state health plans) cover all or part of the cost?
- Will the staff help me with health insurance claims or appeals, if needed?
- What is the average total cost for the complete stroke program (acute rehab, home care, outpatient)?

Customer Service and Satisfaction

- Does the program collect information from patients and their families about satisfaction with the care received?

- If so, is the feedback generally positive?

- Can I talk to other people who have used the services?

- How long do most stroke survivors stay in the program?

Chapter 58

Improving Brain Function in Postrehab Stroke Survivors

After years of researching and developing stroke rehabilitation techniques, Rafael H. Llinas, M.D., assistant professor of neurology at the Johns Hopkins Bayview Medical Center, has concluded that "the brain is a very lazy organ."

He doesn't mean to be disparaging. Rather, his view signals a fundamental shift in how physicians and researchers now view the long-term consequences of stroke. For years, it was thought that stroke victims reached a plateau in their recovery within three to six months because vital neural connections had been lost forever. But the last decade has seen researchers embracing the idea of "neuroplasticity"—the concept that the brain can continue changing and rewiring if patients are challenged and stimulated in new ways.

Too often, however, the demands of managed care lengths-of-stay means that standard therapy has to focus on getting patients to work around motor impairments instead of trying to improve them, an approach that researchers now think lulls the brain into "laziness."

As a result, researchers now are working on ways to galvanize the brain and get it to reorganize, either by using existing pathways for new purposes or creating new pathways even years after a stroke occurs. Their methods run the gamut from physical therapy techniques, to electrical stimulation of the brain, to robotics, to medications generally used to treat other neurological disorders. Here's a look at some of the most promising developments.

"Waking up the brain after stroke," by Yasmine Iqbal, *ACP Observer,* July-August 2007. © 2007 American College of Physicians. All rights reserved.

New Rehabilitative Techniques

Constraint-induced movement therapy (CIMT) involves intensively exercising an impaired limb while restraining the unaffected one. Unlike conventional therapy, which might focus on getting patients to rely on their stronger side, CIMT forces them to develop the potential in their weaker areas.

"When we reinforce the notion of 'learned non-use,' by teaching patients to compensate, we squelch the potential of use," said Steven L. Wolf, Ph.D., professor of rehabilitation medicine at the Emory University School of Medicine in Atlanta.

Dr. Wolf was the principal investigator in the EXCITE (Extremity Constraint Induced Therapy Evaluation, published in the Nov. 1, 2006 *Journal of the American Medical Association*) clinical trial, which involved 222 patients who had experienced strokes three to nine months before enrolling in the study. All patients had experienced hemiparesis that resulted in diminished arm or hand movement. During the study, 106 patients wore an immobilizing mitt on their less-impaired hand or arm for 90% of their waking hours for 14 days. These patients received therapy, which included practicing repetitive movements and functional activities (such as eating and writing) for up to six hours a day. The remaining 116 patients received standard care.

In one year, the CIMT patients regained more function than control group patients. They were able to complete a task 52% faster, compared with 26% faster in control group patients, and they increased the proportion of tasks completed with their impaired limb more than 50% of the time by 24%, compared with a 13% increase in the control group.

The EXCITE trial was the first multi-center clinical trial of any rehabilitation method to improve motor function after a stroke. "The EXCITE trial really moved rehabilitation into the Phase 3 clinical trial arena," said Carolee J. Winstein, Ph.D., professor of biokinesiology and physical therapy at the University of Southern California, Los Angeles, the study's co-principal investigator. She noted that although it's clear that CIMT was successful, key questions about what intensity and duration of therapy are needed to make a difference remain unanswered. "We still need to understand what the ingredients are that made this work," she said.

Some researchers suspect that CIMT need not be so intense to be effective. Stephen J. Page, Ph.D., associate professor of physical medicine and rehabilitation at the University of Cincinnati, has developed a modified CIMT regimen that involves therapy sessions of 30 minutes a day, three times a week, for 10 weeks. The less-impaired limb is restrained for five hours a day, five days a week. In his studies, patients show clinically significant motor function gains, and fMRI scans show activity in previously dormant areas of the brain. "Modified CIMT is much less intensive, but compliance is much higher, and evidence suggests that it's just as effective as CIMT," he said.

Dr. Page has also been studying mental practice techniques—simply visualizing the performance of physical movements—which engages the same areas of the brain that would become active if the patient were actually performing the task. In an article published in the April 2007 issue of *Stroke,* Dr. Page and his colleagues demonstrated that patients who underwent 30-minute mental practice sessions directly after physical therapy significantly increased their arm motor function compared to a control group receiving only physical therapy.

"Athletes and musicians often use mental practice and visualization to help them perform," said Dr. Page. "Now we're finding that it's an easy, cost-effective strategy for stroke rehabilitation, as well."

Robot-Assisted Physical Therapy

Experts agree that patients make the most progress when working one-on-one with a therapist. But sometimes, patients can experience even better results when their human therapists work in tandem with a robotic device. Examples of robot-assisted therapy include:

- The **Lokomat**, manufactured by Hocoma, a Swiss-based company, assists with partial body-weight supported treadmill training to help patients with walking and gait problems. Patients are strapped into a modified parachute harness while the legs are guided through walking motions by two brace-like components. Traditional training of this type required two therapists to move the legs; with the Lokomat, patients can train for longer periods while the device precisely monitors their gait patterns.

- The **KineAssist**, which is being developed at the Rehabilitation Institute of Chicago, is the first over-ground walking and balance exercise system. It's a wheeled device that follows and supports patients from behind, allowing them to walk, climb stairs, and practice turning. It can even nudge patients slightly off balance, allowing them to practice catching themselves before they fall.

- The **Hand-Wrist Assisting Robotic Device**, or HOWARD, developed at the University of California at Irvine, is a splint-like device that fits around the hand and monitors patients' ability to make gripping and grasping movements. If they can't complete the movement, HOWARD uses a pneumatic system to help them the rest of the way, allowing the brain to relearn the activity.

"Many patients don't have access to good rehabilitation programs," said Steven C. Cramer, MD, Co-Director of the University of California Irvine's Stroke and Cerebrovascular Center, who helped develop HOWARD. Although he admitted that it might be a while before robotic therapy is simple and cost-effective, he envisions a time when patients might supplement their outpatient rehabilitation with a therapy robot in the home.

But even the biggest proponents of robot-assisted therapy say that the technology has its limits. "Robots will never completely substitute for therapists," said Elliot J. Roth, MD, Senior Vice President for Medical Affairs at the Rehabilitation Institute of Chicago. "Their main advantages are that they make therapy more consistent, predictable, and measurable."

And there's a danger in allowing patients to rely too much on robot-assisted movement, said George Hornby, Ph.D., a researcher at the Rehabilitation Institute of Chicago. He noted that some studies indicate that locomotion robots are best used only in the initial stages of therapy when patients are very weak. "Patients don't learn as well if they're getting continuous assistance," he said, noting that patients may not become attuned to subtle sensory and balance shifts while walking if a robot is doing much of the work to hold them up and move their limbs. "Robots are like training wheels," he said. "They can get you to a certain point, but after that, you have to learn to correct your own mistakes."

Electrical Stimulation Therapies

For years, researchers have been studying how low levels of electrical or magnetic stimulation can speed brain recovery. Although the exact mechanism for how this works isn't well understood, it's thought that the stimulation somehow enhances the brain's ability to form new neural connections. Therapies include:

Cortical stimulation involves applying targeted electrical stimulation directly to the cerebral cortex adjacent to the damaged areas of the brain. Seattle-based Northstar Neuroscience, Inc. currently has 21 sites enrolled in a trial of its Renova Cortical Stimulation System, which is comprised of an electrode patch that is placed on the brain and connected to an implantable pulse generator in the chest. The device is turned on only during therapy sessions and explanted after a number of weeks. Previous studies of cortical stimulation suggest that once the device induces neuroplasticity, motor function improvements are permanent, even after the hardware is removed.

Repetitive transcranial magnetic stimulation (rTMS) involves a less-invasive method that uses magnetic fields generated by passing electrical current through a conducting coil held close to the skull. The magnetic pulses can be used to slow activity on the undamaged side of the brain, forcing the damaged portion to work harder during therapy (a concept similar to CIMT). It can also be used to stimulate the damaged portion of the brain. Transcranial direct current stimulation (tDCS), which applies a weak direct current through the scalp, is also being studied for its potential to jump-start neural activity.

Finding New Uses for Common Medications

Researchers are studying how medications used to treat other conditions can be used to relieve stroke symptoms. For example, antidepressants, such as selective serotonin reuptake inhibitors, might help relieve pain as well as depression; amphetamines might be used to increase cortical excitability; and Botox has been shown to help with spasticity. Investigators are also examining whether medications used to treat Parkinson's disease, including carbidopa-levodopa and ropinirole, might be used to improve motor function and aphasia. Modafinil, generally used to treat narcolepsy, has been used with some success to treat patients with brainstem strokes who suffer from sleep disorders and apathy.

All the newest therapies, technologies, and drugs won't make any difference, experts say, if physicians, therapists, patients and patients' families don't commit to the idea that stroke rehabilitation is an ongoing process. But Richard D. Zorowitz, M.D., visiting associate professor and chairman of the department of physical medicine and rehabilitation at Johns Hopkins Bayview Medical Center, noted that for most patients, the rehab period is shorter than ever. "Inpatient therapy has gradually shifted focus from getting patients to being functional to just getting them to be safe at home," he said. "And insurance companies continue to mandate that we send patients home earlier and earlier." Dr. Winstein added that "a big problem is that there's limited continuity between inpatient and outpatient programs."

Another challenge is getting therapists to try innovative but sometimes time-consuming strategies, such as CIMT. "People are dying to learn effective rehabilitation techniques, because conventional therapies often aren't effective," said Dr. Page. "But it takes a while for these things to trickle down to the average therapist in the field." Dr. Roth added that robotic technology might be a particularly tough sell. "Therapists are conditioned to work with their hands and rely on their interpersonal skills," he said. "They don't always accept that technology might help them."

"There are always going to be more 'techie' things in stroke rehabilitation," said Dr. Llinas. "But the most important development will be in how these advancements change our entire concept of care." He pointed out, for example, that the advent of tPA therapy, although it's not appropriate for every kind of stroke, helped people to understand that they needed to get treatment for stroke as soon as possible. Now that treatments for chronic stroke are proliferating, they will hopefully raise awareness that stroke rehabilitation can continue to be effective long after the actual event.

"It's great that all these advancements are putting more focus on the problem of stroke itself," said Dr. Llinas. "The more we learn about stroke and its effects, the more we realize that rehabilitation will almost always provide the potential for improvement."

Chapter 59

Regaining Muscle
Strength and Control

Chapter Contents

Section 59.1

Strengthening Exercises for Stroke Survivors

Excerpted from "Hope: The Stroke Recovery Guide,"
Copyright © 2007 National Stroke Association. Reprinted with permission.

Moving around safely and easily may not be something you think about, unless you've had a stroke. Many stroke survivors have trouble moving around. These problems range from balance issues to arm or leg paralysis. As a result, about 40 percent of stroke survivors have serious falls within a year of their strokes. But, there is good news. Rehab and therapy may improve your balance and ability to move.

Movement

The most common physical effect of stroke is muscle weakness and having less control of an affected arm or leg. Survivors often work with therapists to restore strength and control through exercise programs. They also learn skills to deal with the loss of certain body movements.

Paralysis and Spasticity

Paralysis is the inability of muscle or group of muscles to move on their own. After stroke, signals from the brain to the muscles often don't work right. This is due to stroke damage to the brain. This damage can cause an arm or leg to become paralyzed and/or to develop spasticity.

Spasticity is a condition where muscles are stiff and resist being stretched. It can be found throughout the body but may be most common in the arms, fingers, or legs. Depending on where it occurs, it can result in an arm being pressed against the chest, a stiff knee, or a pointed foot that interferes with walking. It can also be accompanied by painful muscle spasms.

Treatment Options for Spasticity

- Treatment for spasticity is often a combination of therapy and medicine. Therapy can include range-of-motion exercises, gentle stretching, and splinting or casting.

- Medicine can treat the general effects of spasticity and act on multiple muscle groups in the body.

- Injections or shots of botulinum toxin (Botox® or Myobloc®) or phenol relax stiff muscles by blocking the nerve activity that makes them tight.

- ITB℠ Therapy (Intrathecal Baclofen Therapy) is a treatment option for the management of severe spasticity. This involves the delivery of the drug baclofen directly into the spinal fluid using a surgically placed pump.

- Surgery is the last option to treat spasticity. It can be done on the brain or the muscles and joints. Surgery may block pain and restore some movement.

Exercise

Walking, bending, and stretching are forms of exercise that can help strengthen your body and keep it flexible. Mild exercise, which should be undertaken every day, can take the form of a short walk or a simple activity like sweeping the floor. Stretching exercises, such as extending the arms or bending the torso, should be done regularly. Moving weakened or paralyzed body parts can be done while seated or lying down. Swimming is another beneficial exercise if the pool is accessible and a helper is available. Use an exercise program that is written down, with illustrations and guidelines for a helper if necessary.

Fatigue

Fatigue while exercising is to be expected. Like everyone else, you will have good and bad days. You can modify these programs to accommodate for fatigue or other conditions. Avoid overexertion and pain. However, it may be necessary to tolerate some discomfort to make progress.

Sample Exercise Programs

There are two exercise programs in the following text. The first is for the person whose physical abilities have been mildly affected by the stroke. The second is for those with greater limitations. If you are not sure which one is appropriate, consult the profile that precedes each program.

All of the exercises may be performed alone if you are able to do so safely. However, for many stroke survivors, it is advisable for someone to stand nearby while an exercise session is in progress. Your caregiver should watch for errors in judgment that could affect safety. For instance, some stroke survivors are not aware that their balance is unsteady, nor can they tell left from right. Others may have lost the ability to read the exercise instructions, or may need assistance to remember a full sequence of movements.

In general, each exercise is performed five to 10 times daily, unless otherwise directed. The exercise session should be scheduled for a time of day when you feel alert and well. You might have these ups and downs frequently. If the exercises are too tiring, divide them into two sessions—perhaps once in the morning and again in the afternoon.

Because the effects of stroke vary, it is impossible to devise a single exercise program suitable for everyone. The two programs detailed here are general and are intended to serve as a guide. You should consult an occupational therapist and/or physical therapist, who can help in selecting the specific exercises that will benefit you, and who will provide instruction for both you and your caregiver.

Resources

For referral to an occupational or physical therapist, consult your doctor or contact a home health agency, a family service agency, or the physical therapy department of your community hospital. You may also try contacting the American Occupational Therapy Association at 301-652-2682 or the American Physical Therapy Association at 800-999-2782 for a referral in your area.

As with any exercise program, consult with your doctor and/or therapist before beginning this program. If any exercises are too difficult and cause pain or increased stiffness in your limbs, do not do them.

Exercise Program I: For Those Mildly Affected by Stroke

If you were mildly affected by stroke, you may still have some degree of weakness in the affected arm and leg, but generally have some ability to control your movements. You may also have some obvious stiffness or muscle spasms, particularly with fatigue or stress.

You may be able to walk without someone's assistance, but may use a walker, cane, or brace. For managing longer distances or uneven terrain, you may require some minimal assistance from another person, a more supportive walking aid, or a wheelchair.

Abnormalities may be present when you walk, but may be corrected by exercise and by fitting shoes with lifts or wedges. A prescription for these shoe modifications can be obtained from a doctor following evaluation by a physical therapist. You can usually use the stairs with or without handrails, with a helper close by or with very minimal assistance.

Clothing that does not restrict movement is appropriate for exercising. It is not necessary to wear shorts. Leisure clothing such as sweat suits or jogging suits is appropriate. Sturdy, well-constructed shoes with non-skid soles, such as athletic shoes, are recommended at all times. It is important that your foot on the affected side be checked periodically for reddened areas, pressure marks, swelling, or blisters—especially when there is poor sensation or a lack of sensation. Reddened areas and pressure marks should be reported to a doctor or physical therapist.

The following exercises can help you:

- require less assistance for stair climbing;
- move more steadily when you walk;
- improve balance and endurance;
- strengthen and refine movement patterns; and
- improve the coordination and speed of movement necessary for fine motor skills, such as fastening buttons or tying shoelaces.

Note: The word "floor" has been used to simplify the instructions; the exercises can be performed on the floor, on a firm mattress, or on any appropriate supportive surface.

Exercise 1. To strengthen the muscles that stabilize the shoulder:

1. Lie on your back with your arms resting at your sides.

2. Keep your elbow straight, lift your affected arm to shoulder level with your hand pointing to the ceiling.

3. Raise your hand toward the ceiling, lifting your shoulder blade from the floor.

4. Hold for three to five seconds, and then relax, allowing your shoulder blade to return to the floor.

5. Slowly repeat the reaching motion several times.

6. Lower your arm to rest by your side.

Exercise 2. To strengthen the shoulder muscles as well as those which straighten the elbow:

1. Lying on your back, grasp one end of an elasticized band* in each hand with enough tension to provide light resistance to the exercise, but without causing undue strain.

2. To start, place both hands alongside the unaffected hip, keeping your elbows as straight as possible.

3. Move your affected arm upward in a diagonal direction, reaching out to the side, above your head, keeping your elbow straight.** Your unaffected arm should remain at your side throughout the exercise.

4. During the exercise, stretch the band so that it provides resistance.

*Elasticized bands are marketed as Thera-Band. They are available in varying strengths (color-coded) to provide progressive resistance. Initially, a three or four foot length band—perhaps with the ends knotted together to improve grip—is sufficient for the exercise. To increase resistance as strength improves, the next density of Thera-Band can be purchased, or two or more bands of the original density can be used at once. Thera-Band can be obtained from a medical supply company. Similar elastic bands or cords are also available at many sporting goods stores where exercise equipment is sold.

**If it is too difficult to keep the elbow straight, the exercise can be done with the elbow bent. If you cannot grip with your hand, a loop can be tied at the end to slip your hand partially through the loop, leaving the thumb out to "catch" the loop during upward movement.

Exercise 3. To strengthen the muscles which straighten the elbow:

1. Lie on your back with your arms resting at your sides and a rolled towel under the affected elbow.

2. Bend affected elbow and move your hand up toward your shoulder. Keep your elbow resting on the towel.

3. Hold for a few seconds.

4. Straighten your elbow and hold.

5. Slowly repeat several times.

Note: Try not to let the hand roll in towards your midsection/stomach.

Exercise 4. To improve hip control in preparation for walking activities:

1. Start with your unaffected leg flat on the floor and your affected leg bent.

2. Lift your affected foot and cross your affected leg over the other leg.

3. Lift your affected foot and un-cross, resuming the position of step 2.

4. Repeat the crossing and un-crossing motion several times.

Exercise 5. To enhance hip and knee control:

1. Start with your knees bent, feet resting on the floor.

2. Slowly slide the heel of your affected leg down so that the leg straightens.

3. Slowly bring the heel of your affected leg along the floor, returning to the starting position. Keep your heel in contact with the floor throughout the exercise.

Note: Your foot will slide more smoothly if you do this exercise without shoes.

Exercise 6. To improve control of knee motions for walking:

1. Lie on your unaffected side with the bottom knee bent for stability and your affected arm placed in front for support.

2. Starting with your affected leg straight, bend your affected knee, bringing the heel toward your buttocks, then return to the straightened position.

3. Concentrate on bending and straightening your knee while keeping your hip straight.

Exercise 7. To improve weight shift and control for proper walking technique:

1. Start with your knees bent, feet flat on the floor and knees close together.

2. Lift your hips from the floor and keep them raised in the air.

3. Slowly twist your hips side to side. Return to center and lower your hips to the floor.

4. Rest. Repeat motion.

Note: This exercise may be difficult for some stroke survivors and it may worsen back problems. Do not do it if you experience pain.

Exercise 8. To improve balance, weight shift, and control to prepare for walking activities:

1. The starting position is on your hands and knees. Weight should be evenly distributed on both arms and both legs.

2. Rock in a diagonal direction back toward your right heel as far as possible, then as far forward toward your left hand as possible.

3. Repeat motion several times, slowly rocking as far as possible in each direction.

4. Return to center.

5. Rock in a diagonal direction toward your right hand. Move as far back as possible in each direction slowly.

Note: For safety, an assistant may be nearby to prevent loss of balance. This position may not be appropriate or safe for elderly stroke survivors. Consult your doctor and/or physical therapist before attempting this exercise.

Exercise 9. To simulate proper weight shift and knee control necessary for walking:

1. Stand with your unaffected side next to a countertop or other firm surface. Rest your unaffected arm on the surface for support.

2. Lift your unaffected foot from the floor so that you are standing on your affected leg.

3. Slowly bend and straighten the leg on which you are standing through a small range of motion. Try to move smoothly, not allowing your knee to buckle when you bend, or to snap back when you straighten.

4. Repeat the knee bending and straightening several times, slowly.

Exercise 10. To simulate proper weight shift while strengthening hip and pelvis muscles:

1. Stand facing a countertop or other firm surface for support.

2. Shift your weight onto your right leg and lift your knee straight.

3. Return to center with both feet on the floor.

4. Shift your weight onto your left leg and lift your right leg out to the side keeping your back and knee straight.

5. Repeat several times, alternating lifts.

Exercise Program II: For the Person Moderately Affected by Stroke

If you were moderately affected by your stroke, you may use a wheelchair most of the time. You are probably able to walk—at least around the house—with the aid of another person or by using a walking aid. A short leg brace may be needed to help control foot drop or inward turning of the foot. A sling may be used to help the arm and aid in shoulder positioning for controlling pain. Your affected arm and leg may be stiff or may assume a spastic posture that is difficult to control. The toe may turn inward or the foot may drag. When walking, you may "lead" with the unaffected side, leaving the other side behind. Often there are balance problems and difficulty shifting weight toward the affected side.

Clothing that does not restrict movement is appropriate for exercising. It is not necessary to wear shorts. Leisure clothing such as sweat suits or jogging suits is appropriate. Sturdy, well-constructed shoes with non-skid soles, such as athletic shoes, are recommended at all times. It is important that your foot on the affected side be checked periodically for reddened areas, pressure marks, swelling, or blisters—especially when there is poor sensation or a lack of sensation. Reddened areas and pressure marks should be reported to a doctor or physical therapist.

The purpose of this exercise program is to:

- promote flexibility and relaxation of muscles on the affected side;
- help return to more normal movement;
- improve balance and coordination;
- decrease pain and stiffness; and
- maintain range of motion in the affected arm and leg.

For the Stroke Survivor

Begin with exercises done lying on your back, and then move on to those performed lying on your unaffected side, then sitting, and then standing. Make sure that the surface on which you lie is firm and provides good support. Take your time when you exercise. Don't rush the movements or strain to complete them.

Note: The word "floor" has been used to simplify the instructions; the exercises can be performed on the floor, on a firm mattress or on any appropriate supporting surface.

For the Helper

There may be no need to assist the stroke survivor in the exercises, but you should be nearby during the exercise session. If the survivor has difficulty reading or remembering the sequence of movements, you can repeat the instructions one by one. You can also offer physical assistance and encouragement when needed.

Exercise 1. To enhance shoulder motion and possibly prevent shoulder pain:

1. Lie on your back on a firm bed. Interlace your fingers with your hands resting on your stomach.

2. Slowly raise your arms to shoulder level, keeping your elbows straight.

3. Return your hands to resting position on your stomach.

Note: If pain occurs, it may be reduced by working within the range of motion that is relatively pain-free, then going up to the point where pain is felt. The arm should not be forced if pain is excessive, but effort should be made to daily increase the range of pain-free motion.

Exercise 2. To maintain shoulder motion (may be useful for someone who has difficulty rolling over in bed):

1. Lie on your back on a firm bed. Interlace your fingers, with your hands resting on your stomach.

2. Slowly raise your hands directly over your chest, straightening your elbows.

3. Slowly move your hands to one side and then the other.

4. When all repetitions have been completed, bend your elbows and return your hands to resting position on your stomach.

Note: If shoulder pain occurs, move only to the point where it begins to hurt. If the pain continues, don't do this exercise.

Exercise 3. To promote motion in the pelvis, hip and knee (can help to reduce stiffness and is also useful for rolling over and moving in bed):

1. Lie on your back on a firm bed. Keep your interlaced fingers resting on your stomach.

2. Bend your knees and put your feet flat on the bed.

3. Holding your knees tightly together, slowly move them as far to the right as possible. Return to center.

4. Slowly move your knees as far as possible to the left, still keeping them together. Return to center.

Note: The helper may provide assistance or verbal cues to help you keep your knees together during this exercise.

Exercise 4. To improve motion at the hip and knee, simulating the movements needed for walking (can be useful when moving toward the edge of the bed before coming to a sitting position):

1. Lie on your unaffected side, with your legs together.

2. Bend and move your affected knee as far as possible toward your chest. You may need your helper's assistance to support the leg you're exercising.

3. Return to starting position.

503

Exercise 5. To strengthen the muscles that straighten the elbow (necessary for getting up from a lying position):

1. Sitting on a firm mattress or sofa, put your affected forearm flat on the surface with your palm facing down if possible. You may want to place a firm pillow under your elbow.

2. Slowly lean your weight onto your bent elbow. You may need your helper's assistance to maintain your balance.

3. Push your hand down against the support surface, straightening your elbow and sitting more upright. (Assistance may be required to prevent sudden elbow collapse).

4. Slowly allow your elbow to bend, returning your forearm to the support surface.

5. Work back and forth between the two extremes (completely bent or completely straight) in a slow, rhythmical manner.

Note: This exercise should not be performed if your shoulder is not yet stable and/or will not support your upper body weight. Consult your doctor and/or physical therapist before attempting this exercise.

Exercise 6. To reduce stiffness in the trunk and promote the body rotation needed for walking:

1. Sit on a firm straight chair with both feet flat on the floor. If necessary, a firm mattress, sofa, or wheelchair may be used.

2. Interlace your fingers.

3. Bend forward and reach with your hands toward the outside of your right foot, rotating your trunk.

4. Move your hands upward in a diagonal direction toward your left shoulder, keeping your elbows as straight as possible.

5. Repeat the motions, moving your hands from your left foot to your right shoulder.

Note: Only individuals with good balance who can sit fairly independently should do this exercise. If balance is impaired, an assistant may stand in front, guiding the arms through the motions.

Exercise 7. Movements needed to rise from a sitting position:

1. Sit on a firm chair that has been placed against the wall to prevent slipping.

2. Interlace your fingers. Reach forward with your hands.

3. With your feet slightly apart and your hips at the edge of the seat, lean forward, lifting your hips up slightly from the seat.

4. Slowly return to sitting.

Note: In a progression of the exercise, try to rise to a complete standing position (see step 3) and return to sitting. However, this should only be done by someone with good balance who can come to a standing position safely.

Exercise 8. To maintain the ankle motion needed for walking (also maintains motion at the wrist and elbow):

1. Stand at arm's length from the wall, knees straight, feet planted slightly apart and flat on the floor with equal weight on both feet.

2. With your unaffected hand, hold your affected hand in place against the wall at chest level.

3. Slowly bend your elbows, leaning into the wall. This places a stretch on the back of your lower legs. Keep your heels on the floor.

4. Straighten your elbows, pushing your body away from the wall.

Note: If the stroke survivor's affected arm is very involved, he or she may find this exercise too difficult. Consult your doctor and/or physical therapist before attempting this exercise.

Section 59.2

New Treatments Open Doors for People with Spasticity

"Intrathecal Baclofen Treatment for Spasticity,"
© 2008 University of Pittsburgh Department of Neurological Surgery
(www.neurosurgery.pitt.edu). Reprinted with permission.

ITB [intrathecal baclofen treatment] is indicated to treat spasticity that is severe or moderately severe in most of the body (arms and legs, and often the trunk), which cannot be adequately treated with oral medications and Botox.

There is no age limitation to ITB, although most people treated with it are four years old or older.

Screening

Patients with spasticity rarely undergo screening. The experience of the team was that > 95% of patients had a good response to the trial and proceeded with the pump. For this reason trials are not routinely performed on patients with spasticity related to CP [cerebral palsy]. In other patients with less common causes for their spasticity a trial may be performed. Patients are admitted to the hospital. Once they are admitted, they are evaluated by a physical therapist to obtain baseline scores (measurements) of the muscle tone. After the evaluation, they are given a test dose of baclofen. That test dose involves numbing the skin on the back with EMLA [eutectic mixture of local anesthetic] cream, and injection of a local anesthetic, or both and injecting a dose of baclofen (usually 50 micrograms) into the spinal fluid. The patient is then evaluated every two hours for 4–8 hours to determine if there has been a significant reduction in their tone. If a significant change has been noticed, the pump is usually inserted the following day.

Surgery

The procedure for insertion of an intrathecal baclofen pump lasts 1–1.5 hours. The pump is inserted under the covering of the abdominal muscles while the patient is under a general anesthetic. A small catheter is inserted through a needle into the spinal fluid and is threaded upward toward the neck. The catheter is tunneled under the skin to the abdomen and is connected to the pump. The pump is filled with the drug baclofen and is programmed by a computer to continuously release a specified dose that is determined by the physician.

Expectations (In Hospital and Immediately Following)

Patients are usually kept at bed rest for 2–3 days after pump insertion. During that time, their baclofen dose is increased every day as needed and they are given intravenous antibiotics for one day. Usually by the fourth or fifth day, spasticity is distinctly better. Patients are often discharged 4–6 days postoperatively. Those who live nearby go home but we ask families who live a considerable distance away from the hospital (e.g., more than a 4–5 hour drive) to stay nearby for an additional 3–4 days to make sure they are well before returning home.

Follow-Up

The pump needs to be refilled every two to six months, depending on the pump size, concentration, and dose. Refills are done in the office (or occasionally by visiting nurses) using a syringe and needle and take approximately 15 minutes to complete. At that time, baclofen doses are adjusted depending on the effects that are being seen. Doses typically increase slowly during the first year, then remain at that level for years thereafter. The battery in the pump lasts seven to eight years at which time the pump needs to be replaced. Baclofen has been used for more than 15 years with no long-term complications being reported.

Myths/Facts

Myth: A test dose of baclofen into the spinal fluid is a good test of how a person's spasticity would be changed if a baclofen pump were inserted.

Fact: The test dose is given to answer one question: does it relieve spasticity? The test dose often produces more relaxation than would be desired day after day.

Myth: A baclofen pump improves spasticity in the legs but not in the arms.

Fact: The amount of spasticity reduction in the arms depends on where the catheter is positioned in the spinal fluid. When baclofen was first given, catheters were placed low (T10-12) and improved mainly the legs; now, catheters are positioned higher (e.g., T 1-2) and arm spasticity is improved much more.

Section 59.3

Chemodenervation Treatment for Spasticity

"Spasticity Treatment with Botulinum Toxins," by
Christina Marciniak, M.D. © 2008 Rehabilitation Institute of Chicago
(www.lifecenter.ric.org). All rights reserved. Reprinted with permission.

Chemodenervation is a treatment for spasticity that involves injections into the muscle or nerve. This treatment is used when spasticity is severe and may include one or more injections of medicine into the affected muscles. Botulinum toxins (Botox® and Myobloc®) are the medicines most commonly used. Phenol, a type of alcohol, and sometimes ethyl alcohol are also used, particularly when multiple, large muscles are affected. Phenol may be injected into nerves or into the area where the nerve connects with the muscle.

What is botulinum toxin?

Botulinum toxin is produced by bacteria, *Clostridium botulinum*. This bacteria causes muscle weakness and when injected in tiny amounts into muscle, it makes the muscles relax. This occurs because botulinum blocks the nerve from receiving a signal from acetylcholine, a chemical substance which normally causes the muscle to tighten.

What kinds of medical conditions may be helped by botulinum toxin?

They have been used for many causes of spasticity as the result of:

- stroke
- multiple sclerosis
- spinal cord injury
- traumatic brain injury
- cerebral palsy

Although the Food and Drug Administration (FDA) has not approved either drug for the treatment of spasticity, they are commonly used for this purpose. This is termed "off-label" use.

Injections may also be used in treating involuntary continuous tightening of the neck or limbs, a condition called cervical dystonia or limb dystonia.

How soon do the injections work and how long do they last?

Gradual relaxation of the muscles begins one to three days after the injection. Effects are strongest at about two to four weeks and wear off in about three to six months. This means that the treatment needs to be repeated, sometimes as often as every three months.

How is the medicine given?

The botulinum toxins are injected directly into the muscles that are tight. If more than one muscle is tight, then more than one injection is given. Larger muscles may require more than one injection. In order for the physician to locate the correct place to inject, an EMG [electromyography] machine may be used to record the electrical activity of the muscle. Sometimes stimulation of the nerves and ultrasound (sound waves) are used to locate the muscle.

Does botulinum toxin interfere with other medicines?

Botulinum toxins do not generally interfere with other medicines, but some considerations are necessary.

- Those taking medicine for myasthenia gravis should not undergo chemodenervation injections.
- Individuals taking blood thinning medication (Coumadin®/warfarin) must have regular blood tests reviewed. It is helpful for patients to bring these results to each appointment.

What are the most common side effects?

- The most common side effects are soreness, stiffness, slight redness, or swelling at the injection site.

- Mild swallowing problems sometimes occur if the injection is given in the neck.

- People taking medicine to prevent strokes, such as aspirin, or medicines that affect blood clotting are more likely to have bruising from the injections.

- Myobloc®, but not Botox®, may burn while being injected.

- Myobloc® and to a lesser extent Botox® may cause dryness in the mouth.

Are there other side effects?

A number of other side effects have been reported but are very rare. These include:

- headache

- seizures have been reported in stroke patients, but not any more often than in those stroke patients not receiving the injections

- flu-like muscle ache

These other, very rare side effects are also possible. Anyone experiencing any of the following should contact their doctor immediately:

- Swallowing problems following neck injection, if they occur, are generally mild, but sometimes patients have to change their diet for a while or have a feeding tube. Swallowing problems can also lead to serious pneumonia.

- blood clot (hematoma) or infection at the injection site

- generalized muscle weakness including swallowing problems, from injections in the limbs

- rash

- eye movement problems

- difficulty talking or breathing

References

Botulinum toxin type A injections: Adverse events reported to the U.S. Food and Drug Administration in therapeutic and cosmetic cases. Cote, TR et al. *J Am Acad Dermatol* 2005;53:407–15.

Early Communication about an Ongoing Safety Review Botox and Botox Cosmetic (Botulinum toxin Type A) and Myobloc (Botulinum toxin Type B). U.S. Food and Drug Administration Center for Drug Evaluation and Research. February, 2008.

Section 59.4

Neural Clamps Help Restore Function after Neurological Damage

From "Tiny Neural Clamps Make Connections," published in *e-Advances,* by the National Institute of Biomedical Imaging and Bioengineering (NIBIB, www.nibib.nih.gov), part of the National Institutes of Health, April 26, 2006.

Active nerves enable limbs to move, the bladder to empty at appropriate times, and hundreds of other bodily feats that we take for granted. Thanks to girls' hair barrettes, researchers at Arizona State University have developed a device that may revolutionize ways to communicate with the peripheral nervous system, the body's nerve network that sends messages to and from the brain and spinal cord. The neural clamp, which resembles a tiny circuit board, could impact how electrical systems are used to record or stimulate nerve activity to restore limb movement in people with spinal cord injuries, amputees, and others with neurological movement disorders.

A Case of Open and Shut

Dr. Ranu Jung, co-director of the Center for Adaptive Neural Systems at Arizona State University's Biodesign Institute, got the idea for the neural clamp after observing that girls quickly reposition locks

511

of their hair with barrettes that easily pop open or shut with slight bending. Jung, along with collaborator Stephen Phillips, chair of ASU's Department of Electrical Engineering, determined that temperature changes would cause the clamp to open or shut. At body temperature, the device closes. Add a squirt of saline and the clamp opens.

The key to the clamp is its ability to directly connect to nerves as they first emerge from the spine. These nerves or rootlets are about as thick and as long as a standard paper staple. During implantation surgery a surgeon would fit the neural clamp onto the spinal roots and reposition it as needed until a robust nerve signal emerges. Electronic circuitry connected to electrodes on the clamp would record ongoing nerve activity or stimulate missing nerve activity.

No Bulky Electrodes

The neural clamp would be a vast improvement over currently available systems used to activate nerve function lost to stroke and spinal cord injuries. Often multiple electrodes are placed on the skin to stimulate movement in those with spinal cord injuries. Electricity delivered via the electrodes prompts nerves to signal muscle movement. But multiple attachments make them awkward to use and it is difficult to reliably place all the electrodes at the same location again and again.

Implanted electrodes overcome these problems but the devices used today are large and often hand made. However, because Jung's neural clamp relies on fabrication techniques used to mass produce computer chips, large quantities of the micro-component can be readily made.

Refining Movement

Current systems to control movement in people with spinal cord injuries or prostheses of amputees also lack adaptive capabilities needed for smooth or precise actions. The temperature-sensitive clamp could provide an effective interface between nerves and electronic control systems. A system for recording nerve activity based on neural clamps would provide feedback about the status of the nervous system by sensing signals coming from the spinal roots. These signals would be used for adaptive stimulation of nerves and muscles downstream from the spinal roots for people with spinal cord injuries or adaptive control of the motors of artificial limbs for amputees, adjusting stimulation accordingly. Over time as a person recovers from incomplete spinal cord injury or improves their ability to control prostheses, feedback of neural signals recorded with the clamps would provide less stimulation.

A Bionic Future?

Dr. Jung and her colleagues hope to start testing the neural clamp this year in animal models. The team still must find a way to make the clamp durable and unlikely to damage nerves. Jung notes that the clamp's design may be altered to improve durability and make it flexible enough to provide long-term electrical connections with nerves without damaging them in the process. Human testing is still another 10 or more years away.

The potential for this device to revolutionize rehabilitative medicine helps keep the research team on task. "We are very much driven by the needs of the patients. We are trying to find ways to repair or replace lost neural function using adaptive interfaces. The bottom line is, 'Can we get function back?'" Dr. Jung says.

Will this research lead us on a path to realizing the fictional bionic woman or six-million-dollar-man whose artificial parts gave each super powers? "We are all bionic more or less," says Dr. Jung. "Many of us have pacemakers, hip replacements, or insulin pumps. We are becoming more and more integrated with technology. Why not take advantage of the capabilities of advanced technology to help us get back or improve function?"

Development of the neural clamp is supported by the National Institute of Biomedical Imaging and Bioengineering and spinal cord injury research support is provided by the National Institute of Child Health and Human Development.

Reference: Venkatasubramanian, G., R. Jung, J. D. Sweeney. "Functional Electrical Stimulation", In: *The Wiley Encyclopedia of Medical Devices and Instrumentation,* 2nd Edition, Editor. J. G. Webster, Wiley, March 2006.

Chapter 60

Skin Care after Stroke

After a stroke, skin problems become more common since paralysis causes decreased movement and feeling. People who can't move run into problems when they lay or sit in one spot for long periods of time. And those who have lost feeling don't get the signals that help prevent burns and bruises. A person who has bladder or bowel accidents also has special concerns with keeping the skin clean, dry, and free of irritation. Older people tend to have greater skin problems after a stroke, since skin becomes less elastic with age. The most important thing to remember about skin problems is that they can be prevented. The first step is knowing what you can do to keep your skin healthy.

Normal Function of the Skin

Your skin is an important part of your body that works in many ways to keep you healthy. Here are a few of its jobs:

- protects you from outside injury or illness;
- prevents germs from entering your body;
- keeps fluids and nutrients inside your body; and
- helps to control your body temperature in hot and cold weather.

Skin has several layers of tissue that cover your body. Some tissues are filled with tiny blood vessels that move oxygen and nutrients to the skin. The skin also has nerves, which send messages from different parts of your body to your brain. These make you aware of touch, pain, and temperature. Other nerves give you information about where your body and body parts (arms, legs) are positioned in space and whether you are lying on an object.

Keeping Skin Healthy

Healthy skin is intact, well lubricated with natural oils, and nourished by a good blood supply. Skin stays healthy with a balanced diet, good hygiene, regular skin checks, and pressure relief. By relieving pressure and checking your skin, you will ensure a good blood supply and improve the health of your skin. Here are a few ideas for keeping your skin healthy.

Hygiene

- Keep skin clean and dry. Skin that is wet from urine, sweat, or stool is more likely to break down.

- Dry skin well after bathing, but don't rub hard with a towel since rubbing can hurt the skin.

- Do not bathe everyday unless it is really needed. Daily baths wash away natural oils that lubricate the skin.

- Do not use skin drying alcohol massages over bony areas of your body. If a back rub helps you to relax, ask that a massage be done with a gentle lotion.

Nutrition

- Eat a healthy diet. Protein, vitamins, and iron are especially important. Consult with a nutrition professional to plan a diet that will meet your needs.

- Drink 6–8 glasses of fluid every day.

- Pureeing or chopping foods does not change the nutritional value. If you are on tube feedings, the formula chosen will provide the nutrients you need for healthy skin.

Skin Inspection

- Check your skin to spot sores when they are just starting.

516

- Don't depend on others to tell you how your skin looks. If you need help, however, clearly tell others what warning signs they should try to look for.

- Remember to check your entire body, especially bony areas.

- Check skin at least twice a day in the morning and evening. Check skin more often if you are increasing sitting or turning times. It should be done when you change position.

- Use a long handled mirror to help you check areas.

- Be alert to areas that have been broken and healed. Scar tissue breaks very easily.

- Look for red areas, blisters, openings in the skin, or rashes. In red areas, use the back of your strong hand to feel for heat.

- Check your groin area. Men who wear an external catheter should check their penis for sores or other problems.

Chapter 61

Coping with Emotions Following a Disabling Illness

Chapter Contents

Section 61.1

Depression and Anxiety

"Depression and Anxiety," by Robert J. Hartke, Ph.D.
© 2008 Rehabilitation Institute of Chicago (www.lifecenter.ric.org).
All rights reserved. Reprinted with permission.

Mental health problems such as depression and anxiety can accompany an illness. The following information includes information on signs, symptoms, and treatment.

Symptoms of Depression

Depression is characterized by feelings of sadness, despair, and discouragement. It often follows a personal loss or injury. It is not a sign of weakness nor does it represent a moral failing.

Sadness that lasts a long time and a loss of enjoyment in almost all activities are the central features of depression. Sadness is a symptom, but not the same thing as depression. Everyone is sad sometimes. The type of sadness that occurs in depression lasts all day or most of the day, every day for a long time (at least two weeks). Other symptoms include feelings of worthlessness or guilt, suicidal thoughts, loss of concentration, decreased energy, slowed thinking and movement, appetite loss, and sleep problems.

It is important to remember that many of these symptoms can occur with illnesses such as brain injury or stroke or even less serious problems like a cold or flu, but may not indicate depression. Even if you have trouble sleeping, lack of appetite, and problems concentrating, there is no reason to be concerned about a separate mental health condition unless you also feel sad most of the time or rarely find enjoyment in life.

What is the difference between normal grief and depression?

Some symptoms of depression as described above are normal after any kind of loss including the onset of a disability or severe illness. If you have had these symptoms for a long time it may be helpful to talk with a mental health professional. It is also helpful to talk to someone if you have other symptoms such as feeling guilty or worthless, or if sadness interferes with the ability to do important life tasks (take medication; go to therapies, work, or school).

Symptoms of Anxiety

Following a major life-changing event like a disabling illness, it is normal to feel a great deal of stress. Stress can build up over time and can lead to anxiety. Anxiety can be a response to a specific situation such as learning to walk all over again; it can also be more generalized such as not wanting to leave the house after being discharged from the hospital.

The most common symptoms of anxiety are fear and worry. Anxiety can also cause restlessness, and difficulty concentrating and sleeping. Sometimes people will express anxiety by being irritable, tired, or even stubborn. Anxiety can cause physical symptoms like muscle tension, shortness of breath, or even feelings of panic. Nearly everyone feels anxiety when faced with a bad physical problem. Anxiety becomes a concern when these feelings are very strong and interfere with important tasks in life.

Can anxiety or depression be different depending on age?

Children and older adults often show anxiety and depression differently. Children may misbehave either at school or at home. Older adults might report vague physical problems when there is no clear medical cause.

Treatment

Both depression and anxiety can go away over time but without treatment the symptoms last longer and may return. Chronic depression or anxiety can cause low self-esteem and poor quality of life.

Anxiety and depression are usually treated with medication and/ or psychotherapy (counseling) by a trained professional. Treatment is usually quite successful, so there is little reason to delay seeking help.

If feeling anxious or depressed, it is important to admit to it and get help. Even when family and friends are around for support, professional attention is best. A good first step is to discuss concerns with your regular doctor. He or she can provide advice about the best treatment and suggest a qualified therapist. There are several types of mental health

521

professionals who can provide psychotherapy (counselors, social workers, and psychologists), but any medications must be prescribed by a physician (your regular doctor or a psychiatrist). It is important to select a therapist with whom you feel comfortable and can talk honestly about your feelings. Psychotherapy can be done individually, with other family members, or in a group.

Sometimes it is best to both take medication and see a therapist. Medications can be helpful in many cases. Sometimes people are afraid of acting and thinking strangely, or becoming dependent on drugs used to treat anxiety and depression. When these medications are taken as prescribed by a doctor, bad side effects can be reduced or eliminated and there is little risk of becoming addicted to them. Remember that these medications are not the same as street drugs to get high.

Tips for Coping with Anxiety and Depression While in the Hospital

There is no single, simple way to adjust to a disability, but there are a few tips to keep in mind.

- Follow a routine. Aside from the regular therapy schedule, try to go to bed the same time each night, and to set aside time for relaxing and visiting (either in person or on the phone).

- Be open with staff, family, and friends regarding your needs.

- Ask questions about any aspect of your care that is unclear.

- Share things that worry you with others. Keeping feelings bottled up often makes being in the hospital more difficult. Sometimes people have problems admitting anything bad has happened as a way to be protected from depression and anxiety. It is healthier to admit you may not be able to do everything you used to do.

- Acknowledge that you will be sad about this for a while until you find new things to do that you enjoy. Try not to exaggerate these losses with thoughts such as "I can't do anything anymore;" "I'll never be able to find anything worthwhile to do again."

Tips for Coping with Anxiety and Depression after Leaving the Hospital

Sometimes people have prejudices about physical disability that make them feel like "second class citizens" when they become disabled themselves. Sometimes people with a disability get into the habit of letting other people do things for them and as a result they start to feel helpless. Sometimes people with a disability start to avoid situations that make them nervous (for example going out in public where others can see that they look or act differently). This makes those situations much more scary or upsetting when they can no longer be avoided.

- Set up a routine and stay with it to work on your recovery after leaving the hospital.

- Stay involved in life. Find enjoyable activities—either ones from before or new ones.

- Acknowledge improvements. This decreases the risk of boredom and depression and will boost self-confidence.

- This is a stressful time, so be open to the support of others. Healthy relationships with family, friends, or others with a disability can go a long way in preventing depression and anxiety.

- There is also evidence that a strong spiritual life can help keep you healthier and hopeful.

Special Tips for Parents

Parents may need to provide more comfort and support than usual for their children. It is not unusual for a child to regress to an earlier stage of development following a traumatic event. Children may find it hard to separate from parents, become clingy or emotionally needy during a hospital stay. Children usually show signs of greater independence by the time of discharge. Please talk to your physician if these problems do not improve.

Section 61.2

Strokes and Sexuality

A stroke can change many aspects of life including the ability to walk, talk, think, and care for oneself. It can also affect the ability to have sex and how you and your partner feel about sex. Sex is an important aspect of life. The following describes some of the sexual concerns experienced by stroke patients.

A common fear is that having sex can cause another stroke. There are many activities that can cause the heart to beat faster and to increase breathing without causing another stroke. Ask your physician if you are worried about whether or not it is all right to engage in sexual activity.

Talk with your partner, take your time, and share your feelings and concerns. This will help you enjoy each other and your time together. Choose a quiet, familiar place. Use music if you enjoy it.

Try something as simple as putting on makeup or perfume or having your hair done, which may help you feel better about yourself and feel more attractive. Keeping a sense of humor that is considerate of your partner's feelings may lighten the mood.

If the stroke affected movement on one side of your body, it may be necessary to try new positions. Try using pillows to support weak arms and legs, or having sex in a shower. Also using medicine to prevent spasms may help.

The feeling on one side of your body may be different. Try touching, caressing and kissing on the stronger side or increasing the touch on the weaker side. If you are the partner, approach your mate from the stronger side. Describing what you are doing may also help.

Sexual experience can be affected due to problems with memory and concentration. Let your partner help you through short familiar steps. The ability to understand what is being said and the ability to say what you would like can be affected. Both partners should focus on facial expressions and gestures to exchange thoughts and feelings.

Touching and helping each other is the best way to share what you both want.

One of the most embarrassing things that can happen is having a bowel or bladder accident during sex. Make sure you empty beforehand. Indwelling catheters can be taped out of the way or removed for a short time during sexual activity. Have clean-up items nearby just in case.

It is normal to lack interest in sex right after a stroke. It may take a lot of energy just to get through the day, leaving little for anything else. Sometimes people feel down or depressed which can affect the desire for sex. Also aging itself causes changes that can lessen sexual desire.

Certain medicines affect the desire for sex, and switching medication may help. Discuss this with your doctor. Never change or stop taking medications without first consulting your doctor.

Finally, it is important to practice safe sex and contraceptive methods the same as before having the stroke. If you are a woman and able to become pregnant, talk to your doctor about birth control; some birth control methods may be easier or safer to use with other medicines. Also speak to your doctor about any risks you may have if you decide to become pregnant.

Chapter 62

Managing Life at Home after Stroke

Managing life at home is an important part of stroke recovery. Whether your "home" is a house, apartment, assisted living facility, or retirement home, you still want some independence in your everyday activities.

Stroke affects each survivor differently. To live well after stroke, you may need to make some changes in your home and daily routine. A few simple changes can help you keep up your energy level for therapy and the activities you enjoy.

Preparing to Go Home

Ask your doctor to arrange a home visit by an occupational therapist (OT), who is trained to help you manage daily activities and regain your independence.

- The OT will check your home and may suggest simple changes to make everyday living easier.

- Arrange for changes to be finished before you return home.

The OT may suggest some of the following:

- Change areas of your home to allow for a wheelchair (front door, bathrooms, or areas where you spend time).

- Move extra furniture out of the way to make room for a wheelchair or for walking with a walker or cane.

- Add or adjust lighting throughout your home to decrease glare and help you see better in low-lit areas.

- Obtain and use equipment to make getting into and out of the shower or bathtub easier.

- Keep telephones or call devices within easy reach.

Also talk to your OT about your everyday activities before you return home.

- Make a safety checklist of different situations and possible solutions.

- You may want to make a short home visit with the OT before you leave the hospital—if allowed by your health insurance company. This will help you find out what changes are needed and give you time to arrange for them to be made before you go home.

Staying Safe and Connected

- Write out emergency phone numbers in large print on index cards and keep them in handy locations all over your home.

- Arrange for people to check in with you regularly.

- Accept help with household chores such as cleaning, meals, and errands. Allow family and friends to drive you places.

- Allow loved ones to support your recovery goals by going to therapy with you, helping with exercises, and playing cards or doing puzzles together.

- Encourage your friends and family to visit or call when they can.

- Plan outings with your friends when you are ready. They will be eager to see you and to celebrate your recovery.

Getting around Safely

Forty percent (40%) of stroke survivors suffer serious falls within a year after their strokes. The following tips may help you avoid falling in your home:

- Move extra furniture out of the way, either to corners or another room.

- Clear paths to the kitchen, bedroom, and bathroom.

- Move electrical cords out of pathways.

- Wear non-skid shoes and avoid slick surfaces.

- Remove loose carpets and runners in hallways and stairwells or fasten them with non-skid tape to improve traction.

- Replace thick carpeting with lower pile carpeting to make wheelchair or walker movement easier.

- Install handrails for support in going up and down stairs. Check to make sure they're securely fastened to the wall.

- Consider stair glides, stair lifts, and platform lifts if you need to use the stairs many times during the day.

Cleaning Up

To make cleaning and other household chores easier:

- Use simple cleaning products such as disposable wipes and mop heads.

- Choose one multipurpose cleaning solution for most of your cleaning.

- Use smaller, lightweight containers, wheeled push carts, and cleaning tools with long handles or extensions.

- Work on small areas.

- Take frequent breaks.

- Let your friends, family, neighbors, or even a maid or cleaning service do some of the work for you.

- Consider a home health aide to help you with daily chores.

Doing Laundry

Doing laundry will be less challenging if you make a few simple changes.

- Move laundry machines to a place where you can easily get to them.

- Stackable, front-loading machines may be easier to reach and take up less space.

- Use easy-to-reach, labeled detergents and laundry supplies.

- Have easy-to-read markings for wash settings.

- Use a nearby table or cart at the right height for you to sort and fold clothes.

- Use an ironing board that folds down from the wall.

Using the Bathroom

Bathrooms are usually tight places and can pose challenges. To make bathing both simple and safe, consider the following:

- Sturdy hand rails

- Grab bars in the tub or shower

- Non-slip flooring strips installed inside and outside of the tub

- Bathtub benches and toilet chairs

- Easy-to-use water control knobs with easily seen settings or long-handled levers

- An adjustable or handheld showerhead

- Bathing supplies that are easy to reach and use

To make toileting safer:

- Use a cane, walker, wheelchair, or grab bars to stabilize and balance yourself whenever you get on or off the toilet.

- Install a raised toilet seat or toilet seat riser to reduce the distance and difficulty in sitting down and getting up.

- Try a three-in-one commode chair with a raised seat, grab bars, and a removable bucket. It can be kept near a bed or chair or used over an existing toilet with the bucket removed.

- Use disposable underpants.

- Keep a change of clothing handy in the bathroom for the unexpected.

Some bathroom sinks can be tough to use and hard to access. Faucets can be hard to turn and bathroom products hard to use. To make your time at the sink easier, think about getting some of these products:

- A one-piece faucet that has lever handles or long extensions, allowing you to turn water on and off with a fist or arm movement.

- A cut-out or roll-under sink, which allows room for your legs underneath the sink while you are sitting down—especially useful if you are in a wheelchair or are seated while washing.

- Squeeze bottles and soap pumps, which may be easier to use than original containers.

- Suction pads to hold grooming tools or bottles in place on a counter, requiring just one hand to pick up or use.

- A flip-top toothpaste tube.

- A toothbrush with a larger handle.

- An electric razor (if you shave), which may be simpler and safer to handle than a regular razor.

- Ask your occupational therapist and/or physical therapist for more tips.

Making the Bedroom Safe and Comfortable

Your bedroom is a place where you should feel safe and comfortable and have a sense of privacy.

To make it safer:

- Make sure that help is easily and quickly within reach via telephone.

- Have a light switch near your bed.

- Move and reorganize clothes and personal items to make them easier to access. This may involve putting the clothes you wear most often in a place where you can easily reach them, lowering closet rods or shelves and replacing drawer handles with ones that you can easily open.

- Use a nightlight and clear a path for easy access to the toilet at night. To avoid accidents at night, keep a commode chair near the bed.

- Since some accidents are unavoidable, consider placing disposable "blue pads" underneath your sheets. With cloth on one side

531

and waterproof material on the other, blue pads can prevent bed staining. Some blue pads are disposable and others are washable and reusable.

Getting Dressed

To make dressing yourself easier:

- Avoid tight-fitting sleeves, armholes, pant legs, and waist-lines.

- Select clothes with fasteners in the front.

- Replace buttons, zippers, and laces with Velcro fasteners.

- Speak with other stroke survivors for ideas and resources.

- Try out dressing aids (things that make dressing easier) and adaptable clothing.

You can find them on internet sites and at health supply stores. Check out the following websites for adaptable clothing:

- www.makoa.org/clothing.htm

- www.professionalfit.com

Taking Care in the Kitchen

To get back into your own kitchen, you may need to adjust to a small space where things can be hard to reach.

And if you have less sensitivity in your hands and arms, you must learn how to manage many sharp or hot objects that pose serious dangers in the kitchen.

To work independently and accident-free in the kitchen, plan ahead for cooking tasks.

- Consider the control buttons you use to turn your stove on and off and change the temperature from low to high. Controls at the front of the stove are easier and safer to use than the traditional back-of-the-stove controls. Also, push-button controls typically are easier to use than those that turn.

- Automatic shut-off controls can be installed for safety.

- Consider an over-the-stove mirror to help you see stovetop contents if cooking while seated.

- Keep a clear space near the stove where you can place a hot pot or pan quickly.

- Make sure you have oven mitts on hand.

- Keep a fire extinguisher nearby.

- The kitchen table should be at the right height for a wheelchair or for a chair with arms that supports your posture.

What Can Help

- Ask your doctors and therapists to help you solve everyday living issues.

- New resources, equipment, and therapies are available each year. Take advantage of them to improve your quality of life.

- Continue to set new goals for your stroke recovery.

- Be creative.

- Get information on stroke recovery from National Stroke Association. Visit www.stroke.org or call 800-STROKES (800-787-6537).

- Contact your local stroke association.

- Subscribe to *Stroke Smart* magazine at www.stroke.org to view the latest gears and gadgets to assist you. It's free!

- Join a stroke support group. Other survivors will understand, validate your issues, and offer encouragement and ideas for managing life at home.

- Speak honestly with your family and caregivers about your home living needs. They'll be glad you did, and, together, you can often work out the best solution.

- Check out many helpful products at: www.familyvillage.wisc.edu/at/adaptive-devices.html

Professionals Who Can Help

- Occupational therapist, who helps stroke survivors manage daily activities.

- Physical therapist, who assesses problems with moving, balance, and coordination.

Rehabilitation is a lifetime commitment and an important part of recovering from a stroke. Through rehabilitation, you relearn basic skills such as talking, eating, dressing, and walking. Rehabilitation can also improve your strength, flexibility, and endurance. The goal is to regain as much independence as possible.

Remember to ask your doctor, "Where am I on my stroke recovery journey?"

Chapter 63

Driving after Stroke

For most people, being able to drive is a sign of independence and freedom. Driving enables people to get to the places they want to go and do what they want to do. It is something that many of us have done for much, if not most, of our lives. Nevertheless, driving is a very complex skill. Our ability to drive safely can be affected by changes in our physical, emotional, and medical condition. The goal of this chapter is to:

- assist you, your family, your physician, and other health care professionals address how a stroke may affect your ability to drive; and

- describe the role of a driver's rehabilitation program.

How can having a stroke affect my driving?

A stroke can affect your strength, your coordination, or your ability to use or move different body parts. It can also affect your thinking skills such as memory, concentration, or ability to make safe judgments and problem solve. In some instances, it may even affect your vision (double vision, blurry vision, or the inability to see out of the corners of your eyes). Due to these impairments, you may:

- Have trouble using the gas and brake pedals with your right foot.

"Driving after a Stroke," by Jillian Dworak, Ph.D. © 2008 Rehabilitation Institute of Chicago (www.lifecenter.ric.org). All rights reserved. Reprinted with permission.

- Have difficulty turning the steering wheel.
- Become easily frustrated or confused when driving.
- Not remember the location of familiar places.
- Have difficulty seeing or being aware of traffic around you.

Can I still drive after a stroke?

Most stroke survivors can return to independent and safe driving. As part of the rehabilitation process, it is important to discuss with your physician and other health care professionals your goals for returning to driving. Depending on the severity of the stroke, your doctor may refer you to a driver rehabilitation program.

What is a driver rehabilitation program?

A driver rehabilitation program provides a comprehensive driving evaluation which includes both clinical and Behind the Wheel (BTW) components. A driver rehabilitation specialist assesses your ability to return to safe driving and recommends the use of specific equipment if necessary.

In order to be seen in a driver rehabilitation program you will need a referral from your doctor, a valid driver's license (or permit), and payment.

During the clinical evaluation, an occupational therapist talks with you about your medical history, current condition, and your goals for returning to driving. The therapist evaluates your vision, thinking skills, and overall strength, movement, and coordination. You may also be asked questions about your driving history and tested on your driving knowledge. If you need any special equipment for driving, it may also be introduced to you at this time. The clinical evaluation usually takes about one hour.

The Behind the Wheel evaluation consists of driving in a vehicle with a driving instructor in different types of traffic and driving situations. Adaptive equipment may also be introduced to you at this time. Certain types of driving equipment such as hand controls or left foot accelerators will require additional training sessions after your evaluation. The BTW evaluation takes about two hours.

What happens after the evaluation?

After the evaluation, results as well as any recommendations are given to both you and your doctor. These results will allow you and your doctor to decide whether driving is a feasible option at that time.

Although everyone is eager to return to driving, it is important to deal with driving at the most appropriate time in the healing process. We often encourage patients to wait until they are at their highest level of functioning (physically, mentally, and emotionally) before addressing driving. Your doctor and your health care team can help you decide when this time might be.

Does insurance cover the driving evaluation?

Most insurance providers including private insurance companies and Medicare/Medicaid will cover the clinical evaluation but will not cover any of the BTW cost, additional training, or equipment. Ask your health care team or call a driver rehabilitation program in regards to possible additional sources of funding.

Chapter 64

Stroke, Diet, and Poststroke Nutrition

Introduction

A well balanced diet including protein, carbohydrates, vegetables, and fruit is a vital part of stroke risk reduction. Healthy eating habits may help lower blood pressure rates, cholesterol levels, and reduce complications from diabetes.

Eat Your Vegetables

A recent Harvard University study concluded that eating five daily servings of fruits and vegetables might lower your risk for a clot-caused stroke by 30 percent. Citrus fruits and vegetables such as broccoli or Brussels sprouts are particularly beneficial. Their higher concentrations of folic acid, fiber, and potassium, may be a key to reducing heart disease and stroke risk.

Unfortunately, most individuals eat only half of the recommended servings. Increasing your intake can be easy. For example:

- Drink a glass of orange or vegetable juice.

- Buy pre-sliced vegetables or fruit for easy snacking or cooking.

- For flavor, use a variety of herbs and spices on vegetables. Add basil or dill to green beans or tomatoes.

"Nutrition Guide," © 2006 North Carolina Stroke Association (www.ncstroke .org). Reprinted with permission.

- Add grated vegetables to casseroles, spaghetti sauces or meat patties.

Eat a Low-Fat Diet

Eating and cooking in a low-fat manner reduces your waistline and decreases stroke and heart attack risk. Taking a few minutes to think through your food choices and how you cook them can make a difference.

For instance, grilling a piece of chicken instead of frying it reduces your fat intake significantly. Adding the following foods to your regular diet may also help:

- fruits and vegetables

- lean meats such as chicken, turkey, and fish

- lean cuts of beef (round or sirloin steak) or pork (pork chops, pork loin)

- low-fat dairy products (skim milk, 2% fat cottage cheese)

- egg substitutes or a maximum of four egg yolks per week

- fiber, including whole grain breads, cereal products, or dried beans

Watch Your Homocysteine Levels

Homocysteine is an amino acid (a building block of protein) that is produced naturally in the body and then changed into other amino acids for the body's use. Researchers recently found that too much homocysteine in the blood may increase a person's chance of developing heart disease, stroke, or other blood flow disorders.

Homocysteine levels are determined by two key factors: genetics and lifestyle. Genetic factors affect the speed homocysteine is processed in your body. Lifestyle factors, such as diet, affect homocysteine levels in another manner. For example, people with a high homocysteine level may have a low dietary intake of vitamins B6, B12, and folic acid. Replacing these vitamins helps levels return to normal. Low thyroid hormone levels, kidney disease, psoriasis, or some medications may also cause abnormally high homocysteine levels.

Folic acid is another part of the homocysteine puzzle. Most Americans do not get enough folic acid from their diets. Eating more fruits and vegetables including lentils, chickpeas, and asparagus increases folic acid levels and decreases health risks. Grain products, including ready-to-eat cereals and enriched products such as bread, pasta, and rice, are also good sources of folic acid.

Vitamins B6 and B12 are essential in controlling homocysteine levels and maintaining good health. As a person's body ages, the ability to absorb B12 is reduced. This may cause a variety of health problems including an increased risk for heart disease. Eating more foods containing vitamin B12 such as cereals, low-fat meat, fish, poultry, milk, or milk products may help. In some instances of vitamin B12 deficiency, more proactive steps may be needed, including B12 injections

Additional B6 can be easily added to your diet by eating fortified cereals and grains, bananas, baked potatoes, watermelon, meats, fish, and poultry.

Adjusting your diet may not be enough to lower your homocysteine to a desirable level. Vitamins may also be needed. Speak with your healthcare provider before starting any vitamin regimen. Taking high doses of vitamins is not generally recommended. Rechecking your homocysteine levels after you've taken vitamins is essential. If your homocysteine remains high, your doctor will modify your treatment.

Nutrition Care

Drink Alcohol Only in Moderation

Recent studies indicate that drinking a daily four ounce glass of wine or a 12 ounce can of beer or one drink made with spirits or liquor (1 1/4 ounce) may lower your risk for stroke (provided that there is no other medical reason you should avoid alcohol). Remember that alcohol is a drug and can interact with other drugs you are taking. It is harmful if taken in large doses. Speak with your physician before consuming alcoholic beverages on a regular basis. If you don't drink, don't start.

Poststroke Nutrition to Help Restore Health

Normal nutritional requirements are altered with any trauma or illness. After a stroke, modifying your diet may be necessary. The focus in early treatment and throughout rehabilitation is to meet daily energy needs and basic nutritional demands.

Although each individual has specific needs, stroke survivors may have additional considerations including:

541

- **Ability to Eat:** Chewing or swallowing difficulties will interfere with adequate intake. Often a stroke patient's is the same easy-to-eat foods repeatedly (mashed potatoes, pudding, etc.) A registered dietitian can help ensure that a variety of foods meet daily nutrition requirements.

- **Poor Appetite:** Food and eating may become unappealing after a stroke for many reasons including: lack of desire for food, lack of taste sensation, fear of choking due to swallowing and chewing problems, mouth discomfort from ill-fitting dentures, and/or medication. Constant encouragement may help increase the desire to eat and improve health.

- **Visual Perception:** Vision problems that may occur after stroke can affect food intake. For instance, food items on a plate or tray may be out of the field of vision and may not be eaten. Special assistance during meals may teach survivors to finish their meals and "look" for all the food.

- **Length of Time:** Eating may take more time after a stroke. If assistance is not always available, smaller, more frequent feedings should be used with a focus on foods high in nutritional value.

- **Medical Considerations:** High blood pressure, diabetes, bowel and bladder function, and other medical complications will also require dietary modification.

Diet in Rehabilitation

Being aware of the following nutritional needs will enhance the recovery/rehabilitation process:

- **Malnourishment**—Survivors who demonstrate low motivation, apathy, or excessive fatigue may not be getting the nourishment they need. Increased monitoring of food intake may help.

- **Overweight/Obesity**—Reducing calorie intake, but maintaining daily nutrients is essential for stroke survivors who are overweight or obese. It is possible to be overweight and be malnourished. Statements such as, "It's all right that she hasn't eaten for five days, she needs to lose weight," are inaccurate. A registered dietitian can help create a balanced diet and weight-loss plan.

Nutritional Care

Dietary management is an essential part of care giving, whether performed by the dietitian, nurse, or family members. A nutritional care plan should include the following components:

- **Individual Needs**—No standard menu or diet will apply to everyone.

- **Relevant Background Information**—Many social/cultural factors affect eating habits. Consider adapting the diet to the survivor's preference.

- **Intake Monitoring**—Observe and record the survivor's acceptance and tolerance of food items.

- **Diet Instruction**—Teach the survivor how to follow the diet makes compliance easier.

Chapter 65

Tips for Caregivers of Chronically Ill or Disabled People

Introduction

Research studies confirm what anyone who has cared for a chronically ill or disabled relative or friend knows firsthand—such a labor of love can exact an enormous physical, emotional, social, and financial toll. All too often those who provide care to others neglect their own need for self-care. Taking care of oneself is essential if the best care is to be provided to another person. Caregivers must learn how to balance their own needs with the needs of someone who needs care. There is no single recipe for ensuring that one remains a healthy caregiver but the following basic ingredients appear central.

Educate Yourself about the Disease or Medical Condition

Whether you care for someone with heart disease, stroke, or dementia or whether care takes place in your own home or at a distance, many of the daily challenges are similar.

- Learn new information and skills and learn how to adapt to the challenges you encounter.

- Get up-to-date and accurate information through books, fact sheets, and brochures regarding your relative's condition.

"Taking Care of Yourself" is from the Administration on Aging (AOA, www.aoa.gov), 2004.

- Contact the appropriate disease-related organization, that can guide you to other resources such as hospital-based education programs and support groups.

Find a Doctor or Another Health Professional Who Understands the Disease

Armed with some knowledge, you are capable of asking the right questions of the patient's doctor.

- Make a short list of questions and assert that you need such questions answered before you leave.

- Good doctors understand the impact of caregiving on you and should be willing to involve you in health care decisions that affect both your relative and you.

Consult with Other Experts

You may need additional professional help to plan for the future. For instance:

- You may need legal authority to make health care and financial decisions on behalf of your relative.

- A certified financial planner may help you prepare for the possibility of expensive care for your relative in an assisted living facility or other chronic-care facility.

- Getting experts involved as soon as possible may save you a lot of worry later.

- If you are too busy to attend to this matter, make sure someone acts in your behalf to handle it.

Tap Your Social Resources

Other family members and friends can play key roles in helping you to share in the care.

- Organize a family meeting so that everyone can get on the same page and find out what each person may or may not be able to offer. All potential sources of help need to be informed about the tasks at hand for both you and the relative in need of care.

- Make a plan with the family and then meet again a month later to evaluate progress.

Find a Confidante

Providing care can indeed be stressful at times and having some-one to talk with about your frustrations can be helpful. A person who needs care can sometimes be angry or depressed about being depen-dent and you make an easy target for the venting of negative emo-tions. It is difficult to be compassionate if the person you care for is upset with you. It is seldom helpful to confront your disabled rela-tive about the ill effects of his or her disability on you. Find a confi-dante such as a good friend or counselor to share your own emotional burden and learn ways to cope effectively.

Take Time for Relaxation and Exercise

Let's face it—helping another person can be hard work.

- Set aside time every day from the work of caregiving or you risk losing yourself to the exclusive needs of another person.

- Diversions are necessary in order to be renewed. Enjoy a hobby, see a movie, take a walk, ride a bike, or take part in any number of leisure time activities. You deserve a sense of normalcy. Some-thing enjoyable should be built into every day, if even for just ten minutes, that reminds you that your needs are important, too. Take care of yourself in ways that are meaningful to you.

Use Community Resources

Unfortunately, most caregivers delay looking for help outside their social network until they are virtually exhausted.

- Check the local Area Agency on Aging, which administers state and federal funds to help older chronically ill persons and their family caregivers. To find your local Area Agency on Aging, contact the Eldercare Locator (800-677-1116 or go to www.eldercare.gov).

- Other local agencies target the needs of younger disabled people and their families. Such agencies can help you get a well-deserved break by paying for occasional in-home services by someone to re-lieve you or providing adult day services for your relative.

Maintain Your Sense of Humor

There is nothing funny about a chronic illness, but being able to see humor in difficult situations can bring about much relief. Taking a lighthearted view can alter the meaning of a situation that might otherwise appear overwhelmingly depressing. Jokes, comics, and funny movies can fill the void if you cannot find something funny on your own.

Explore Religious Beliefs and Spiritual Values

Caring for someone with a chronic illness often evokes questions about faith, hope, God, and the meaning of life.

- Organized religion may offer a fresh perspective, but spirituality runs deeper than any particular tenet or belief system.

- Individual and group prayer, rituals, meditation, inspirational reading, and spiritual direction may shed light on matters of the soul.

Set Realistic Goals

Accustomed to doing things in a hurry, you may be surprised to find out how little you can accomplish when you are responsible for another person.

- Be patient. Set small goals for yourself each day or week and build upon your successes instead of thinking about your failings.

- Learn to appreciate that you are making progress in ensuring that both you and your loved one are getting the best possible care. Finally, celebrate your achievements.

Chapter 66

Complementary and Alternative Stroke Therapies

A stroke occurs when the blood supply to part of the brain is suddenly interrupted due to the presence of a blood clot (ischemic stroke) or when a blood vessel in the brain bursts, spilling blood into the spaces surrounding brain cells (hemorrhagic stroke). Brain cells die when they no longer receive oxygen and nutrients from the blood or when they are damaged by sudden bleeding into or around the brain. This results in temporary or permanent neurologic impairment. Ischemic stroke, also known as cerebral infarction, accounts for 80–85% of all strokes, while hemorrhagic stroke accounts for the other 15–20%. Prior to a stroke, some people suffer transient ischemic attacks (TIAs), mini-strokes that generally last only 5–20 minutes but can linger for up to 24 hours before the symptoms go away completely. Many times, a TIA is a warning of an impending stroke. An estimated 700,000 people in the United States suffer a stroke each year, making this one of the most serious of all health problems. Half of stroke sufferers are left disabled, with many undergoing years of rehabilitation.

Nutrition and Dietary Supplements

Potentially beneficial nutritional supplements include the following:

Alpha-lipoic acid. Alpha-lipoic acid works together with other antioxidants, such as vitamins C and E. It is important for growth, helps to prevent cell damage, and helps the body rid itself of harmful

---

Excerpted from "Alternative Medicine: Stroke" © 2008 A.D.A.M., Inc. Reprinted with permission.

substances. Because alpha-lipoic acid can pass easily into the brain, it has protective effects on brain and nerve tissue and shows promise as a treatment for stroke and other brain disorders involving free radical damage. Animals treated with alpha-lipoic acid, for example, suffered less brain damage and had a four times greater survival rate after a stroke than the animals who did not receive this supplement, especially when alpha-lipoic acid is combined with vitamin E. While animal studies are encouraging, more research is needed to understand whether this benefit applies to people as well.

Calcium. In a population based study (one in which large groups of people are followed over time), women who take in more calcium, both through the diet and with added supplements, were less likely to have a stroke over a 14 year time course. More research is needed to fully assess the strength of the connection between calcium and risk of stroke.

Folic Acid, Vitamin B6, Vitamin B12, Betaine. Many clinical studies indicate that patients with elevated levels of the amino acid homocysteine are as much as 2.5 times more likely to suffer from a stroke than those with normal levels. Homocysteine levels are strongly influenced by dietary factors, particularly vitamin B9 (folic acid), vitamin B6, vitamin B12, and betaine. These substances help break down homocysteine in the body. Some studies have even shown that healthy individuals who consume higher amounts of folic acid and vitamin B6 are less likely to develop atherosclerosis than those who consume lower amounts of these substances. Despite these findings, the American Heart Association (AHA) reports that there is insufficient evidence to suggest that supplementation with betaine and B vitamins reduce the risk of atherosclerosis or that taking these supplements prevents the development or recurrence of heart disease. The AHA does not currently recommend population-wide homocysteine screening, and suggests that folic acid, as well as vitamin B6, B12, and betaine requirements be met through diet alone. Individuals at high risk for developing atherosclerosis, however, should be screened for blood levels of homocysteine. If elevated levels are detected, a health care provider may recommend supplementation.

Magnesium. Population based information suggests that people with low magnesium in their diet may be at greater risk for stroke. Some preliminary scientific evidence suggests that magnesium sulfate may be helpful in the treatment of a stroke or transient ischemic attack. More research is needed to know for certain if use of this mineral following a stroke or TIA is helpful.

Omega-3 Fatty Acids. Strong evidence from population-based studies suggests that omega-3 fatty acid intake (primarily from fish), helps protect against stroke caused by plaque buildup and blood clots in the arteries that lead to the brain. In fact, eating at least two servings of fish per week can reduce the risk of stroke by as much as 50%. However, people who eat more than 3 grams of omega-3 fatty acids per day (equivalent to 3 servings of fish per day) may be at an increased risk for hemorrhagic stroke, a potentially fatal type of stroke in which an artery in the brain leaks or ruptures. Omega-3 fatty acids may increase the chances of bleeding, especially in those taking anticoagulant medications such as warfarin (Coumadin) or even aspirin.

Pregnant women and women of childbearing age, who may become pregnant, however, are advised by the U.S. Food and Drug Administration (FDA), to limit their consumption of shark, tuna, and swordfish to no more than once a month. These fish have much higher levels of methyl mercury than other commonly consumed fish. Since the fetus may be more susceptible than the mother to the adverse effects of methyl mercury, FDA experts say that it is prudent to minimize the consumption of fish that have higher levels of methyl mercury, like shark, tuna, and swordfish.

Potassium. Although low levels of potassium in the blood may be associated with stroke, taking potassium supplements does not seem to reduce the risk of having a stroke.

Vitamin C. Having low levels of vitamin C contributes to the development of atherosclerosis and other damage to blood vessels and the consequences such as stroke. Vitamin C supplements may also improve cognitive function if you have suffered from multiple strokes.

Vitamin E. Eating plenty of foods rich in vitamin E, along with other antioxidants like vitamin C, selenium, and carotenoids, reduces your risk for stroke. In addition, low levels of vitamin E in the blood may be associated with risk of dementia (memory impairment) following stroke. Animal studies also suggest that vitamin E supplements, possibly in combination with alpha-lipoic acid, may reduce the amount of brain damaged if taken prior to the actual stroke.

Researchers suggest testing this theory in people who are at high risk for stroke. Thus far, however, some large and well-designed studies of people suggest that it is safest and best to obtain this antioxidant via food sources and that supplements do not bring about any added benefit.

Others. Additional supplements that require further research but may be useful as part of the treatment or prevention of stroke include:

- **Coenzyme Q10**—works as an antioxidant and may reduce damage following a stroke.

- **Selenium**—low levels can worsen atherosclerosis and its consequences. However, it is not known if taking selenium supplements will help.

Herbs

The use of herbs is a time-honored approach to strengthening the body and treating disease. Herbs, however, contain active substances that can trigger side effects and interact with other herbs, supplements, or medications. For these reasons, herbs should be taken with care and only under the supervision of a practitioner knowledgeable in the field.

Bilberry *(Vaccinium myrtillus).* A close relative of the cranberry, bilberry fruits contain flavonoid compounds called anthocyanidins. Flavonoids are plant pigments that have excellent antioxidant properties. This means that they scavenge damaging particles in the body known as free radicals and may help prevent a number of long-term illnesses, such as heart disease.

Garlic *(Allium sativum).* Clinical studies suggest that fresh garlic and garlic supplements may prevent blood clots and destroy plaque. Blood clots and plaque block blood flow and contribute to the development of heart attack and stroke. Garlic may also be beneficial for reducing risk factors for heart disease and stroke like high blood pressure, high cholesterol, and diabetes. Homocysteine, similar to cholesterol, may contribute to increasing amounts of blood clots and plaque in blood vessels. If you take aspirin or other blood thinners [like warfarin (Coumadin)}, ACE [angiotensin-converting enzyme] inhibitors (a class of blood pressure medications), sulfonylureas for diabetes, or statins for high cholesterol, talk to your doctor before using garlic supplements.

Ginkgo *(Ginkgo biloba).* Ginkgo may reduce the likelihood of dementia following multiple strokes (often called multi-infarct dementia). The protection from ginkgo may be related to the prevention of platelet adhesion which can help prevent blood clot formation. Ginkgo may also decrease the amount of brain damage following a stroke. While animal studies support these possible benefits of ginkgo, more research in people is needed. Also, ginkgo should not be used with the blood thinner warfarin (Coumadin) unless specifically instructed by your health care provider.

Ginseng *(Panax ginseng)*. Asian ginseng may decrease endothelial cell dysfunction. Endothelial cells line the inside of blood vessels. When these cells are disturbed, referred to as dysfunction, it may lead to a heart attack or stroke. The potential for ginseng to quiet down the blood vessels may prove to be protective against these conditions. Much more research is needed before this use can be recommended. Ginseng may also thin your blood and, therefore, should be used only under the supervision of a doctor if you are taking blood-thinning medication warfarin (Coumadin).

Turmeric *(Curcuma longa)*. Early studies suggest that turmeric may prove helpful in preventing heart attack or stroke in one of two ways. First, in animal studies an extract of turmeric lowered cholesterol levels and inhibited the oxidation of LDL (low density lipoprotein, or "bad") cholesterol. Oxidized LDL deposits in the walls of blood vessels and contributes to the formation of atherosclerotic plaque and other damage to the vessels. Turmeric may also prevent platelet build up along the walls of an injured blood vessel. Platelets collecting at the site of a damaged blood vessel cause blood clots to form and blockage of the artery as well. Clinical studies of the use of turmeric to prevent or treat stroke in people would be interesting in terms of determining if these mechanisms discovered in animals apply to people at risk for this condition.

Homeopathy

Although an experienced homeopath might prescribe a regimen for treating stroke that includes one of the following remedies, the scientific evidence to date does not confirm the value of homeopathy for this purpose.

- *Aconitum napellus* for numbness or paralysis after a cerebral accident
- **Belladonna** for stroke that leaves person very sensitive to any motion, with vertigo and trembling
- *Kali bromatum* for stroke resulting in restlessness, wringing of the hands or other repeated gestures, insomnia, and night terrors

553

- *Nux vomica* for cerebral accident with paresis (muscular weakness caused by disease of the nervous system), expressive aphasia (language disorder), convulsions, and great irritability

Acupuncture

Many studies have been conducted on the effects of acupuncture during stroke rehabilitation. These studies have found that acupuncture reduces hospital stays and improves recovery speed. Acupuncture has been shown to help stroke patients regain motor and cognitive skills and to improve their ability to manage daily functioning. Based on the available data, the National Institutes of Health recommended acupuncture as an alternative or supplemental therapy for stroke rehabilitation. In general, the evidence indicates that acupuncture is most effective when initiated as soon as possible after a stroke occurs, but good results have been found for acupuncture started as late as 6 months following a stroke.

People who have suffered a stroke often have a deficiency of qi in the liver meridian and a relative excess in the gallbladder meridian. In addition to a primary needling treatment on the liver meridian and the supporting kidney meridians, moxibustion (a technique in which the herb mugwort is burned over specific acupuncture points) may be used to enhance therapy. Treatment may also include performing acupuncture on affected limbs. Certain scalp acupuncture techniques that have been developed by Chinese, Korean, and Japanese practitioners also show promise.

Chiropractic

Chiropractors **do not** treat stroke, and high velocity manipulation of the upper spine is considered inappropriate in individuals who are taking blood-thinning medications or other medications used to reduce the risk of stroke. It should also be noted that chiropractic spinal manipulation of the neck is associated with an exceedingly small risk of causing stroke (reports range from 1 per 400,000 to 1 per 2,000,000).

Traditional Chinese Medicine

In Traditional Chinese Medicine, there are reports of over 100 substances that have been used to treat stroke. In fact, pharmacologic research of these substances is focused on understanding the ingredients and their mechanisms of action in order to develop new drugs.

Chapter 67

Return to Work after Stroke Depends on Job Demands

Job characteristics may be a key determinant in how soon an individual returns to work after having a stroke, according to research presented on February 15, 2001 at the American Stroke Association's 26th International Stroke Conference. The American Stroke Association is a division of the American Heart Association.

It was the first study to examine job characteristics and compare them with the time stroke survivors take to return to work or whether they return at all.

"The type and characteristics of the job are very important in determining who will return to work," says lead researcher Marcella A. Wozniak, M.D., Ph.D., an associate professor of neurology at the University of Maryland School of Medicine in Baltimore.

"By understanding why some individuals do not return to work, we can develop programs to help more people get back to their jobs. Similarly, we can learn to identify those who will have great difficulty resuming work."

Researchers found that both the physical and mental demands of the job were important in predicting patients' return. Individuals who were back to work within 12 months had significantly less physically and psychologically demanding jobs. They felt their jobs were very

"Job Demands Sway Speed of Return to Work after Stroke," February 15, 2001, reprinted with permission from the University of Maryland Medical Center (www.umm.edu). This document was reviewed by David A. Cooke, M.D., February 25, 2008.

secure, felt more job satisfaction, and believed they had more authority to make decisions on the job.

"Survivors who felt their job was secure returned to work significantly sooner than those who felt they were at risk of losing their job," says Wozniak. "Those with authority to make decisions about their job and with supportive coworkers and employers also tended to return to work sooner."

The results are important in light of the aging of America's workforce. Wozniak notes that the risk of stroke increases dramatically with age, that the average age of workers is increasing, and that the Social Security Administration recently has changed its policies.

"They've increased the minimum retirement age to 67 for people born after 1959," says Wozniak. "For people born between 1934 and 1959, a sliding scale to determine retirement age is in place. Therefore, more people will be working at the time of stroke and, as more effective treatments are developed, more survivors will be facing the possibility of reemployment."

The study, conducted at the University of Maryland Medical Center, recruited patients who had their first ischemic stroke (a stroke due to blood-vessel blockage) between the ages of 24 and 64 and were employed full-time outside of the home. Of 150 patients, 64 percent were male and 48 percent were black. They were all able to go home or to a rehabilitation center immediately after their stroke.

Six weeks later, study participants completed standardized questionnaires that measured their perceptions of their jobs. These questionnaires have been used in other studies examining the association of heart disease and other illnesses with employment. Patients were asked to rate their agreement or disagreement with statements about their job such as: "My job is very hectic;" "I have a lot to say about what happens on my job;" "My prospects for career development and promotions are good;" and "I can take it easy and still get my work done."

Patients were phoned at six and 12 months after the stroke to determine when they returned to work.

"Our prior analysis and work by others had found that white-collar, more educated, and wealthier patients were more likely to return to work," says Wozniak. "On one level, this seems obvious because blue-collar jobs are more likely to be physically demanding. On other levels, white-collar jobs would have more cognitive demands, and educated patients with higher-paying jobs would be more likely to have disability insurance and other financial resources to retire early. These factors should make it less likely for white-collar workers to return."

Other factors that may help employees make the decision to return to work could include their perceived ability to change or modify their job environment, their assessment of how easily they could be replaced at work, how likely they feel they are to lose the job, and their social support network at work.

"How the other factors play into what is clearly a complex relationship is mostly speculation right now," says Wozniak. "It is interesting that even in people who regain their independence in daily activities, only about 60 percent return to work."

The research team plans further study of this issue.

Other researchers are Melissa McCarthy, Ph.D.; Patricia Langenberg, Ph.D.; Thomas R. Price, M.D.; and Steven J. Kittner, M.D., M.P.H.

Chapter 68

Social Security Disability Benefits: What You Need to Know

Disability is something most people do not like to think about. But the chances that you will become disabled probably are greater than you realize. Studies show that a 20-year-old worker has a 3 in 10 chance of becoming disabled before reaching retirement age.

This text provides basic information on Social Security disability benefits and is not intended to answer all questions. For specific information about your situation, you should talk with a Social Security representative.

We pay disability benefits through two programs: the Social Security disability insurance program and the Supplemental Security Income (SSI) program. Publications are available at www.socialsecurity .gov.

Who Can Get Social Security Disability Benefits?

Social Security pays benefits to people who cannot work because they have a medical condition that is expected to last at least one year or result in death. Federal law requires this very strict definition of disability. While some programs give money to people with partial disability or short-term disability, Social Security does not.

Certain family members of disabled workers also can receive money from Social Security.

Excerpted from "Disability Benefits," by the Social Security Administration (SSA, www.ssa.gov), SSA Publication No. 05-10029, January 2006.

In general, to get disability benefits, you must meet two different earnings tests:

1. A "recent work" test based on your age at the time you became disabled; and

2. A "duration of work" test to show that you worked long enough under Social Security.

Certain blind workers have to meet only the "duration of work" test.

Table 68.1 shows the rules for how much work you need for the "recent work" test based on your age when your disability began. The rules in this table are based on the calendar quarter in which you turned or will turn a certain age.

The calendar quarters are:

• First Quarter: January 1 through March 31

• Second Quarter: April 1 through June 30

• Third Quarter: July 1 through September 30

• Fourth Quarter: October 1 through December 31

Table 68.1. Rules for Work Needed for the "Recent Work Test"

If you become disabled . . .	Then you generally need:
In or before the quarter you turn age 24	1.5 years of work during the 3-year period ending with the quarter your disability began.
In the quarter after you turn age 24 but before the quarter you turn age 31	Work during half the time for the period beginning with the quarter after you turned 21 and ending with the quarter you became disabled.
	Example: If you become disabled in the quarter you turned age 27, then you would need three years of work out of the 6-year period ending with the quarter you became disabled.
In the quarter you turn age 31 or later	Work during 5 years out of the 10-year period ending with the quarter your disability began.

Table 68.2 shows examples of how much work you need to meet the "duration of work test" if you become disabled at various selected ages. For the "duration of work" test, your work does not have to fall

within a certain period of time. Note: This table does not cover all situations.

How Do I Apply for Disability Benefits?

There are two ways that you can apply for disability benefits. You can:

1. Apply at www.socialsecurity.gov; or

2. Call our toll-free number, 800-772-1213, to make an appointment to file a disability claim at your local Social Security office or to set up an appointment for someone to take your claim over the telephone. The disability claims interview lasts about one hour. If you are deaf or hard of hearing, you may call our toll-free TTY number, 800-325-0778, between 7 a.m. and 7 p.m. on business days. If you schedule an appointment, a Disability Starter Kit will be mailed to you. The Disability Starter Kit will help you get ready for your disability claims interview. If you

Table 68.2. Examples of Work Needed for the "Duration of Work" Test

If you become disabled . . .	Then you generally need:
Before age 28	1.5 years of work
Age 30	2 years
Age 34	3 years
Age 38	4 years
Age 42	5 years
Age 44	5.5 years
Age 46	6 years
Age 48	6.5 years
Age 50	7 years
Age 52	7.5 years
Age 54	8 years
Age 56	8.5 years
Age 58	9 years
Age 60	9.5 years

apply online, the Disability Starter Kit is available at www .socialsecurity.gov/disability.

Who Decides If I Am Disabled?

We will review your application to make sure you meet some basic requirements for disability benefits. We will check whether you worked enough years to qualify. Also, we will evaluate any current work activities. If you meet these requirements, we will send your application to the Disability Determination Services office in your state.

This state agency completes the disability decision for us. Doctors and disability specialists in the state agency ask your doctors for information about your condition. They will consider all the facts in your case. They will use the medical evidence from your doctors and hospitals, clinics, or institutions where you have been treated and all other information. They will ask your doctors:

- what your medical condition is;
- when your medical condition began;
- how your medical condition limits your activities;
- what the medical tests have shown; and
- what treatment you have received.

They also will ask the doctors for information about your ability to do work-related activities, such as walking, sitting, lifting, carrying and remembering instructions. Your doctors are not asked to decide if you are disabled.

The state agency staff may need more medical information before they can decide if you are disabled. If more information is not available from your current medical sources, the state agency may ask you to go for a special examination. We prefer to ask your own doctor, but sometimes the exam may have to be done by someone else. Social Security will pay for the exam and for some of the related travel costs.

Chapter 69

Health Insurance Concerns during Stroke Recovery

Stroke recovery can require lots of time and medical attention. Ideally, some of that medical care is covered by health insurance. Dealing with health insurance companies, however, can be a challenge. But, taking the time to understand the specific benefits of your health care plan will help you manage your stroke recovery.

Dealing with Insurance Companies

Rehab programs can be costly. So it is important to know what portion of the bill your health insurance will pay and what you will have to pay "out-of-pocket." It is also good to know if you can choose any doctor you want. Some plans require that you choose a doctor or specialist in a particular "network."

There are two main types of health plans: Indemnity plans and managed care plans.

Traditional "Indemnity Insurance"

This type of health insurance usually:

- involves a deductible, or amount you must pay toward your medical expenses before the insurance company will pay anything at all on your behalf;

"Recovery after Stroke: Health Insurance," Copyright © 2006 National Stroke Association. Reprinted with permission.

- pays part of your expense (usually 80%), once your deductible is met;

- pays only for "covered" services listed in material sent by the insurance company;

- allows you the flexibility to go to any doctor or rehab facility you choose;

- requires more paperwork than other plans because you have to fill out and submit claim forms to receive your insurance benefits; and

- involves higher payments by you.

Managed Care

Managed care plans provide complete health services at reduced prices for their members, who agree to use doctors and facilities that belong to their plan. Under managed care plans:

- all medical costs are covered except for a small co-payment that you have to pay each time you are seen by a doctor or therapist;

- your out-of-pocket expenses are often less; and

- your choice of providers, facilities, and services is usually limited to those within the network of health care providers. If you see a doctor or therapist that is not in the network you may have to pay full price.

There are different kinds of managed care plans. The two most common are:

- **Health maintenance organization (HMO).** With an HMO, you usually have to get a referral from your doctor in order to see a specialist.

- **Preferred provider organization (PPO).** With a PPO, no referrals are necessary. You can go to any specialist in the network or pay more to go to a specialist that is not in the network.

Settings and Services

Stroke recovery may require extensive rehabilitation. This may include many services in different settings. Check with your health insurance company to make sure you are covered under the following settings and services.

- **acute care (inpatient) and rehab hospitals**—provide 24-hour medical care and a full range of rehab services in a hospital setting.

- **sub-acute facilities**—provide daily nursing care and a fairly wide range of rehab services.

- **long-term care facilities or "skilled nursing homes"**—provide rehab services several times per week to long-term and short-term residents.

- **outpatient facilities**—provide a wide range of rehab services for people who live at home and can come to the center for treatment several times a week.

- **home health agencies**—provide rehab services to stroke survivors in their own homes.

It is important to remember that there are inpatient and outpatient settings and services.

Inpatient services are those that are given to hospital residents who get treatments while they are staying in the hospital. Outpatient services arc those given to patients who live in their own homes. These patients come into an office to see a doctor or therapist. Insurance companies sometimes pay different rates/benefits for these two types of services.

Key Questions on Coverage

Figuring out what your insurance plan pays for requires that you ask a lot of questions. Examples include:

- Does the plan cover rehabilitation services? Which services?

- Does the plan require me to pay more for rehab services than for regular doctor visits?

- Are my doctors and facilities in the provider network?

- Does the plan require my primary care doctor to give me a referral to see a specialist?

- Does the plan provide coverage for prescription drugs?

- What medical equipment is covered by the plan (power wheelchair, adaptive equipment, braces, equipment to continue therapy at home)? How much of the equipment cost is paid by health insurance? How much do I pay?

- Does the plan limit the number of days for rehab program visits (either inpatient days in a facility or outpatient days/doctor visits, or combined)?

- If days are limited, are they renewed from year to year?

- Does the plan limit coverage, or require special referrals for treatment of a preexisting condition or a repeat experience, such as a stroke?

- Does the plan require me to have speech therapy in order to receive occupational therapy (help with performing daily activities)?

- Does the plan cover outpatient speech therapy?

- Does the plan limit the dollar amount it will pay for a particular setting or service?

- Can the plan suddenly remove my doctor or therapist from the network, leaving me without coverage to continue with them? Can the plan decide I will no longer be covered? In either situation, how much advance notice would I receive?

- What are the procedures to appeal a decision made by the health insurance plan? Does the insurance company or an independent reviewer handle an appeal?

- Does the plan exclude "cognitive therapy" (a form of treatment used to change patterns of thinking, such as depression)?

- What type of home care is covered? What do I pay for home care?

Disability Benefits

If you are working in a place where you are covered by the Family Medical Leave Act (FMLA), you must apply as soon as possible. For one, FMLA will protect your job. Also, you often have to apply for FMLA before you can apply for short-term and long-term disability from an employer sponsored plan.

It is important that you apply for disability benefits shortly after your stroke. These benefits can assist you financially until you are able to go back to work.

There are several types of disability benefits that may apply to you, including private disability insurance or government disability benefits. Private disability insurance benefits are provided by an employer or through a disability insurance plan you purchased on your own. If you have private disability insurance, take these steps to apply:

- If your disability insurance is through your employer, contact human resources to assist you in applying for benefits.

- Check with your employer to see if you will have to pay taxes on the money received.

- If you have your own disability insurance policy, call your insurance agent to help you apply for benefits.

- Not all disability plans are the same. Some will pay if you cannot do your current job. Others will only pay if you cannot do any job at all. Check to see which applies to your situation.

- Check your life insurance policies because they may pay your premiums while you are disabled.

Government Disability Benefits

The Social Security Administration (SSA) has two programs that provide money to people who are disabled and unable to work.

- Social Security Disability Insurance (SSDI)
- Supplemental Security Income (SSI)

You can learn more about Social Security programs on the web at www.ssa.gov or by calling 800-772-1213. There are a few things to consider:

- If you are already retired and receive a Social Security benefit, you will not be eligible to receive additional benefits.

- SSA's definition of disability is a physical or mental condition that lasts for at least 12 months and keeps you from working.

- Apply for benefits even if you plan to go back to work.

- You will need to describe to them the impact the stroke has had on you physically—they need to know why you can't work.

Because of the time needed to process the paperwork, be sure to contact them as soon as possible. Also, make and keep copies of all the documents you send to them and letters they have sent to you. Keep track of the names of all the people you talked to, dates, and what they told you.

Changes in Your Abilities

After stroke, what you are able to do may change many times. For example, you may start walking after years of using a wheelchair. Or you may regain sensation in an arm or leg. You may even lose the ability to do something that you once could do. Changes may happen shortly after stroke or take place years later. Either way, they generally require new rehab treatments.

Under Medicare and many private health plans, you are entitled to "re-enter" the system at any time if you experience a change in your abilities. This means that you can re-apply for added rehab benefits based on the change.

What Can Help

Every health insurance plan has coverage limitations. But you may have options for getting the rehab services you need.

- Try contacting the "exceptions" department of your health plan.

- Ask to work with a case manager for chronic or catastrophic illness.

- Seek help from your employer in dealing with the plan.

- Trade inpatient rehab days for outpatient days. Some plans have short inpatient coverage but longer home care/outpatient coverage.

- File an appeal if you feel you are being denied payment or a medical service to which you are entitled.

- If you need help talking to your insurance company about your health care and recovery, consider contacting resources in your community, including vocational rehabilitation services, aging agencies, disability law/elder law projects, and the Social Security Administration Office of Disability (http://www.ssa.gov/disability).

- For more information on Medicare coverage for stroke rehab, call 800-MEDICARE or visit www.medicare.gov

- For information on your specific private health insurance plan, contact your insurance company or your employer's benefits administrator.

Rehabilitation is a lifetime commitment and an important part of recovering from a stroke. Through rehabilitation, you relearn basic skills such as talking, eating, dressing, and walking. Rehabilitation can also improve your strength, flexibility, and endurance. The goal is to regain as much independence as possible.

Remember to ask your doctor, "Where am I on my stroke recovery journey?"

Chapter 70

Finding and Evaluating Assisted-Living Centers

What is an assisted living residence?

An assisted living residence is a special combination of housing, personalized supportive services, and health care designed to meet the needs—both scheduled and unscheduled—of those who need help with activities of daily living.

What is the philosophy of assisted living?

ALFA members subscribe to a 10-point philosophy of care:

- Offering cost-effective quality care that is personalized for individual needs
- Fostering independence for each resident
- Treating each resident with dignity and respect
- Promoting the individuality of each resident
- Allowing each resident choice of care and lifestyle
- Protecting each resident's right to privacy
- Nurturing the spirit of each resident
- Involving family and friends, as appropriate, in care planning and implementation

"About Assisted Living," © 2008 Assisted Living Federation of America (www.alfa.org). Reprinted with permission.

- Providing a safe, residential environment
- Making the assisted living residence a valuable community asset

Who lives in assisted living residences?

Currently, more than a million Americans live in an estimated 20,000 assisted living residences. Assisted living residents can be young or old, affluent or low income, frail or disabled. A typical resident is a woman in her eighties and is either widowed or single. Residents may suffer from Alzheimer's disease or other memory disorders. Residents may also need help with incontinence or mobility.

What does an assisted living residence look like?

Assisted living residences can range from a high-rise apartment complex to a converted Victorian home to a renovated school. Residences may be free standing or housed with other residential options, such as independent living or nursing care. They may be operated by non-profit or for-profit companies. Most facilities have between 25 and 120 units. There is no single blueprint, because consumers' preferences and needs vary widely. Units may vary in size from one room to a full apartment.

How is assisted living regulated?

Licensing and other assisted living regulations vary from state to state contributing to the wide range of senior housing models considered assisted living. Most providers and their staff have special training as a result of either state requirements or company policy. Some states require special staff certification and training. Residences must comply with local building codes and fire safety regulations. ALFA believes the most successful regulations are consumer driven, balancing the safety concerns we all share with the consumers' desires to retain their independence and freedom of choice.

What types of services are offered in assisted living residences?

Services provided in assisted living residences usually include:

- three meals a day served in a common dining area;
- housekeeping services;

- transportation;
- assistance with eating, bathing, dressing, toileting, and walking;
- access to health and medical services;
- 24-hour security and staff availability;
- emergency call systems for each resident's unit;
- health promotion and exercise programs;
- medication management;
- personal laundry services; and
- social and recreational activities.

What about costs?

Costs vary with the residence, room size, and the types of services needed by the residents. Across the nation, the median monthly rate per resident is $2,350 (source: 2006 Overview of Assisted Living)—generally less than the cost of home health services and nursing home care. A basic assisted living fee may cover all services or there may be additional charges for special services. Most assisted living residences charge month-to-month rates, but a few residences require long-term arrangements.

Who pays the bill for an assisted living residence?

Residents or their families generally pay the cost of care from their own financial resources. Depending on the nature of an individual's health insurance program or long-term care insurance policy, costs may be reimbursed. In addition, some residences have their own financial assistance programs. Government payments for assisted living residences have been limited. Some state and local governments offer subsidies for rent or services for low income elders. Others may provide subsidies in the form of an additional payment for those who receive Supplemental Security Income or Medicaid. Some states also utilize Medicaid waiver programs to help pay for assisted living services.

How to find an assisted living residence?

- Call the national Eldercare locator service at 800-677-1116. Calls are accepted between 9 a.m. through 5 p.m. Monday through Friday.

- Contact your local area agency on aging. These agencies are generally listed in the blue pages of your telephone directory.

- Check your library for the *National Directory of Retirement Facilities*.

Chapter 71

Preparing for Catastrophic Medical Events: Advance Directives and Living Wills

Advance Preparation

Experience shows that a catastrophic medical event, such as an accident or a stroke, can leave a person incapacitated and unable to make decisions or to communicate with others. That leaves treatment decisions concerning what is in your best interest up to family members, significant others, health care providers, or the judicial system. In order to avoid this difficult situation, all adults—not just the adults with chronic diseases or other medical conditions—should plan for their future health care treatment preferences and complete an Advance Directive document that specifies personal preferences regarding acceptable and unacceptable medical treatments.

There is a fairly easy way to stay in control—to "have your say"— about these events that are often fraught with emotions. An Advance Directive document can provide specific guidance regarding a person's treatment preferences in a situation such as an irreversible coma following a debilitating stroke.

Typically, a person may not know what medical treatments he or she may prefer or reject. The advantage of preparing an Advance Directive is that the process serves as a guide for those who may need

---

"Having Your Say: Advance Directives, A Consumer's Guide," is reprinted with permission from the American Health Care Association, © 2005. For additional information, visit http://www.longtermcareliving.com.

to make informed decisions regarding major treatments such as tube feeding or ventilator care. You decide in different scenarios how you wish to be treated and even "if" you wish to be treated. Since an Advance Directive prescribes your care plan if you are incapacitated, it may be wise to involve family, significant others, a religious advisor, your physician, other medical professionals, or an attorney (however, an attorney may not be required to complete this document).

Each state government may regulate the preparation of an Advance Directive differently. This makes it important to work within a state's framework to ensure that health care providers, including nursing facilities and assisted living residences, honor your choices regarding, for example, situations involving permanent coma, persistent vegetative state, brain death, and comfort care.

Two Types of Advance Directives

There are two legal forms of an Advance Directive: 1) a Living Will; and, 2) a Medical Power of Attorney (which may also be called a "durable power of attorney for health care" or "health care proxy").

An Advance Directive allows you to state your choices for health care or to name someone to make those choices for you if you become unable to make decisions about your medical treatment or to communicate your preferences. It is best to complete an Advance Directive as part of a strategy for financial planning, retirement, or long term health care. Preparation avoids having to deal with this matter in the event of unexpected serious illness or debilitation.

Living Will

A Living Will generally states the kind of medical care you prefer (or do not want) if you become unable to make your own decision or cannot communicate. It is called a "Living Will" because it takes effect while you are still living.

Most states have their own Living Will forms, each somewhat different. It may also be possible to complete and sign a preprinted Living Will form available in your own community, draw up your own form, or simply write a statement of your preferences for treatment. Generally a Living Will needs to be signed in the presence of two witnesses, and in some states it must also be notarized. You may also wish to speak to an attorney, your physician, or health care or long term health care provider to be certain the Living Will is properly prepared to ensure that your wishes are understood and followed. An Advance

Directive should be completed prior to there being any question about competency of the individual, as when diseases such as Alzheimer's or other dementias are present.

Medical Power of Attorney

A Medical Power of Attorney is a signed, dated, and witnessed document—some states require notarization too—naming another person, such as a husband, wife, daughter, son, or significant other as your "agent" or "proxy" to make medical decisions for you if you are no longer capable of making them or unable to communicate your preferences. You can include instructions about any treatment you wish to avoid.

In selecting your health care agent, it is important to communicate with this person in advance and that they agree to the designation; they could be the ones making treatment decisions for you if future medical situations require it. The agent needs to have reached majority age for your jurisdiction, and not be a health care provider that is treating you. Be sure to verify any other exclusion in your jurisdiction.

Note that a Medical Power of Attorney and the more commonly known "Power of Attorney"—often referred to as Non-Durable Power of Attorney—are not the same. Power of Attorney allows a person to act on matters you specify, such as financial matters. Generally speaking, the person holding the Power of Attorney cannot also be designated as the Medical Power of Attorney. Again, this information needs to be confirmed for your state.

Living Will Vs. Medical Power of Attorney

It might be best to have a Living Will and appoint a health care agent or proxy. However, in some states, laws may make it better to have one or the other. It may also be possible to combine both documents into a single document that describes treatment choices in a variety of situations—you might want to seek medical advice about these situations and choices—and names your health care agent.

Designating a health care agent as part of a Medical Power of Attorney provides more flexibility for future decisions unanticipated in a Living Will. A health care agent, along with a written Living Will, can provide guidance in the absence of the health care agent or support decisions made by the health care agent based on knowledge of your wishes.

577

Modifying an Advance Directive

You may modify, update, or even cancel an Advance Directive at any time in accordance with state law. Any change or cancellation should be written, signed, and dated in accordance with state law, and copies should be given to your doctor or to others to whom you may have given copies of the original documents. Be sure to notify your health care agent of any changes. Some states allow an Advance Directive to be changed by oral statement but, if possible, it is always preferable to put your changes in writing.

If you change or cancel an Advance Directive while you are in any health care setting, the provider of those services should be advised of your decision with new documents to replace any outdated ones.

Even without a change in writing, your wishes stated verbally to your doctor may carry more weight than a Living Will or Medical Power of Attorney, as long as you are competent to make decisions and can communicate your wishes. Again, be sure to clearly express your wishes and be sure that they are understood. It is always better if there are witnesses to your statements.

Retrieving the Advance Directive

Make sure that someone, such as a close family member, legal advisor etc., knows that you have an Advance Directive and knows where it is located. In the case of a health care proxy be sure that person has a current copy. You should also consider the following:

If you spend a great deal of time in more than one state, you should consider having an Advance Directive in each state. Be sure to keep a copy in each location that you reside.

- If you have an Advance Directive—that is, a Living Will or Medical Power of Attorney—give a copy to your health care agent or health care proxy among others.

- Give your physician and the long term health care facility (e.g., a nursing facility or assisted living residence) or other health care provider, a copy of your Advance Directive and advise them to make it part of your permanent medical record.

- Keep a second copy of your Advance Directive in a safe place where it can be found easily if it is needed. However do not keep in a safe deposit box, as that is not easily accessible to others.

- Keep a small card on your person that states that you have an Advance Directive, where it is located, and who your agent or proxy is if you have one.

Under federal law, when you are admitted to most health care settings you will be asked if you have an Advance Directive. If so, the facility will want a copy as part of your medical record.

Finally, as you've read in this text, an Advance Directive may prevent anguish and turmoil within families and provide clear guidance to health care and long term care providers. An Advance Directive should be considered an essential component of future planning just as much as financial planning, life or disability insurance, or drawing up a will.

Part Six

Additional Help and Information

Chapter 72

Glossary of Terms Related to Stroke

Acute stroke: A stage of stroke starting at the onset of symptoms and lasting for a few hours thereafter.

Agnosia: A cognitive disability characterized by ignorance of or inability to acknowledge one side of the body or one side of the visual field.

Aneurysm: A weak or thin spot on an artery wall that has stretched or ballooned out from the wall and filled with blood, or damage to an artery leading to pooling of blood between the layers of the blood vessel walls.

Anoxia: A state of almost no oxygen delivery to a cell, resulting in low energy production and possible death of the cell; see hypoxia.

Anticoagulants: A drug therapy used to prevent the formation of blood clots that can become lodged in cerebral arteries and cause strokes.

Antiplatelet agents: A type of anticoagulant drug therapy that prevents the formation of blood clots by preventing the accumulation of platelets that form the basis of blood clots; some common antiplatelets include aspirin and ticlopidine; see anticoagulants.

This glossary contains terms excerpted from "Stroke: Hope Through Research," by the National Institute of Neurological Disorders and Stroke (NINDS, www.ninds.nih.gov), September 11, 2007.

Antithrombotics: A type of anticoagulant drug therapy that prevents the formation of blood clots by inhibiting the coagulating actions of the blood protein thrombin; some common antithrombotics include warfarin and heparin; see anticoagulants.

Aphasia: The inability to understand or create speech, writing, or language in general due to damage to the speech centers of the brain.

Apoplexy: A historical, but obsolete term for a cerebral stroke, most often intracerebral hemorrhage, that was applied to any condition that involved disorientation and/or paralysis.

Apoptosis: A form of cell death involving shrinking of the cell and eventual disposal of the internal elements of the cell by the body's immune system. Apoptosis is an active, non-toxic form of cell suicide that does not induce an inflammatory response. It is often called pro-grammed cell death because it is triggered by a genetic signal, involves specific cell mechanisms, and is irreversible once initiated.

Apraxia: A movement disorder characterized by the inability to per-form skilled or purposeful voluntary movements, generally caused by damage to the areas of the brain responsible for voluntary movement.

Arteriography: An x-ray of the carotid artery taken when a special dye is injected into the artery.

Arteriovenous malformation (AVM): A congenital disorder char-acterized by a complex tangled web of arteries and veins.

Atherosclerosis: A blood vessel disease characterized by deposits of lipid material on the inside of the walls of large- to medium-sized ar-teries, which make the artery walls thick, hard, brittle, and prone to breaking.

Atrial fibrillation: Irregular beating of the left atrium, or left up-per chamber, of the heart.

Blood-brain barrier: An elaborate network of supportive brain cells, called glia, that surrounds blood vessels and protects neurons from the toxic effects of direct exposure to blood.

Carotid artery: An artery, located on either side of the neck, that supplies the brain with blood.

Carotid endarterectomy: Surgery used to remove fatty deposits from the carotid arteries.

Central stroke pain (central pain syndrome): Pain caused by damage to an area in the thalamus. The pain is a mixture of sensations, including heat and cold, burning, tingling, numbness, and sharp stabbing and underlying aching pain.

Cerebral blood flow (CBF): The flow of blood through the arteries that lead to the brain, called the cerebrovascular system.

Cerebrospinal fluid (CSF): Clear fluid that bathes the brain and spinal cord.

Cerebrovascular disease: A reduction in the supply of blood to the brain either by narrowing of the arteries through the buildup of plaque on the inside walls of the arteries, called stenosis, or through blockage of an artery due to a blood clot.

Cholesterol: A waxy substance, produced naturally by the liver and also found in foods, that circulates in the blood and helps maintain tissues and cell membranes. Excess cholesterol in the body can contribute to atherosclerosis and high blood pressure.

Clipping: Surgical procedure for treatment of brain aneurysms, involving clamping an aneurysm from a blood vessel, surgically removing this ballooned part of the blood vessel, and closing the opening in the artery wall.

Computed tomography (CT) scan: A series of cross-sectional x-rays of the brain and head; also called computerized axial tomography or CAT scan.

Coumadin®: A commonly used anticoagulant, also known as warfarin.

Cytokines: Small, hormone-like proteins released by leukocytes, endothelial cells, and other cells to promote an inflammatory immune response to an injury.

Cytotoxic edema: A state of cell compromise involving influx of fluids and toxic chemicals into a cell causing subsequent swelling of the cell.

Detachable coil: A platinum coil that is inserted into an artery in the thigh and strung through the arteries to the site of an aneurysm. The coil is released into the aneurysm creating an immune response from the body. The body produces a blood clot inside the aneurysm, strengthening the artery walls and reducing the risk of rupture.

Duplex Doppler ultrasound: A diagnostic imaging technique in which an image of an artery can be formed by bouncing sound waves off the moving blood in the artery and measuring the frequency changes of the echoes.

Dysarthria: A disorder characterized by slurred speech due to weakness or incoordination of the muscles involved in speaking.

Dysphagia: Trouble swallowing.

Edema: The swelling of a cell that results from the influx of large amounts of water or fluid into the cell.

Embolic stroke: A stroke caused by an embolus.

Embolus: A free-roaming clot that usually forms in the heart.

Endothelial wall: A flat layer of cells that make up the innermost lining of a blood vessel.

Excitatory amino acids: A subset of neurotransmitters; proteins released by one neuron into the space between two neurons to promote an excitatory state in the other neuron.

Extracranial/intracranial (EC/IC) bypass: A type of surgery that restores blood flow to a blood-deprived area of brain tissue by rerouting a healthy artery in the scalp to the area of brain tissue affected by a blocked artery.

Functional magnetic resonance imaging (fMRI): A type of imaging that measures increases in blood flow within the brain.

Glia: Also called neuroglia; supportive cells of the nervous system that make up the blood-brain barrier, provide nutrients and oxygen to the vital neurons, and protect the neurons from infection, toxicity, and trauma.

Glutamate: Also known as glutamic acid, an amino acid that acts as an excitatory neurotransmitter in the brain.

Hemiparesis: Weakness on one side of the body.

Hemiplegia: Complete paralysis on one side of the body.

Hemorrhagic stroke: Sudden bleeding into or around the brain.

Heparin: A type of anticoagulant.

High-density lipoprotein (HDL): Also known as the good cholesterol; a compound consisting of a lipid and a protein that carries a small percentage of the total cholesterol in the blood and deposits it in the liver.

Homeostasis: A state of equilibrium or balance among various fluids and chemicals in a cell, in tissues, or in the body as a whole.

Hypertension (high blood pressure): Characterized by persistently high arterial blood pressure defined as a measurement greater than or equal to 140 mm/Hg systolic pressure over 90 mm/Hg diastolic pressure.

Hypoxia: A state of decreased oxygen delivery to a cell so that the oxygen falls below normal levels; see anoxia.

Incidence: The extent or frequency of an occurrence; the number of specific new events in a given period of time.

Infarct: An area of tissue that is dead or dying because of a loss of blood supply.

Infarction: A sudden loss of blood supply to tissue, causing the formation of an infarct.

Interleukins: A group of cytokine-related proteins secreted by leukocytes and involved in the inflammatory immune response of the ischemic cascade.

Intracerebral hemorrhage: Occurs when a vessel within the brain leaks blood into the brain.

Ischemia: A loss of blood flow to tissue, caused by an obstruction of the blood vessel, usually in the form of plaque stenosis or a blood clot.

Ischemic cascade: A series of events lasting for several hours to several days following initial ischemia that results in extensive cell death and tissue damage beyond the area of tissue originally affected by the initial lack of blood flow.

Ischemic penumbra: Areas of damaged, but still living, brain cells arranged in a patchwork pattern around areas of dead brain cells.

Ischemic stroke: Ischemia in the tissues of the brain.

Lacunar infarction: Occlusion of a small artery in the brain resulting in a small area of dead brain tissue, called a lacunar infarct; often caused by stenosis of the small arteries, called small vessel disease.

Large vessel disease: Stenosis in large arteries of the cerebrovascular system.

Leukocytes: Blood proteins involved in the inflammatory immune response of the ischemic cascade.

Lipoprotein: Small globules of cholesterol covered by a layer of protein; produced by the liver.

Low-density lipoprotein (LDL): Also known as the bad cholesterol; a compound consisting of a lipid and a protein that carries the majority of the total cholesterol in the blood and deposits the excess along the inside of arterial walls.

Magnetic resonance angiography (MRA): An imaging technique involving injection of a contrast dye into a blood vessel and using magnetic resonance techniques to create an image of the flowing blood through the vessel; often used to detect stenosis of the brain arteries inside the skull.

Magnetic resonance imaging (MRI) scan: A type of imaging involving the use of magnetic fields to detect subtle changes in the water content of tissues.

Mitochondria: The energy producing organelles of the cell.

Mitral annular calcification: A disease of the mitral valve of the heart.

Mitral valve stenosis: A disease of the mitral heart valve involving the buildup of plaque-like material on and around the valve.

Necrosis: A form of cell death resulting from anoxia, trauma, or any other form of irreversible damage to the cell; involves the release of toxic cellular material into the intercellular space, poisoning surrounding cells.

Neuron: The main functional cell of the brain and nervous system, consisting of a cell body, an axon, and dendrites.

Neuroprotective agents: Medications that protect the brain from secondary injury caused by stroke.

Oxygen-free radicals: Toxic chemicals released during the process of cellular respiration and released in excessive amounts during necrosis of a cell; involved in secondary cell death associated with the ischemic cascade.

Plaque: Fatty cholesterol deposits found along the inside of artery walls that lead to atherosclerosis and stenosis of the arteries.

Plasticity: The ability to be formed or molded; in reference to the brain, the ability to adapt to deficits and injury.

Platelets: Structures found in blood that are known primarily for their role in blood coagulation.

Prevalence: The number of cases of a disease in a population at any given point in time.

Recombinant tissue plasminogen activator (rtPA): A genetically engineered form of tPA, a thrombolytic, anti-clotting substance made naturally by the body.

Small vessel disease: A cerebrovascular disease defined by stenosis in small arteries of the brain.

Stenosis: Narrowing of an artery due to the buildup of plaque on the inside wall of the artery.

Stroke belt: An area of the southeastern United States with the highest stroke mortality rate in the country.

Stroke buckle: Three southeastern states, North Carolina, South Carolina, and Georgia, that have an extremely high stroke mortality rate.

Subarachnoid hemorrhage: Bleeding within the meninges, or outer membranes, of the brain into the clear fluid that surrounds the brain.

Thrombolytics: Drugs used to treat an ongoing, acute ischemic stroke by dissolving the blood clot causing the stroke and thereby restoring blood flow through the artery.

Thrombosis: The formation of a blood clot in one of the cerebral arteries of the head or neck that stays attached to the artery wall until it grows large enough to block blood flow.

Thrombotic stroke: A stroke caused by thrombosis.

Tissue necrosis factors: Chemicals released by leukocytes and other cells that cause secondary cell death during the inflammatory immune response associated with the ischemic cascade.

Total serum cholesterol: A combined measurement of a person's high-density lipoprotein (HDL) and low-density lipoprotein (LDL).

tPA: See recombinant tissue plasminogen activator.

Transcranial magnetic stimulation (TMS): A small magnetic current delivered to an area of the brain to promote plasticity and healing.

Transient ischemic attack (TIA): A short-lived stroke that lasts from a few minutes up to 24 hours; often called a mini-stroke.

Vasodilators: Medications that increase blood flow to the brain by expanding or dilating blood vessels.

Vasospasm: A dangerous side effect of subarachnoid hemorrhage in which the blood vessels in the subarachnoid space constrict erratically, cutting off blood flow.

Vertebral artery: An artery on either side of the neck; see carotid artery.

Warfarin: A commonly used anticoagulant, also known as Coumadin®.

Chapter 73

Directory of Organizations That Provide Information to Stroke Survivors and Their Families

Government Agencies That Provide Information about Stroke

Administration on Aging
Washington, DC 20201
Toll-Free: 800-677-1116
(Eldercare Locator)
Phone: 202-619-0724
Website: www.aoa.gov
E-mail: aoainfo@aoa.hhs.gov

Agency for Healthcare Research and Quality
Office of Communications and Knowledge Transfer
540 Gaither Road, Suite 2000
Rockville, MD 20850
Phone: 301-427-1364
Website: www.ahrq.gov

Center for Medicare and Medicaid Services
Toll-Free: 800-MEDICARE
(633-4227)
TTY: 877-486-2048
Website: www.cms.hhs.gov

Centers for Disease Control and Prevention
1600 Clifton Road
Atlanta, GA 30333
Toll-Free: 800-311-3435
Phone: 404-639-3311
Website: www.cdc.gov
E-mail: cdcinfo@cdc.gov

Resources in this chapter were compiled from several sources deemed reliable; all contact information was verified and updated in March 2008.

591

Equal Employment Opportunity Commission
1801 L Street, NW
Washington, DC 20507
Toll-Free: 800-669-4000
Phone: 202-663-4900
TTY: 202-663-4494
Website: www.eeoc.gov
E-mail: info@eeoc.gov

Healthfinder®
National Health Information Center
P.O. Box 1133
Washington, DC 20013-1133
Toll-Free: 800-336-4797
Phone: 301-565-4167
Fax: 301-984-4256
Website: www.healthfinder.gov
E-mail: healthfinder@nhic.org

National Cancer Institute
Cancer Information Service
6116 Executive Boulevard
Room 3036A
Bethesda, MD 20892-8322
Toll-Free: 800-4-CANCER
(422-6237)
TTY Toll-Free: 800-332-8615
Website: www.cancer.gov
E-mail:
cancergovstaff@mail.nih.gov

National Center for Complementary and Alternative Medicine
NCCAM Clearinghouse
P.O. Box 7923
Gaithersburg, MD 20898-7923
Toll-Free: 888-644-6226
Phone: 301-519-3153
Fax: 866-464-3616
TTY: 866-464-3615
Website: nccam.nih.gov
E-mail: info@nccam.nih.gov

National Center for Health Statistics
3311 Toledo Road
Hyattsville, MD 20782
Phone: 301-458-4000
Phone: 301-458-4636
Website: www.cdc.gov/nchs
E-mail: nchsquery@cdc.gov

National Heart, Lung and Blood Institute
NHLBI Health Information Center
P.O. Box 30105
Bethesda, MD 20824-0105
Phone: 301-592-8573
TTY: 240-629-3255
Fax: 301-592-8563
Website: www.nhlbi.nih.gov
E-mail: nhlbiinfo@nhlbi.nih.gov

National Human Genome Research Institute
National Institutes of Health
Building 31, Room 4B09
Bethesda, MD 20892-2152
Phone: 301-402-0911
Fax: 301-402-0837
Website: www.genome.gov

National Institute of Neurological Disorders and Stroke
NIH Neurological Institute
P.O. Box 5801
Bethesda, MD 20824
Toll-Free: 800-352-9424
Phone: 301-496-5751
TTY: 301-468-5981
Website: www.ninds.nih.gov
E-mail: braininfo@ninds.nih.gov

National Institute on Aging
Building 31, Room 5C27
31 Center Drive, MSC 2292
Bethesda, MD 20892
Publications Toll-Free:
800-222-2225
Phone: 301-496-1752
TTY: 800-222-4225
Fax: 301-496-1072
Websites: www.nia.nih.gov
Publications Website:
www.niapublications.org
E-mail: niainfo@nia.nih.gov

National Institutes of Health
9000 Rockville Pike
Bethesda, MD 20892
Phone: 301-496-4000
TTY: 301-402-9612
Website: www.nih.gov
E-mail: NIHinfo@od.nih.gov

National Women's Health Information Center
8270 Willow Oaks Corporate Dr.
Fairfax, VA 22031
Toll-Free: 800-994-9662
TDD: 888-220-5446
Website: www.4women.gov

Social Security Administration
Office of Public Inquiries
Windsor Park Building
6401 Security Boulevard
Baltimore, MD 21235
Toll-Free: 800-772-1213
Website: www.socialsecurity.gov

U.S. Department of Health and Human Services
200 Independent Avenue, SW
Washington, DC 20201
Toll-Free: 877-696-6775
Phone: 202-619-0257
Website: www.hhs.gov

U.S. Food and Drug Administration
5600 Fishers Lane
Rockville, MD 20857-0001
Toll-Free: 888-463-6332
Phone: 301-827-4420
Fax: 301-443-9767
Website: www.fda.gov

U.S. National Library of Medicine
8600 Rockville Pike
Bethesda, MD 20894
Toll-Free: 888-346-3656
Phone: 301-594-5983
TDD: 800-735-2258
Website: www.nlm.nih.gov
E-mail: custserv@nlm.nih.gov

Private Agencies That Provide Information about Stroke

American Academy of
Family Physicians
P.O. Box 11210
Shawnee Mission, KS 66207-1210
Toll-Free: 800-274-2237
Phone: 913-906-6000
Website: www.aafp.org
E-mail: fp@aafp.org

American Academy of
Neurology
1080 Montreal Avenue
Saint Paul, MN 55116
Toll-Free: 800-879-1960
Phone: 651-695-2717
Fax: 651-695-2791
Website: www.aan.com
E-mail:
memberservices@aan.com

American Academy of
Pediatrics
141 Northwest Point Boulevard
Elk Grove Village, IL, 60007
Phone: 847-434-4000
Fax: 847-434-8000
Website: www.aap.org
E-mail: kidsdocs@aap.org

American Academy of
Physical Medicine and
Rehabilitation
330 North Wabash Avenue
Suite 2500
Chicago, IL 60611-7617
Phone: 312-464-9700
Fax: 312-464-0227
Website: www.aapmr.org
E-mail: info@aapmr.org

American Association of
Neurological Surgeons
5550 Meadowbrook Drive
Rolling Meadows, IL 60008
Toll-Free: 888-566-2267
Phone: 847-378-0500
Fax: 847-378-0600
Website: www.aans.org
E-mail: info@aans.org

American College of Obste-
tricians and Gynecologists
409 12th Street, SW
P.O. Box 96920
Washington, DC 20090-6920
Phone: 202-638-5577
Website: www.acog.org
E-mail: resources@acog.org

American Congress of
Rehabilitation Medicine
6801 Lake Plaza Drive
Suite B-205
Indianapolis, IN 46220
Phone: 317-915-2250
Fax: 317-915-2245
Website: www.acrm.org

American Heart
Association/American
Stroke Association
National Center
7272 Greenville Avenue
Dallas, TX 75231
Toll-Free: 800-AHA-USA-1
(242-8721)
Websites:
www.americanheart.org;
www.strokeassociation.org

American Medical Association/Medem
100 Pine Street, 3rd Floor
San Francisco, CA 94111
Toll-Free: 877-926-3336
Phone: 415-644-3800
Fax: 415-644-3950
Website: www.medem.com
E-mail: info@medem.com

American Occupational Therapy Association
4720 Montgomery Lane
P.O. Box 31220
Bethesda, MD 20824-1220
Toll-Free: 800-377-8555
Phone: 301-652-2682
Fax: 301-652-7711
Website: www.aota.org

American Physical Therapy Association
1111 North Fairfax Street
Alexandria, VA 22314-1488
Toll-Free: 800-999-2782
Phone: 703-684-2782
TDD: 703-683-6748
Fax: 703-684-7343
Website: www.apta.org

American Society of Neurorehabilitation
5841 Cedar Lake Road
Suite 204
Minneapolis, MN 55416
Phone: 952-545-6324
Fax: 952-545-6073
Website: www.asnr.com
E-mail: asnr@llmsi.com

American Speech-Language-Hearing Association (ASHA)
2200 Research Boulevard
Rockville, MD 20850-3289
Toll-Free: 800-638-8255
Fax: 301-296-8580
Website: www.asha.org
E-mail: actioncenter@asha.org

Association for Driver Rehabilitation Specialists (ADED)
2424 N. Center Street, #369
Hickory, NC 28601
Toll-Free: 877-529-1830
Phone: 828-855-1623
Fax: 828-855-1672
Website: www.driver-ed.org
E-mail: info@driver-ed.org

Brain Aneurysm Foundation, Inc.
269 Hanover Street, Building 3
Hanover, MA 02339
Toll-Free: 888-272-4602
Phone: 617-269-3870
Website: www.bafound.org
E-mail: office@bafound.org

Brain Injury Association of America
8201 Greensburro, Suite 611
McLane, VA 22102
Toll-Free: 800-444-6443
Phone: 703-761-0750
Fax: 703-761-0755
Website: www.biausa.org

Brain Injury Recovery Network
840 Central Avenue
Carlisle, OH 45005
Toll-Free: 877-810-2100
Fax: 877-810-2100
Website: www.tbirecovery.org

Brain Injury Resource Center
P.O. Box 84151
Seattle, WA 98124-5451
Phone: 206-621-8558
Website: www.headinjury.com
E-mail: brain@headinjury.com

Children's Hemiplegia and Stroke Association (CHASA)
4101 W. Green Oaks
Suite 305, #149
Arlington, TX 76016
Websites: www.chasa.org;
www.pediatricstroke.org

Cleveland Clinic
9500 Euclid Avenue
Cleveland, OH 44195
Toll-Free: 800-223-2273
Phone: 216-444-2200
TTY: 216-444-0261
Website: www.clevelandclinic.org

Family Caregiver Alliance
180 Montgomery Street
Suite 1100
San Francisco, CA 94104
Toll-Free: 800-445-8106
Phone: 415-434-3388
Fax: 415-434-3508
Website: www.caregiver.org
E-mail: info@caregiver.org

Hazel K. Goddess Fund for Stroke Research in Women
785 Park Avenue
New York, NY 10021-3552
Phone: 212-713-6789
Fax: 212-288-2160
Website:
www.thegoddessfund.org
E-mail:
davonna@thegoddessfund.org

Internet Stroke Center
Washington University School of Medicine
Department of Neurology
660 South Euclid
P.O. Box 8111
St. Louis, MO 63110
Phone: 314-362-3868
Website: www.strokecenter.org

Job Accommodation Network (JAN)
P.O. Box 6080
224 Spruce Street
Morgantown, WV 26506-6080
Toll-Free: 800-526-7234
TTY: 877-781-9403
Fax: 304-293-5407
Website: www.jan.wvu.edu

National Alliance for Caregiving
4720 Montgomery Lane
5th Floor, Suite 205
Bethesda, MD 20814
Phone: 301-718-8444
Fax: 301-951-9067
Website: www.caregiving.org
E-mail: info@caregiving.org

National Aphasia Association
350 Seventh Avenue, Suite 902
New York, NY 10001
Toll-Free: 800-922-4622
Website: www.aphasia.org
E-mail:
responsenter@aphasia.org

National Brain Tumor Foundation
22 Battery Street, Suite 612
San Francisco, CA 94111
Toll-Free: 800-934-2873
Phone: 415-834-9970
Fax: 415-834-9980
Website: www.braintumor.org
E-mail: nbtf@braintumor.org

National Center for Learning Disabilities
381 Park Avenue South
Suite 1401
New York, NY 10016
Toll-Free: 888-575-7373
Phone: 212-545-7510
Fax: 212-545-9665
Website: www.ncld.org

National Family Caregivers Association
10400 Connecticut Avenue,
Suite 500
Kensington, MD 20895-3944
Toll-Free: 800-896-3650
Phone: 301-942-6430
Fax: 301-942-2302
Website: www.nfcacares.org
E-mail:
info@thefamilycaregiver.org

National Information Center for Children and Youth with Disabilities (NICHCY)
P.O. Box 1492
Washington, DC 20013
Toll-Free: 800-695-0285
Fax: 202-884-8441
Website: www.nichcy.org
E-mail: nichcy@aed.org

National Rehabilitation Information Center
8201 Corporate Drive, Suite 600
Landover, MD 20785
Toll-Free: 800-346-2742
Phone: 301-459-5900
TTY: 301-459-5984
Website: www.naric.com
E-mail:
naricinfo@heitechservices.com

National Stroke Association
9707 E. Easter Lane Building B
Centennial, CO 80112
Toll-Free: 800-787-6537
Fax: 303-649-1328
Website: www.stroke.org
E-mail: info@stroke.org

Nemours Foundation Center for Children's Health Media
1600 Rockland Road
Wilmington, DE 19803
Phone: 302-651-4000
Fax: 302-651-4055
Website: www.kidshealth.org
E-mail: info@kidshealth.org

Rehabilitation Institute of Chicago

345 E. Superior Street
First Floor
Chicago, IL 60611
Phone: 312-238-5433
Fax: 312-238-2860
Website: lifecenter.ric.org
E-mail: lifecenter@ric.org

Society for Vascular Surgery

633 N. St. Clair, 24th Floor
Chicago, IL 60611
Toll-Free: 800-258-7188
Phone: 312-334-2300
Fax: 312-334-2320
Website: www.vascularweb.org
E-mail:
vascular@vascularsociety.org

Stroke Association UK

Stroke House, 240 City Road
London, EC1V 2PR
United Kingdom
Phone: 020 7566 0300
Helpline: 0845 3033 100
Fax: 020 7490 2686
Website: www.stroke.org.uk
E-mail: info@stroke.org.uk

Stroke Awareness Foundation

c/o The Health Trust
2105 S. Bascom Avenue
Campbell, CA 95008
Phone: 408-879-8433
Fax: 408-559-9515
Website: www.strokeinfo.org
E-mail: sherry@strokeinfo.org

Stroke Network

P.O. Box 492
Abingdon, MD 21009
Website: www.strokenetwork.org

Well Spouse Foundation

63 West Main Street, Suite H
Freehold, NJ 07728
Toll-Free: 800-838-0879
Phone: 732-577-8899
Fax: 732-577-8644
Website: www.wellspouse.org
E-mail: info@wellspouse.org

Index

Index

Page numbers followed by 'n' indicate a footnote. Page numbers in *italics* indicate a table or illustration.

A

AAA *see* abdominal aortic aneurysm
AAFP *see* American Academy of Family Physicians
AAN *see* American Academy of Neurology
abdominal aortic aneurysm (AAA)
  described 39
  diagnosis 44
  symptoms 42
"About Assisted Living" (ALFA) 571n
ABPM machine *see* Ambulatory Blood Pressure Monitoring machine
ACAS *see* Asymptomatic Carotid Atherosclerosis Trial
ACE inhibitors *see* angiotensin converting enzyme inhibitors
Aconitum napellus 553
acquired brain injury
  see traumatic brain injury
Activase (tissue plasminogen activator)
  described 324
  stroke prevention *318*

activities of daily living (ADL)
  cognitive deficits 415–16
  stroke patients 23
acupuncture 554
acute stroke
  defined 583
  therapies 19
A.D.A.M., Inc., publications
  alternative medicine 549n
  carotid stenosis 117n
  fibromuscular dysplasia 161n
  syphilis 244n
adenoviruses, gene therapy 391
ADL *see* activities of daily living
Administration on Aging
  caregiver tips publication 545n
  contact information 591
advance directives, overview 575–78
age factor
  access to care 97–99
  aneurysm 41
  atherosclerosis 105–6
  atrial fibrillation 14, 126
  carotid artery problems 351
  carotid stenosis 118
  diabetes mellitus 155
  peripheral artery disease 200

601

617

Health Reference Series
COMPLETE CATALOG
List price $87 per volume. **School and library price $78 per volume.**

Adolescent Health Sourcebook, 2nd Edition

Basic Consumer Health Information about the Physical, Mental, and Emotional Growth and Development of Adolescents, Including Medical Care, Nutritional and Physical Activity Requirements, Puberty, Sexual Activity, Acne, Tanning, Body Piercing, Common Physical Illnesses and Disorders, Eating Disorders, Attention Deficit Hyperactivity Disorder, Depression, Bullying, Hazing, and Adolescent Injuries Related to Sports, Driving, and Work

Along with Substance Abuse Information about Nicotine, Alcohol, and Drug Use, a Glossary, and Directory of Additional Resources

Edited by Joyce Brennfleck Shannon. 683 pages. 2006. 978-0-7808-0943-7.

"It is written in clear, nontechnical language aimed at general readers. . . . Recommended for public libraries, community colleges, and other agencies serving health care consumers."
— *American Reference Books Annual, 2003*

"Recommended for school and public libraries. Parents and professionals dealing with teens will appreciate the easy-to-follow format and the clearly written text. This could become a 'must have' for every high school teacher." — *E-Streams, Jan '03*

"A good starting point for information related to common medical, mental, and emotional concerns of adolescents." — *School Library Journal, Nov '02*

"This book provides accurate information in an easy to access format. It addresses topics that parents and caregivers might not be aware of and provides practical, useable information."
— *Doody's Health Sciences Book Review Journal, Sep-Oct '02*

"Recommended reference source."
— *Booklist, American Library Association, Sep '02*

■

AIDS Sourcebook, 3rd Edition

Basic Consumer Health Information about Acquired Immune Deficiency Syndrome (AIDS) and Human Immunodeficiency Virus (HIV) Infection, Including Facts about Transmission, Prevention, Diagnosis, Treatment, Opportunistic Infections, and Other Complications, with a Section for Women and Children, Including Details about Associated Gynecological Concerns, Pregnancy, and Pediatric Care

Along with Updated Statistical Information, Reports on Current Research Initiatives, a Glossary, and Directories of Internet, Hotline, and Other Resources

Edited by Dawn D. Matthews. 664 pages. 2003. 978-0-7808-0631-3.

"The 3rd edition of the *AIDS Sourcebook*, part of Omnigraphics' *Health Reference Series*, is a welcome update. . . . This resource is highly recommended for academic and public libraries."
— *American Reference Books Annual, 2004*

"Excellent sourcebook. This continues to be a highly recommended book. There is no other book that provides as much information as this book provides."
— *AIDS Book Review Journal, Dec-Jan '00*

"Recommended reference source."
— *Booklist, American Library Association, Dec '99*

■

Alcoholism Sourcebook, 2nd Edition

Basic Consumer Health Information about Alcohol Use, Abuse, and Dependence, Featuring Facts about the Physical, Mental, and Social Health Effects of Alcohol Addiction, Including Alcoholic Liver Disease, Pancreatic Disease, Cardiovascular Disease, Neurological Disorders, and the Effects of Drinking during Pregnancy

Along with Information about Alcohol Treatment, Medications, and Recovery Programs, in Addition to Tips for Reducing the Prevalence of Underage Drinking, Statistics about Alcohol Use, a Glossary of Related Terms, and Directories of Resources for More Help and Information

Edited by Amy L. Sutton. 653 pages. 2006. 978-0-7808-0942-0.

"This title is one of the few reference works on alcoholism for general readers. For some readers this will be a welcome complement to the many self-help books on the market. Recommended for collections serving general readers and consumer health collections."
— *E-Streams, Mar '01*

"This book is an excellent choice for public and academic libraries."
— *American Reference Books Annual, 2001*

"Recommended reference source."
— *Booklist, American Library Association, Dec '00*

"Presents a wealth of information on alcohol use and abuse and its effects on the body and mind, treatment, and prevention." — *SciTech Book News, Dec '00*

"Important new health guide which packs in the latest consumer information about the problems of alcoholism." — *Reviewer's Bookwatch, Nov '00*

SEE ALSO Drug Abuse Sourcebook

Allergies Sourcebook, 3rd Edition

Basic Consumer Health Information about Allergic Disorders, Such as Anaphylaxis, Hives, Eczema, Rhinitis, Sinusitis, and Conjunctivitis, and Their Triggers, Including Pollen, Mold, Dust Mites, Animal Dander, Insects, Chemicals, Food, Food Additives, and Medications;

Along with Advice about the Diagnosis and Treatment of Allergy Symptoms, a Glossary of Related Terms, a Directory of Resources for Help and Information, and Suggestions for Additional Reading

Edited by Amy L. Sutton. 598 pages. 2007. 978-0-7808-0950-5.

"This book brings a great deal of useful material together. . . . This is an excellent addition to public and consumer health library collections."
— *American Reference Books Annual, 2003*

"This second edition would be useful to laypersons with little or advanced knowledge of the subject matter. This book would also serve as a resource for nursing and other health care professions students. It would be useful in public, academic, and hospital libraries with consumer health collections." — *E-Streams, Jul '02*

■

Alternative Medicine Sourcebook

SEE Complementary & Alternative Medicine Sourcebook

■

Alzheimer's Disease Sourcebook, 3rd Edition

Basic Consumer Health Information about Alzheimer's Disease, Other Dementias, and Related Disorders, Including Multi-Infarct Dementia, AIDS Dementia Complex, Dementia with Lewy Bodies, Huntington's Disease, Wernicke-Korsakoff Syndrome (Alcohol-Related Dementia), Delirium, and Confusional States

Along with Information for People Newly Diagnosed with Alzheimer's Disease and Caregivers, Reports Detailing Current Research Efforts in Prevention, Diagnosis, and Treatment, Facts about Long-Term Care Issues, and Listings of Sources for Additional Information

Edited by Karen Bellenir. 645 pages. 2003. 978-0-7808-0666-5.

"This very informative and valuable tool will be a great addition to any library serving consumers, students and health care workers."
— *American Reference Books Annual, 2004*

"This is a valuable resource for people affected by dementias such as Alzheimer's. It is easy to navigate and includes important information and resources."
— *Doody's Review Service, Feb '04*

"Recommended reference source."
— *Booklist, American Library Association, Oct '99*

SEE ALSO *Brain Disorders Sourcebook*

Arthritis Sourcebook, 2nd Edition

Basic Consumer Health Information about Osteoarthritis, Rheumatoid Arthritis, Other Rheumatic Disorders, Infectious Forms of Arthritis, and Diseases with Symptoms Linked to Arthritis, Featuring Facts about Diagnosis, Pain Management, and Surgical Therapies

Along with Coping Strategies, Research Updates, a Glossary, and Resources for Additional Help and Information

Edited by Amy L. Sutton. 593 pages. 2004. 978-0-7808-0667-2.

"This easy-to-read volume is recommended for consumer health collections within public or academic libraries." — *E-Streams, May '05*

"As expected, this updated edition continues the excellent reputation of this series in providing sound, usable health information. . . . Highly recommended."
— *American Reference Books Annual, 2005*

"Excellent reference." — *The Bookwatch, Jan '05*

■

Asthma Sourcebook, 2nd Edition

Basic Consumer Health Information about the Causes, Symptoms, Diagnosis, and Treatment of Asthma in Infants, Children, Teenagers, and Adults, Including Facts about Different Types of Asthma, Common Co-Occurring Conditions, Asthma Management Plans, Triggers, Medications, and Medication Delivery Devices

Along with Asthma Statistics, Research Updates, a Glossary, a Directory of Asthma-Related Resources, and More

Edited by Karen Bellenir. 609 pages. 2006. 978-0-7808-0866-9.

"A worthwhile reference acquisition for public libraries and academic medical libraries whose readers desire a quick introduction to the wide range of asthma information." — *Choice, Association of College & Research Libraries, Jun '01*

"Recommended reference source."
— *Booklist, American Library Association, Feb '01*

"Highly recommended." — *The Bookwatch, Jan '01*

"There is much good information for patients and their families who deal with asthma daily."
— *American Medical Writers Association Journal, Winter '01*

"This informative text is recommended for consumer health collections in public, secondary school, and community college libraries and the libraries of universities with a large undergraduate population."
— *American Reference Books Annual, 2001*

■

Attention Deficit Disorder Sourcebook

Basic Consumer Health Information about Attention Deficit/Hyperactivity Disorder in Children and Adults,

628

Including Facts about Causes, Symptoms, Diagnostic Criteria, and Treatment Options Such as Medications, Behavior Therapy, Coaching, and Homeopathy

Along with Reports on Current Research Initiatives, Legal Issues, and Government Regulations, and Featuring a Glossary of Related Terms, Internet Resources, and a List of Additional Reading Material

Edited by Dawn D. Matthews. 470 pages. 2002. 978-0-7808-0624-5.

"Recommended reference source."
— *Booklist, American Library Association, Jan '03*

"This book is recommended for all school libraries and the reference or consumer health sections of public libraries." — *American Reference Books Annual, 2003*

∎

Back & Neck Sourcebook, 2nd Edition

Basic Consumer Health Information about Spinal Pain, Spinal Cord Injuries, and Related Disorders, Such as Degenerative Disk Disease, Osteoarthritis, Scoliosis, Sciatica, Spina Bifida, and Spinal Stenosis, and Featuring Facts about Maintaining Spinal Health, Self-Care, Pain Management, Rehabilitative Care, Chiropractic Care, Spinal Surgeries, and Complementary Therapies

Along with Suggestions for Preventing Back and Neck Pain, a Glossary of Related Terms, and a Directory of Resources

Edited by Amy L. Sutton. 633 pages. 2004. 978-0-7808-0738-9.

"Recommended . . . an easy to use, comprehensive medical reference book." — *E-Streams, Sep '05*

"The strength of this work is its basic, easy-to-read format. Recommended." — *Reference and User Services Quarterly, American Library Association, Winter '97*

∎

Blood & Circulatory Disorders Sourcebook, 2nd Edition

Basic Consumer Health Information about the Blood and Circulatory System and Related Disorders, Such as Anemia and Other Hemoglobin Diseases, Cancer of the Blood and Associated Bone Marrow Disorders, Clotting and Bleeding Problems, and Conditions That Affect the Veins, Blood Vessels, and Arteries, Including Facts about the Donation and Transplantation of Bone Marrow, Stem Cells, and Blood and Tips for Keeping the Blood and Circulatory System Healthy

Along with a Glossary of Related Terms and Resources for Additional Help and Information

Edited by Amy L. Sutton. 659 pages. 2005. 978-0-7808-0746-4.

"Highly recommended pick for basic consumer health reference holdings at all levels."
— *The Bookwatch, Aug '05*

"Recommended reference source."
— *Booklist, American Library Association, Feb '99*

"An important reference sourcebook written in simple language for everyday, non-technical users. "
— *Reviewer's Bookwatch, Jan '99*

∎

Brain Disorders Sourcebook, 2nd Edition

Basic Consumer Health Information about Acquired and Traumatic Brain Injuries, Infections of the Brain, Epilepsy and Seizure Disorders, Cerebral Palsy, and Degenerative Neurological Disorders, Including Amyotrophic Lateral Sclerosis (ALS), Dementias, Multiple Sclerosis, and More

Along with Information on the Brain's Structure and Function, Treatment and Rehabilitation Options, Reports on Current Research Initiatives, a Glossary of Terms Related to Brain Disorders and Injuries, and a Directory of Sources for Further Help and Information

Edited by Sandra J. Judd. 625 pages. 2005. 978-0-7808-0744-0.

"Highly recommended pick for basic consumer health reference holdings at all levels."
— *The Bookwatch, Aug '05*

"Belongs on the shelves of any library with a consumer health collection." — *E-Streams, Mar '00*

"Recommended reference source."
— *Booklist, American Library Association, Oct '99*

SEE ALSO *Alzheimer's Disease Sourcebook*

∎

Breast Cancer Sourcebook, 2nd Edition

Basic Consumer Health Information about Breast Cancer, Including Facts about Risk Factors, Prevention, Screening and Diagnostic Methods, Treatment Options, Complementary and Alternative Therapies, Post-Treatment Concerns, Clinical Trials, Special Risk Populations, and New Developments in Breast Cancer Research

Along with Breast Cancer Statistics, a Glossary of Related Terms, and a Directory of Resources for Additional Help and Information

Edited by Sandra J. Judd. 595 pages. 2004. 978-0-7808-0668-9.

"This book will be an excellent addition to public, community college, medical, and academic libraries."
— *American Reference Books Annual, 2006*

"It would be a useful reference book in a library or on loan to women in a support group."
— *Cancer Forum, Mar '03*

"Recommended reference source."
— *Booklist, American Library Association, Jan '02*

"This reference source is highly recommended. It is quite informative, comprehensive and detailed in na-

ture, and yet it offers practical advice in easy-to-read language. It could be thought of as the 'bible' of breast cancer for the consumer."
— *E-Streams, Jan '02*

"From the pros and cons of different screening methods and results to treatment options, *Breast Cancer Sourcebook* provides the latest information on the subject."
— *Library Bookwatch, Dec '01*

"This thoroughgoing, very readable reference covers all aspects of breast health and cancer. . . . Readers will find much to consider here. Recommended for all public and patient health collections."
— *Library Journal, Sep '01*

SEE ALSO Cancer Sourcebook for Women, Women's Health Concerns Sourcebook

■

Breastfeeding Sourcebook

Basic Consumer Health Information about the Benefits of Breastmilk, Preparing to Breastfeed, Breastfeeding as a Baby Grows, Nutrition, and More, Including Information on Special Situations and Concerns Such as Mastitis, Illness, Medications, Allergies, Multiple Births, Prematurity, Special Needs, and Adoption

Along with a Glossary and Resources for Additional Help and Information

Edited by Jenni Lynn Colson. 388 pages. 2002. 978-0-7808-0332-9.

"Particularly useful is the information about professional lactation services and chapters on breastfeeding when returning to work. . . . *Breastfeeding Sourcebook* will be useful for public libraries, consumer health libraries, and technical schools offering nurse assistant training, especially in areas where Internet access is problematic."
— *American Reference Books Annual, 2003*

SEE ALSO Pregnancy & Birth Sourcebook

■

Burns Sourcebook

Basic Consumer Health Information about Various Types of Burns and Scalds, Including Flame, Heat, Cold, Electrical, Chemical, and Sun Burns

Along with Information on Short-Term and Long-Term Treatments, Tissue Reconstruction, Plastic Surgery, Prevention Suggestions, and First Aid

Edited by Allan R. Cook. 604 pages. 1999. 978-0-7808-0204-9.

"This is an exceptional addition to the series and is highly recommended for all consumer health collections, hospital libraries, and academic medical centers."
— *E-Streams, Mar '00*

"This key reference guide is an invaluable addition to all health care and public libraries in confronting this ongoing health issue."
— *American Reference Books Annual, 2000*

"Recommended reference source."
— *Booklist, American Library Association, Dec '99*

SEE ALSO Dermatological Disorders Sourcebook

Cancer Sourcebook, 5th Edition

Basic Consumer Health Information about Major Forms and Stages of Cancer, Featuring Facts about Head and Neck Cancers, Lung Cancers, Gastrointestinal Cancers, Genitourinary Cancers, Lymphomas, Blood Cell Cancers, Endocrine Cancers, Skin Cancers, Bone Cancers, Metastatic Cancers, and More

Along with Facts about Cancer Treatments, Cancer Risks and Prevention, a Glossary of Related Terms, Statistical Data, and a Directory of Resources for Additional Information

Edited by Karen Bellenir. 1,133 pages. 2007. 978-0-7808-0947-5.

"With cancer being the second leading cause of death for Americans, a prodigious work such as this one, which locates centrally so much cancer-related information, is clearly an asset to this nation's citizens and others."
— *Journal of the National Medical Association, 2004*

"This title is recommended for health sciences and public libraries with consumer health collections."
— *E-Streams, Feb '01*

". . . can be effectively used by cancer patients and their families who are looking for answers in a language they can understand. Public and hospital libraries should have it on their shelves."
— *American Reference Books Annual, 2001*

"Recommended reference source."
— *Booklist, American Library Association, Dec '00*

SEE ALSO Breast Cancer Sourcebook, Cancer Sourcebook for Women, Pediatric Cancer Sourcebook, Prostate Cancer Sourcebook

■

Cancer Sourcebook for Women, 3rd Edition

Basic Consumer Health Information about Leading Causes of Cancer in Women, Featuring Facts about Gynecologic Cancers and Related Concerns, Such as Breast Cancer, Cervical Cancer, Endometrial Cancer, Uterine Sarcoma, Vaginal Cancer, Vulvar Cancer, and Common Non-Cancerous Gynecologic Conditions, in Addition to Facts about Lung Cancer, Colorectal Cancer, and Thyroid Cancer in Women

Along with Information about Cancer Risk Factors, Screening and Prevention, Treatment Options, and Tips on Coping with Life after Cancer Treatment, a Glossary of Cancer Terms, and a Directory of Resources for Additional Help and Information

Edited by Amy L. Sutton. 715 pages. 2006. 978-0-7808-0867-6.

"An excellent addition to collections in public, consumer health, and women's health libraries."
— *American Reference Books Annual, 2003*

"Overall, the information is excellent, and complex topics are clearly explained. As a reference book for the consumer it is a valuable resource to assist them to make informed decisions about cancer and its treatments."
— *Cancer Forum, Nov '02*

"Highly recommended for academic and medical reference collections."   — *Library Bookwatch, Sep '02*

"This is a highly recommended book for any public or consumer library, being reader friendly and containing accurate and helpful information."
     — *E-Streams, Aug '02*

"Recommended reference source."
     —*Booklist, American Library Association, Jul '02*

SEE ALSO *Breast Cancer Sourcebook, Women's Health Concerns Sourcebook*

■

Cancer Survivorship Sourcebook

Basic Consumer Health Information about the Physical, Educational, Emotional, Social, and Financial Needs of Cancer Patients from Diagnosis, through Cancer Treatment, and Beyond, Including Facts about Researching Specific Types of Cancer and Learning about Clinical Trials and Treatment Options, and Featuring Tips for Coping with the Side Effects of Cancer Treatments and Adjusting to Life after Cancer Treatment Concludes

Along with Suggestions for Caregivers, Friends, and Family Members of Cancer Patients, a Glossary of Cancer Care Terms, and Directories of Related Resources

Edited by Karen Bellenir. 6561 pages. 2007. 978-0-7808-0985-7.

■

Cardiovascular Diseases & Disorders Sourcebook, 3rd Edition

Basic Consumer Health Information about Heart and Vascular Diseases and Disorders, Such as Angina, Heart Attacks, Arrhythmias, Cardiomyopathy, Valve Disease, Atherosclerosis, and Aneurysms, with Information about Managing Cardiovascular Risk Factors and Maintaining Heart Health, Medications and Procedures Used to Treat Cardiovascular Disorders, and Concerns of Special Significance to Women

Along with Reports on Current Research Initiatives, a Glossary of Related Medical Terms, and a Directory of Sources for Further Help and Information

Edited by Sandra J. Judd. 713 pages. 2005. 978-0-7808-0739-6.

"This updated sourcebook is still the best first stop for comprehensive introductory information on cardiovascular diseases."
     — *American Reference Books Annual, 2006*

"Recommended for public libraries and libraries supporting health care professionals."
     — *E-Streams, Sep '05*

"This should be a standard health library reference."
     —*The Bookwatch, Jun '05*

"Recommended reference source."
     —*Booklist, American Library Association, Dec '00*

"... comprehensive format provides an extensive overview on this subject."
     —*Choice, Association of College & Research Libraries*

■

Caregiving Sourcebook

Basic Consumer Health Information for Caregivers, Including a Profile of Caregivers, Caregiving Responsibilities and Concerns, Tips for Specific Conditions, Care Environments, and the Effects of Caregiving

Along with Facts about Legal Issues, Financial Information, and Future Planning, a Glossary, and a Listing of Additional Resources

Edited by Joyce Brennfleck Shannon. 600 pages. 2001. 978-0-7808-0331-2.

"Essential for most collections."
     — *Library Journal, Apr 1, 2002*

"An ideal addition to the reference collection of any public library. Health sciences information professionals may also want to acquire the *Caregiving Sourcebook* for their hospital or academic library for use as a ready reference tool by health care workers interested in aging and caregiving."   —*E-Streams, Jan '02*

"Recommended reference source."
     —*Booklist, American Library Association, Oct '01*

■

Child Abuse Sourcebook

Basic Consumer Health Information about the Physical, Sexual, and Emotional Abuse of Children, with Additional Facts about Neglect, Munchausen Syndrome by Proxy (MSBP), Shaken Baby Syndrome, and Controversial Issues Related to Child Abuse, Such as Withholding Medical Care, Corporal Punishment, and Child Maltreatment in Youth Sports, and Featuring Facts about Child Protective Services, Foster Care, Adoption, Parenting Challenges, and Other Abuse Prevention Efforts

Along with a Glossary of Related Terms and Resources for Additional Help and Information

Edited by Dawn D. Matthews. 620 pages. 2004. 978-0-7808-0705-1.

"A valuable and highly recommended resource for school, academic and public libraries whether used on its own or as a starting point for more in-depth research."   — *E-Streams, Apr '05*

"Every week the news brings cases of child abuse or neglect, so it is useful to have a source that supplies so much helpful information. . . . Recommended. Public and academic libraries, and child welfare offices."
     — *Choice, Association of College & Research Libraries, Mar '05*

"Packed with insights on all kinds of issues, from foster care and adoption to parenting and abuse prevention."
     —*The Bookwatch, Nov '04*

SEE ALSO: *Domestic Violence Sourcebook*

Childhood Diseases & Disorders Sourcebook

Basic Consumer Health Information about Medical Problems Often Encountered in Pre-Adolescent Children, Including Respiratory Tract Ailments, Ear Infections, Sore Throats, Disorders of the Skin and Scalp, Digestive and Genitourinary Diseases, Infectious Diseases, Inflammatory Disorders, Chronic Physical and Developmental Disorders, Allergies, and More

Along with Information about Diagnostic Tests, Common Childhood Surgeries, and Frequently Used Medications, with a Glossary of Important Terms and Resource Directory

Edited by Chad T. Kimball. 662 pages. 2003. 978-0-7808-0458-6.

"This is an excellent book for new parents and should be included in all health care and public libraries."
— American Reference Books Annual, 2004

SEE ALSO: Healthy Children Sourcebook

■

Colds, Flu & Other Common Ailments Sourcebook

Basic Consumer Health Information about Common Ailments and Injuries, Including Colds, Coughs, the Flu, Sinus Problems, Headaches, Fever, Nausea and Vomiting, Menstrual Cramps, Diarrhea, Constipation, Hemorrhoids, Back Pain, Dandruff, Dry and Itchy Skin, Cuts, Scrapes, Sprains, Bruises, and More

Along with Information about Prevention, Self-Care, Choosing a Doctor, Over-the-Counter Medications, Folk Remedies, and Alternative Therapies, and Including a Glossary of Important Terms and a Directory of Resources for Further Help and Information

Edited by Chad T. Kimball. 638 pages. 2001. 978-0-7808-0435-7.

"A good starting point for research on common illnesses. It will be a useful addition to public and consumer health library collections."
— American Reference Books Annual, 2002

"Will prove valuable to any library seeking to maintain a current, comprehensive reference collection of health resources. . . . Excellent reference."
— The Bookwatch, Aug '01

"Recommended reference source."
— Booklist, American Library Association, Jul '01

■

Communication Disorders Sourcebook

Basic Information about Deafness and Hearing Loss, Speech and Language Disorders, Voice Disorders, Balance and Vestibular Disorders, and Disorders of Smell, Taste, and Touch

Edited by Linda M. Ross. 533 pages. 1996. 978-0-7808-0077-9.

"This is skillfully edited and is a welcome resource for the layperson. It should be found in every public and medical library." — Booklist Health Sciences Supplement, American Library Association, Oct '97

■

Complementary & Alternative Medicine Sourcebook, 3rd Edition

Basic Consumer Health Information about Complementary and Alternative Medical Therapies, Including Acupuncture, Ayurveda, Traditional Chinese Medicine, Herbal Medicine, Homeopathy, Naturopathy, Biofeedback, Hypnotherapy, Yoga, Art Therapy, Aromatherapy, Clinical Nutrition, Vitamin and Mineral Supplements, Chiropractic, Massage, Reflexology, Crystal Therapy, Therapeutic Touch, and More

Along with Facts about Alternative and Complementary Treatments for Specific Conditions Such as Cancer, Diabetes, Osteoarthritis, Chronic Pain, Menopause, Gastrointestinal Disorders, Headaches, and Mental Illness, a Glossary, and a Resource List for Additional Help and Information

Edited by Sandra J. Judd. 657 pages. 2006. 978-0-7808-0864-5.

"Recommended for public, high school, and academic libraries that have consumer health collections. Hospital libraries that also serve the public will find this to be a useful resource." — E-Streams, Feb '03

"Recommended reference source."
— Booklist, American Library Association, Jan '03

"An important alternate health reference."
— MBR Bookwatch, Oct '02

"A great addition to the reference collection of every type of library." — American Reference Books Annual, 2000

■

Congenital Disorders Sourcebook, 2nd Edition

Basic Consumer Health Information about Nonhereditary Birth Defects and Disorders Related to Prematurity, Gestational Injuries, Congenital Infections, and Birth Complications, Including Heart Defects, Hydrocephalus, Spina Bifida, Cleft Lip and Palate, Cerebral Palsy, and More

Along with Facts about the Prevention of Birth Defects, Fetal Surgery and Other Treatment Options, Research Initiatives, a Glossary of Related Terms, and Resources for Additional Information and Support

Edited by Sandra J. Judd. 647 pages. 2006. 978-0-7808-0945-1.

"Recommended reference source."
— Booklist, American Library Association, Oct '97

SEE ALSO Pregnancy & Birth Sourcebook

■

Contagious Diseases Sourcebook

Basic Consumer Health Information about Infectious Diseases Spread by Person-to-Person Contact through

Direct Touch, Airborne Transmission, Sexual Contact, or Contact with Blood or Other Body Fluids, Including Hepatitis, Herpes, Influenza, Lice, Measles, Mumps, Pinworm, Ringworm, Severe Acute Respiratory Syndrome (SARS), Streptococcal Infections, Tuberculosis, and Others

Along with Facts about Disease Transmission, Antimicrobial Resistance, and Vaccines, with a Glossary and Directories of Resources for More Information

Edited by Karen Bellenir. 643 pages. 2004. 978-0-7808-0736-5.

"This easy-to-read volume is recommended for consumer health collections within public or academic libraries." —E-Streams, May '05

"This informative book is highly recommended for public libraries, consumer health collections, and secondary schools and undergraduate libraries." —American Reference Books Annual, 2005

"Excellent reference." —The Bookwatch, Jan '05

■

Death & Dying Sourcebook, 2nd Edition

Basic Consumer Health Information about End-of-Life Care and Related Perspectives and Ethical Issues, Including End-of-Life Symptoms and Treatments, Pain Management, Quality-of-Life Concerns, the Use of Life Support, Patients' Rights and Privacy Issues, Advance Directives, Physician-Assisted Suicide, Caregiving, Organ and Tissue Donation, Autopsies, Funeral Arrangements, and Grief

Along with Statistical Data, Information about the Leading Causes of Death, a Glossary, and Directories of Support Groups and Other Resources

Edited by Joyce Brennfleck Shannon. 653 pages. 2006. 978-0-7808-0871-3.

"Public libraries, medical libraries, and academic libraries will all find this sourcebook a useful addition to their collections." —American Reference Books Annual, 2001

"An extremely useful resource for those concerned with death and dying in the United States." —Respiratory Care, Nov '00

"Recommended reference source." —Booklist, American Library Association, Aug '00

"This book is a definite must for all those involved in end-of-life care." —Doody's Review Service, 2000

■

Dental Care & Oral Health Sourcebook, 2nd Edition

Basic Consumer Health Information about Dental Care, Including Oral Hygiene, Dental Visits, Pain Management, Cavities, Crowns, Bridges, Dental Implants, and Fillings, and Other Oral Health Concerns, Such as Gum Disease, Bad Breath, Dry Mouth, Genetic and Developmental Abnormalities, Oral Cancers, Orthodontics, and Temporomandibular Disorders

Along with Updates on Current Research in Oral Health, a Glossary, a Directory of Dental and Oral Health Organizations, and Resources for People with Dental and Oral Health Disorders

Edited by Amy L. Sutton. 609 pages. 2003. 978-0-7808-0634-4.

"This book could serve as a turning point in the battle to educate consumers in issues concerning oral health." —American Reference Books Annual, 2004

"Unique source which will fill a gap in dental sources for patients and the lay public. A valuable reference tool even in a library with thousands of books on dentistry. Comprehensive, clear, inexpensive, and easy to read and use. It fills an enormous gap in the health care literature." —Reference & User Services Quarterly, American Library Association, Summer '98

"Recommended reference source." —Booklist, American Library Association, Dec '97

■

Depression Sourcebook

Basic Consumer Health Information about Unipolar Depression, Bipolar Disorder, Postpartum Depression, Seasonal Affective Disorder, and Other Types of Depression in Children, Adolescents, Women, Men, the Elderly, and Other Selected Populations

Along with Facts about Causes, Risk Factors, Diagnostic Criteria, Treatment Options, Coping Strategies, Suicide Prevention, a Glossary, and a Directory of Sources for Additional Help and Information

Edited by Karen Bellenir. 602 pages. 2002. 978-0-7808-0611-5.

"Depression Sourcebook is of a very high standard. Its purpose, which is to serve as a reference source to the lay reader, is very well served." —Journal of the National Medical Association, 2004

"Invaluable reference for public and school library collections alike." —Library Bookwatch, Apr '03

"Recommended for purchase." —American Reference Books Annual, 2003

■

Dermatological Disorders Sourcebook, 2nd Edition

Basic Consumer Health Information about Conditions and Disorders Affecting the Skin, Hair, and Nails, Such as Acne, Rosacea, Dermatitis, Rashes, Pigmentation Disorders, Birthmarks, Skin Cancer, Skin Injuries, Psoriasis, Scleroderma, and Hair Loss, Including Facts about Medications and Treatments for Dermatological Disorders and Tips for Maintaining Healthy Skin, Hair, and Nails

Along with Information about How Aging Affects the Skin, a Glossary of Related Terms, and a Directory of Resources for Additional Help and Information

Edited by Amy L. Sutton. 645 pages. 2005. 978-0-7808-0795-2.

"... comprehensive, easily read reference book."
—*Doody's Health Sciences Book Reviews, Oct '97*

SEE ALSO *Burns Sourcebook*

■

Diabetes Sourcebook, 3rd Edition

Basic Consumer Health Information about Type 1 Diabetes (Insulin-Dependent or Juvenile-Onset Diabetes), Type 2 Diabetes (Noninsulin-Dependent or Adult-Onset Diabetes), Gestational Diabetes, Impaired Glucose Tolerance (IGT), and Related Complications, Such as Amputation, Eye Disease, Gum Disease, Nerve Damage, and End-Stage Renal Disease, Including Facts about Insulin, Oral Diabetes Medications, Blood Sugar Testing, and the Role of Exercise and Nutrition in the Control of Diabetes

Along with a Glossary and Resources for Further Help and Information

Edited by Dawn D. Matthews. 622 pages. 2003. 978-0-7808-0629-0.

"This edition is even more helpful than earlier versions. . . . It is a truly valuable tool for anyone seeking readable and authoritative information on diabetes."
— *American Reference Books Annual, 2004*

"An invaluable reference." — *Library Journal, May '00*

Selected as one of the 250 "Best Health Sciences Books of 1999." — *Doody's Rating Service, Mar-Apr '00*

"Provides useful information for the general public."
— *Healthlines, University of Michigan Health Management Research Center, Sep/Oct '99*

"... provides reliable mainstream medical information . . . belongs on the shelves of any library with a consumer health collection." — *E-Streams, Sep '99*

"Recommended reference source."
— *Booklist, American Library Association, Feb '99*

■

Diet & Nutrition Sourcebook, 3rd Edition

Basic Consumer Health Information about Dietary Guidelines and the Food Guidance System, Recommended Daily Nutrient Intakes, Serving Proportions, Weight Control, Vitamins and Supplements, Nutrition Issues for Different Life Stages and Lifestyles, and the Needs of People with Specific Medical Concerns, Including Cancer, Celiac Disease, Diabetes, Eating Disorders, Food Allergies, and Cardiovascular Disease

Along with Facts about Federal Nutrition Support Programs, a Glossary of Nutrition and Dietary Terms, and Directories of Additional Resources for More Information about Nutrition

Edited by Joyce Brennfleck Shannon. 633 pages. 2006. 978-0-7808-0800-3.

"This book is an excellent source of basic diet and nutrition information." — *Booklist Health Sciences Supplement, American Library Association, Dec '00*

"This reference document should be in any public library, but it would be a very good guide for beginning students in the health sciences. If the other books in this publisher's series are as good as this, they should all be in the health sciences collections."
— *American Reference Books Annual, 2000*

"This book is an excellent general nutrition reference for consumers who desire to take an active role in their health care for prevention. Consumers of all ages who select this book can feel confident they are receiving current and accurate information." — *Journal of Nutrition for the Elderly, Vol. 19, No. 4, 2000*

SEE ALSO *Digestive Diseases & Disorders Sourcebook, Eating Disorders Sourcebook, Gastrointestinal Diseases & Disorders Sourcebook, Vegetarian Sourcebook*

■

Digestive Diseases & Disorders Sourcebook

Basic Consumer Health Information about Diseases and Disorders that Impact the Upper and Lower Digestive System, Including Celiac Disease, Constipation, Crohn's Disease, Cyclic Vomiting Syndrome, Diarrhea, Diverticulosis and Diverticulitis, Gallstones, Heartburn, Hemorrhoids, Hernias, Indigestion (Dyspepsia), Irritable Bowel Syndrome, Lactose Intolerance, Ulcers, and More

Along with Information about Medications and Other Treatments, Tips for Maintaining a Healthy Digestive Tract, a Glossary, and Directory of Digestive Diseases Organizations

Edited by Karen Bellenir. 335 pages. 2000. 978-0-7808-0327-5.

"This title would be an excellent addition to all public or patient-research libraries."
— *American Reference Books Annual, 2001*

"This title is recommended for public, hospital, and health sciences libraries with consumer health collections." — *E-Streams, Jul-Aug '00*

"Recommended reference source."
— *Booklist, American Library Association, May '00*

SEE ALSO *Eating Disorders Sourcebook, Gastrointestinal Diseases & Disorders Sourcebook*

■

Disabilities Sourcebook

Basic Consumer Health Information about Physical and Psychiatric Disabilities, Including Descriptions of Major Causes of Disability, Assistive and Adaptive Aids, Workplace Issues, and Accessibility Concerns

Along with Information about the Americans with Disabilities Act, a Glossary, and Resources for Additional Help and Information

Edited by Dawn D. Matthews. 616 pages. 2000. 978-0-7808-0389-3.

"It is a must for libraries with a consumer health section." — *American Reference Books Annual, 2002*

"A much needed addition to the Omnigraphics *Health Reference Series*. A current reference work to provide people with disabilities, their families, caregivers or those who work with them, a broad range of information in one volume, has not been available until now. . . . It is recommended for all public and academic library reference collections." —*E-Streams, May '01*

"An excellent source book in easy-to-read format covering many current topics; highly recommended for all libraries." —*Choice, Association of College & Research Libraries, Jan '01*

"Recommended reference source."
—*Booklist, American Library Association, Jul '00*

■

Domestic Violence Sourcebook, 2nd Edition

Basic Consumer Health Information about the Causes and Consequences of Abusive Relationships, Including Physical Violence, Sexual Assault, Battery, Stalking, and Emotional Abuse, and Facts about the Effects of Violence on Women, Men, Young Adults, and the Elderly, with Reports about Domestic Violence in Selected Populations, and Featuring Facts about Medical Care, Victim Assistance and Protection, Prevention Strategies, Mental Health Services, and Legal Issues

Along with a Glossary of Related Terms and Resources for Additional Help and Information

Edited by Dawn D. Matthews. 628 pages. 2004. 978-0-7808-0669-6.

"Educators, clergy, medical professionals, police, and victims and their families will benefit from this realistic and easy-to-understand resource."
—*American Reference Books Annual, 2005*

"Recommended for all collections supporting consumer health information. It should also be considered for any collection needing general, readable information on domestic violence." —*E-Streams, Jan '05*

"This sourcebook complements other books in its field, providing a one-stop resource . . . Recommended."
—*Choice, Association of College & Research Libraries, Jan '05*

"Interested lay persons should find the book extremely beneficial. . . . A copy of *Domestic Violence and Child Abuse Sourcebook* should be in every public library in the United States."
—*Social Science & Medicine, No. 56, 2003*

"This is important information. The Web has many resources but this sourcebook fills an important societal need. I am not aware of any other resources of this type." —*Doody's Review Service, Sep '01*

"Recommended reference source."
—*Booklist, American Library Association, Apr '01*

"Important pick for college-level health reference libraries." —*The Bookwatch, Mar '01*

"Because this problem is so widespread and because this book includes a lot of issues within one volume, this work is recommended for all public libraries."
—*American Reference Books Annual, 2001*

SEE ALSO *Child Abuse Sourcebook*

■

Drug Abuse Sourcebook, 2nd Edition

Basic Consumer Health Information about Illicit Substances of Abuse and the Misuse of Prescription and Over-the-Counter Medications, Including Depressants, Hallucinogens, Inhalants, Marijuana, Stimulants, and Anabolic Steroids

Along with Facts about Related Health Risks, Treatment Programs, Prevention Programs, a Glossary of Abuse and Addiction Terms, a Glossary of Drug-Related Street Terms, and a Directory of Resources for More Information

Edited by Catherine Ginther. 607 pages. 2004. 978-0-7808-0740-2.

"Commendable for organizing useful, normally scattered government and association-produced data into a logical sequence."
—*American Reference Books Annual, 2006*

"This easy-to-read volume is recommended for consumer health collections within public or academic libraries." —*E-Streams, Sep '05*

"An excellent library reference."
—*The Bookwatch, May '05*

"Containing a wealth of information, this book will be useful to the college student just beginning to explore the topic of substance abuse. This resource belongs in libraries that serve a lower-division undergraduate or community college clientele as well as the general public." —*Choice, Association of College & Research Libraries, Jun '01*

"Recommended reference source."
—*Booklist, American Library Association, Feb '01*

SEE ALSO *Alcoholism Sourcebook*

■

Ear, Nose & Throat Disorders Sourcebook, 2nd Edition

Basic Consumer Health Information about Disorders of the Ears, Hearing Loss, Vestibular Disorders, Nasal and Sinus Problems, Throat and Vocal Cord Disorders, and Otolaryngologic Cancers, Including Facts about Ear Infections and Injuries, Genetic and Congenital Deafness, Sensorineural Hearing Disorders, Tinnitus, Vertigo, Ménière Disease, Rhinitis, Sinusitis, Snoring, Sore Throats, Hoarseness, and More

Along with Reports on Current Research Initiatives, a Glossary of Related Medical Terms, and a Directory of Sources for Further Help and Information

Edited by Sandra J. Judd. 659 pages. 2006. 978-0-7808-0872-0.

"Overall, this sourcebook is helpful for the consumer seeking information on ENT issues. It is recommended for public libraries."
— *American Reference Books Annual, 1999*

"Recommended reference source."
— *Booklist, American Library Association, Dec '98*

■

Eating Disorders Sourcebook, 2nd Edition

Basic Consumer Health Information about Anorexia Nervosa, Bulimia Nervosa, Binge Eating, Compulsive Exercise, Female Athlete Triad, and Other Eating Disorders, Including Facts about Body Image and Other Cultural and Age-Related Risk Factors, Prevention Efforts, Adverse Health Effects, Treatment Options, and the Recovery Process

Along with Guidelines for Healthy Weight Control, a Glossary, and Directories of Additional Resources

Edited by Joyce Brennfleck Shannon. 585 pages. 2007. 978-0-7808-0948-2.

"Recommended for health science libraries that are open to the public, as well as hospital libraries. This book is a good resource for the consumer who is concerned about eating disorders." — *E-Streams, Mar '02*

"This volume is another convenient collection of excerpted articles. Recommended for school and public library patrons; lower-division undergraduates; and two-year technical program students."
— *Choice, Association of College & Research Libraries, Jan '02*

"Recommended reference source."
— *Booklist, American Library Association, Oct '01*

SEE ALSO *Diet & Nutrition Sourcebook, Digestive Diseases & Disorders Sourcebook, Gastrointestinal Diseases & Disorders Sourcebook*

■

Emergency Medical Services Sourcebook

Basic Consumer Health Information about Preventing, Preparing for, and Managing Emergency Situations, When and Who to Call for Help, What to Expect in the Emergency Room, the Emergency Medical Team, Patient Issues, and Current Topics in Emergency Medicine

Along with Statistical Data, a Glossary, and Sources of Additional Help and Information

Edited by Jenni Lynn Colson. 494 pages. 2002. 978-0-7808-0420-3.

"Handy and convenient for home, public, school, and college libraries. Recommended."
— *Choice, Association of College & Research Libraries, Apr '03*

"This reference can provide the consumer with answers to most questions about emergency care in the United States, or it will direct them to a resource where the answer can be found."
— *American Reference Books Annual, 2003*

"Recommended reference source."
— *Booklist, American Library Association, Feb '03*

■

Endocrine & Metabolic Disorders Sourcebook

Basic Information for the Layperson about Pancreatic and Insulin-Related Disorders Such as Pancreatitis, Diabetes, and Hypoglycemia; Adrenal Gland Disorders Such as Cushing's Syndrome, Addison's Disease, and Congenital Adrenal Hyperplasia; Pituitary Gland Disorders Such as Growth Hormone Deficiency, Acromegaly, and Pituitary Tumors; Thyroid Disorders Such as Hypothyroidism, Graves' Disease, Hashimoto's Disease, and Goiter; Hyperparathyroidism; and Other Diseases and Syndromes of Hormone Imbalance or Metabolic Dysfunction

Along with Reports on Current Research Initiatives

Edited by Linda M. Shin. 574 pages. 1998. 978-0-7808-0207-0.

"Omnigraphics has produced another needed resource for health information consumers."
— *American Reference Books Annual, 2000*

"Recommended reference source."
— *Booklist, American Library Association, Dec '98*

■

Environmental Health Sourcebook, 2nd Edition

Basic Consumer Health Information about the Environment and Its Effect on Human Health, Including the Effects of Air Pollution, Water Pollution, Hazardous Chemicals, Food Hazards, Radiation Hazards, Biological Agents, Household Hazards, Such as Radon, Asbestos, Carbon Monoxide, and Mold, and Information about Associated Diseases and Disorders, Including Cancer, Allergies, Respiratory Problems, and Skin Disorders

Along with Information about Environmental Concerns for Specific Populations, a Glossary of Related Terms, and Resources for Further Help and Information

Edited by Dawn D. Matthews. 673 pages. 2003. 978-0-7808-0632-0.

"This recently updated edition continues the level of quality and the reputation of the numerous other volumes in Omnigraphics' *Health Reference Series.*"
— *American Reference Books Annual, 2004*

"An excellent updated edition."
— *The Bookwatch, Oct '03*

"Recommended reference source."
— *Booklist, American Library Association, Sep '98*

"This book will be a useful addition to anyone's library." — *Choice Health Sciences Supplement, Association of College & Research Libraries, May '98*

". . . a good survey of numerous environmentally induced physical disorders . . . a useful addition to anyone's library."
— *Doody's Health Sciences Book Reviews, Jan '98*

Ethnic Diseases Sourcebook

Basic Consumer Health Information for Ethnic and Racial Minority Groups in the United States, Including General Health Indicators and Behaviors, Ethnic Diseases, Genetic Testing, the Impact of Chronic Diseases, Women's Health, Mental Health Issues, and Preventive Health Care Services

Along with a Glossary and a Listing of Additional Resources

Edited by Joyce Brennfleck Shannon. 664 pages. 2001. 978-0-7808-0336-7.

"Recommended for health sciences libraries where public health programs are a priority."
— *E-Streams, Jan '02*

"Not many books have been written on this topic to date, and the *Ethnic Diseases Sourcebook* is a strong addition to the list. It will be an important introductory resource for health consumers, students, health care personnel, and social scientists. It is recommended for public, academic, and large hospital libraries."
— *American Reference Books Annual, 2002*

"Recommended reference source."
— *Booklist, American Library Association, Oct '01*

"Will prove valuable to any library seeking to maintain a current, comprehensive reference collection of health resources. . . . An excellent source of health information about genetic disorders which affect particular ethnic and racial minorities in the U.S."
— *The Bookwatch, Aug '01*

Eye Care Sourcebook, 2nd Edition

Basic Consumer Health Information about Eye Care and Eye Disorders, Including Facts about the Diagnosis, Prevention, and Treatment of Common Refractive Problems Such as Myopia, Hyperopia, Astigmatism, and Presbyopia, and Eye Diseases, Including Glaucoma, Cataract, Age-Related Macular Degeneration, and Diabetic Retinopathy

Along with a Section on Vision Correction and Refractive Surgeries, Including LASIK and LASEK, a Glossary, and Directories of Resources for Additional Help and Information

Edited by Amy L. Sutton. 543 pages. 2003. 978-0-7808-0635-1.

". . . a solid reference tool for eye care and a valuable addition to a collection."
— *American Reference Books Annual, 2004*

Family Planning Sourcebook

Basic Consumer Health Information about Planning for Pregnancy and Contraception, Including Traditional Methods, Barrier Methods, Hormonal Methods, Permanent Methods, Future Methods, Emergency Contraception, and Birth Control Choices for Women at Each Stage of Life

Along with Statistics, a Glossary, and Sources of Additional Information

Edited by Amy Marcaccio Keyzer. 520 pages. 2001. 978-0-7808-0379-4.

"Recommended for public, health, and undergraduate libraries as part of the circulating collection."
— *E-Streams, Mar '02*

"Information is presented in an unbiased, readable manner, and the sourcebook will certainly be a necessary addition to those public and high school libraries where Internet access is restricted or otherwise problematic." — *American Reference Books Annual, 2002*

"Recommended reference source."
— *Booklist, American Library Association, Oct '01*

"Will prove valuable to any library seeking to maintain a current, comprehensive reference collection of health resources. . . . Excellent reference."
— *The Bookwatch, Aug '01*

SEE ALSO Pregnancy & Birth Sourcebook

Fitness & Exercise Sourcebook, 3rd Edition

Basic Consumer Health Information about the Physical and Mental Benefits of Fitness, Including Cardiorespiratory Endurance, Muscular Strength, Muscular Endurance, and Flexibility, with Facts about Sports Nutrition and Exercise-Related Injuries and Tips about Physical Activity and Exercises for People of All Ages and for People with Health Concerns

Along with Advice on Selecting and Using Exercise Equipment, Maintaining Exercise Motivation, a Glossary of Related Terms, and a Directory of Resources for More Help and Information

Edited by Amy L. Sutton. 663 pages. 2007. 978-0-7808-0946-8.

"This work is recommended for all general reference collections."
— *American Reference Books Annual, 2002*

"Highly recommended for public, consumer, and school grades fourth through college." — *E-Streams, Nov '01*

"Recommended reference source."
— *Booklist, American Library Association, Oct '01*

"The information appears quite comprehensive and is considered reliable. . . . This second edition is a welcomed addition to the series."
— *Doody's Review Service, Sep '01*

Food Safety Sourcebook

Basic Consumer Health Information about the Safe Handling of Meat, Poultry, Seafood, Eggs, Fruit Juices, and Other Food Items, and Facts about Pesticides, Drinking Water, Food Safety Overseas, and the Onset, Duration, and Symptoms of Foodborne Illnesses, Including Types of Pathogenic Bacteria, Parasitic Protozoa, Worms, Viruses, and Natural Toxins

Along with the Role of the Consumer, the Food Handler, and the Government in Food Safety; a Glossary, and Resources for Additional Help and Information

Edited by Dawn D. Matthews. 339 pages. 1999. 978-0-7808-0326-8.

"This book is recommended for public libraries and universities with home economic and food science programs."
— *E-Streams, Nov '00*

"Recommended reference source."
— *Booklist, American Library Association, May '00*

"This book takes the complex issues of food safety and foodborne pathogens and presents them in an easily understood manner. [It does] an excellent job of covering a large and often confusing topic."
— *American Reference Books Annual, 2000*

Forensic Medicine Sourcebook

Basic Consumer Information for the Layperson about Forensic Medicine, Including Crime Scene Investigation, Evidence Collection and Analysis, Expert Testimony, Computer-Aided Criminal Identification, Digital Imaging in the Courtroom, DNA Profiling, Accident Reconstruction, Autopsies, Ballistics, Drugs and Explosives Detection, Latent Fingerprints, Product Tampering, and Questioned Document Examination

Along with Statistical Data, a Glossary of Forensics Terminology, and Listings of Sources for Further Help and Information

Edited by Annemarie S. Muth. 574 pages. 1999. 978-0-7808-0232-2.

"Given the expected widespread interest in its content and its easy to read style, this book is recommended for most public and all college and university libraries."
— *E-Streams, Feb '01*

"Recommended for public libraries."
— *Reference & User Services Quarterly, American Library Association, Spring 2000*

"Recommended reference source."
— *Booklist, American Library Association, Feb '00*

"A wealth of information, useful statistics, references are up-to-date and extremely complete. This wonderful collection of data will help students who are interested in a career in any type of forensic field. It is a great resource for attorneys who need information about types of expert witnesses needed in a particular case. It also offers useful information for fiction and nonfiction writers whose work involves a crime. A fascinating compilation. All levels."
— *Choice, Association of College & Research Libraries, Jan '00*

"There are several items that make this book attractive to consumers who are seeking certain forensic data.... This is a useful current source for those seeking general forensic medical answers."
— *American Reference Books Annual, 2000*

Gastrointestinal Diseases & Disorders Sourcebook, 2nd Edition

Basic Consumer Health Information about the Upper and Lower Gastrointestinal (GI) Tract, Including the Esophagus, Stomach, Intestines, Rectum, Liver, and Pancreas, with Facts about Gastroesophageal Reflux Disease, Gastritis, Hernias, Ulcers, Celiac Disease, Diverticulitis, Irritable Bowel Syndrome, Hemorrhoids, Gastrointestinal Cancers, and Other Diseases and Disorders Related to the Digestive Process

Along with Information about Commonly Used Diagnostic and Surgical Procedures, Statistics, Reports on Current Research Initiatives and Clinical Trials, a Glossary, and Resources for Additional Help and Information

Edited by Sandra J. Judd. 681 pages. 2006. 978-0-7808-0798-3.

"... very readable form. The successful editorial work that brought this material together into a useful and understandable reference makes accessible to all readers information that can help them more effectively understand and obtain help for digestive tract problems."
— *Choice, Association of College & Research Libraries, Feb '97*

SEE ALSO Diet & Nutrition Sourcebook, Digestive Diseases & Disorders Sourcebook, Eating Disorders Sourcebook

Genetic Disorders Sourcebook, 3rd Edition

Basic Consumer Health Information about Hereditary Diseases and Disorders, Including Facts about the Human Genome, Genetic Inheritance Patterns, Disorders Associated with Specific Genes, Such as Sickle Cell Disease, Hemophilia, and Cystic Fibrosis, Chromosome Disorders, Such as Down Syndrome, Fragile X Syndrome, and Turner Syndrome, and Complex Diseases and Disorders Resulting from the Interaction of Environmental and Genetic Factors, Such as Allergies, Cancer, and Obesity

Along with Facts about Genetic Testing, Suggestions for Parents of Children with Special Needs, Reports on Current Research Initiatives, a Glossary of Genetic Terminology, and Resources for Additional Help and Information

Edited by Karen Bellenir. 777 pages. 2004. 978-0-7808-0742-6.

"This text is recommended for any library with an interest in providing consumer health resources."
— *E-Streams, Aug '05*

"This is a valuable resource for anyone wishing to have an understandable description of any of the topics or disorders included. The editor succeeds in making complex genetic issues understandable."
— *Doody's Book Review Service, May '05*

"A good acquisition for public libraries."
— *American Reference Books Annual, 2005*

"Excellent reference." — *The Bookwatch, Jan '05*

"Recommended reference source."
— *Booklist, American Library Association, Apr '01*

"Important pick for college-level health reference libraries." — *The Bookwatch, Mar '01*

■

Head Trauma Sourcebook

Basic Information for the Layperson about Open-Head and Closed-Head Injuries, Treatment Advances, Recovery, and Rehabilitation

Along with Reports on Current Research Initiatives

Edited by Karen Bellenir. 414 pages. 1997. 978-0-7808-0208-7.

Headache Sourcebook

Basic Consumer Health Information about Migraine, Tension, Cluster, Rebound and Other Types of Headaches, with Facts about the Cause and Prevention of Headaches, the Effects of Stress and the Environment, Headaches during Pregnancy and Menopause, and Childhood Headaches

Along with a Glossary and Other Resources for Additional Help and Information

Edited by Dawn D. Matthews. 362 pages. 2002. 978-0-7808-0337-4.

"Highly recommended for academic and medical reference collections." — *Library Bookwatch, Sep '02*

■

Healthy Aging Sourcebook

Basic Consumer Health Information about Maintaining Health through the Aging Process, Including Advice on Nutrition, Exercise, and Sleep, Help in Making Decisions about Midlife Issues and Retirement, and Guidance Concerning Practical and Informed Choices in Health Consumerism

Along with Data Concerning the Theories of Aging, Different Experiences in Aging by Minority Groups, and Facts about Aging Now and Aging in the Future; and Featuring a Glossary, a Guide to Consumer Help, Additional Suggested Reading, and Practical Resource Directory

Edited by Jenifer Swanson. 536 pages. 1999. 978-0-7808-0390-9.

"Recommended reference source."
— *Booklist, American Library Association, Feb '00*

SEE ALSO *Physical & Mental Issues in Aging Sourcebook*

■

Healthy Children Sourcebook

Basic Consumer Health Information about the Physical and Mental Development of Children between the Ages of 3 and 12, Including Routine Health Care, Preventative Health Services, Safety and First Aid,

Healthy Sleep, Dental Care, Nutrition, and Fitness, and Featuring Parenting Tips on Such Topics as Bedwetting, Choosing Day Care, Monitoring TV and Other Media, and Establishing a Foundation for Substance Abuse Prevention

Along with a Glossary of Commonly Used Pediatric Terms and Resources for Additional Help and Information

Edited by Chad T. Kimball. 647 pages. 2003. 978-0-7808-0247-6.

"It is hard to imagine that any other single resource exists that would provide such a comprehensive guide of timely information on health promotion and disease prevention for children aged 3 to 12."
— *American Reference Books Annual, 2004*

"The strengths of this book are many. It is clearly written, presented and structured."
— *Journal of the National Medical Association, 2004*

SEE ALSO *Childhood Diseases & Disorders Sourcebook*

■

Healthy Heart Sourcebook for Women

Basic Consumer Health Information about Cardiac Issues Specific to Women, Including Facts about Major Risk Factors and Prevention, Treatment and Control Strategies, and Important Dietary Issues

Along with a Special Section Regarding the Pros and Cons of Hormone Replacement Therapy and Its Impact on Heart Health, and Additional Help, Including Recipes, a Glossary, and a Directory of Resources

Edited by Dawn D. Matthews. 336 pages. 2000. 978-0-7808-0329-9.

"A good reference source and recommended for all public, academic, medical, and hospital libraries."
— *Medical Reference Services Quarterly, Summer '01*

"Because of the lack of information specific to women on this topic, this book is recommended for public libraries and consumer libraries."
— *American Reference Books Annual, 2001*

"Contains very important information about coronary artery disease that all women should know. The information is current and presented in an easy-to-read format. The book will make a good addition to any library." — *American Medical Writers Association Journal, Summer '00*

"Important, basic reference."
— *Reviewer's Bookwatch, Jul '00*

SEE ALSO *Cardiovascular Diseases & Disorders Sourcebook, Women's Health Concerns Sourcebook*

■

Hepatitis Sourcebook

Basic Consumer Health Information about Hepatitis A, Hepatitis B, Hepatitis C, and Other Forms of Hepatitis, Including Autoimmune Hepatitis, Alcoholic Hepatitis, Nonalcoholic Steatohepatitis, and Toxic Hepatitis, with

Facts about Risk Factors, Screening Methods, Diagnostic Tests, and Treatment Options

Along with Information on Liver Health, Tips for People Living with Chronic Hepatitis, Reports on Current Research Initiatives, a Glossary of Terms Related to Hepatitis, and a Directory of Sources for Further Help and Information

Edited by Sandra J. Judd. 597 pages. 2005. 978-0-7808-0749-5.

"Highly recommended."
— American Reference Books Annual, 2006

■

Household Safety Sourcebook

Basic Consumer Health Information about Household Safety, Including Information about Poisons, Chemicals, Fire, and Water Hazards in the Home

Along with Advice about the Safe Use of Home Maintenance Equipment, Choosing Toys and Nursery Furniture, Holiday and Recreation Safety, a Glossary, and Resources for Further Help and Information

Edited by Dawn D. Matthews. 606 pages. 2002. 978-0-7808-0338-1.

"This work will be useful in public libraries with large consumer health and wellness departments."
— American Reference Books Annual, 2003

"As a sourcebook on household safety this book meets its mark. It is encyclopedic in scope and covers a wide range of safety issues that are commonly seen in the home."
— E-Streams, Jul '02

■

Hypertension Sourcebook

Basic Consumer Health Information about the Causes, Diagnosis, and Treatment of High Blood Pressure, with Facts about Consequences, Complications, and Co-Occurring Disorders, Such as Coronary Heart Disease, Diabetes, Stroke, Kidney Disease, and Hypertensive Retinopathy, and Issues in Blood Pressure Control, Including Dietary Choices, Stress Management, and Medications

Along with Reports on Current Research Initiatives and Clinical Trials, a Glossary, and Resources for Additional Help and Information

Edited by Dawn D. Matthews and Karen Bellenir. 613 pages. 2004. 978-0-7808-0674-0.

"Academic, public, and medical libraries will want to add the Hypertension Sourcebook to their collections."
— E-Streams, Aug '05

"The strength of this source is the wide range of information given about hypertension."
— American Reference Books Annual, 2005

■

Immune System Disorders Sourcebook, 2nd Edition

Basic Consumer Health Information about Disorders of the Immune System, Including Immune System Function and Response, Diagnosis of Immune Disorders, Information about Inherited Immune Disease, Acquired Immune Disease, and Autoimmune Diseases, Including Primary Immune Deficiency, Acquired Immunodeficiency Syndrome (AIDS), Lupus, Multiple Sclerosis, Type 1 Diabetes, Rheumatoid Arthritis, and Graves' Disease

Along with Treatments, Tips for Coping with Immune Disorders, a Glossary, and a Directory of Additional Resources.

Edited by Joyce Brennfleck Shannon. 671 pages. 2005. 978-0-7808-0748-8.

"Highly recommended for academic and public libraries." — American Reference Books Annual, 2006

"The updated second edition is a 'must' for any consumer health library seeking a solid resource covering the treatments, symptoms, and options for immune disorder sufferers. . . . An excellent guide."
— MBR Bookwatch, Jan '06

■

Infant & Toddler Health Sourcebook

Basic Consumer Health Information about the Physical and Mental Development of Newborns, Infants, and Toddlers, Including Neonatal Concerns, Nutrition Recommendations, Immunization Schedules, Common Pediatric Disorders, Assessments and Milestones, Safety Tips, and Advice for Parents and Other Caregivers

Along with a Glossary of Terms and Resource Listings for Additional Help

Edited by Jenifer Swanson. 585 pages. 2000. 978-0-7808-0246-9.

"As a reference for the general public, this would be useful in any library." — E-Streams, May '01

"Recommended reference source."
— Booklist, American Library Association, Feb '01

"This is a good source for general use."
— American Reference Books Annual, 2001

■

Infectious Diseases Sourcebook

Basic Consumer Health Information about Non-Contagious Bacterial, Viral, Prion, Fungal, and Parasitic Diseases Spread by Food and Water, Insects and Animals, or Environmental Contact, Including Botulism, E. Coli, Encephalitis, Legionnaires' Disease, Lyme Disease, Malaria, Plague, Rabies, Salmonella, Tetanus, and Others, and Facts about Newly Emerging Diseases, Such as Hantavirus, Mad Cow Disease, Monkeypox, and West Nile Virus

Along with Information about Preventing Disease Transmission, the Threat of Bioterrorism, and Current Research Initiatives, with a Glossary and Directory of Resources for More Information

Edited by Karen Bellenir. 634 pages. 2004. 978-0-7808-0675-7.

"This reference continues the excellent tradition of the *Health Reference Series* in consolidating a wealth of information on a selected topic into a format that is easy to use and accessible to the general public."
— *American Reference Books Annual, 2005*

"Recommended for public and academic libraries."
— *E-Streams, Jan '05*

■

Injury & Trauma Sourcebook

Basic Consumer Health Information about the Impact of Injury, the Diagnosis and Treatment of Common and Traumatic Injuries, Emergency Care, and Specific Injuries Related to Home, Community, Workplace, Transportation, and Recreation

Along with Guidelines for Injury Prevention, a Glossary, and a Directory of Additional Resources

Edited by Joyce Brennfleck Shannon. 696 pages. 2002. 978-0-7808-0421-0.

"This publication is the most comprehensive work of its kind about injury and trauma."
— *American Reference Books Annual, 2003*

"This sourcebook provides concise, easily readable, basic health information about injuries. . . . This book is well organized and an easy to use reference resource suitable for hospital, health sciences and public libraries with consumer health collections."
— *E-Streams, Nov '02*

"Practitioners should be aware of guides such as this in order to facilitate their use by patients and their families."
— *Doody's Health Sciences Book Review Journal, Sep-Oct '02*

"Recommended reference source."
— *Booklist, American Library Association, Sep '02*

"Highly recommended for academic and medical reference collections."
— *Library Bookwatch, Sep '02*

■

Kidney & Urinary Tract Diseases & Disorders Sourcebook

SEE Urinary Tract & Kidney Diseases & Disorders Sourcebook

■

Learning Disabilities Sourcebook, 2nd Edition

Basic Consumer Health Information about Learning Disabilities, Including Dyslexia, Developmental Speech and Language Disabilities, Non-Verbal Learning Disorders, Developmental Arithmetic Disorder, Developmental Writing Disorder, and Other Conditions That Impede Learning Such as Attention Deficit/Hyperactivity Disorder, Brain Injury, Hearing Impairment, Klinefelter Syndrome, Dyspraxia, and Tourette's Syndrome

Along with Facts about Educational Issues and Assistive Technology, Coping Strategies, a Glossary of Related Terms, and Resources for Further Help and Information

Edited by Dawn D. Matthews. 621 pages. 2003. 978-0-7808-0626-9.

"The second edition of Learning Disabilities Sourcebook far surpasses the earlier edition in that it is more focused on information that will be useful as a consumer health resource."
— *American Reference Books Annual, 2004*

"Teachers as well as consumers will find this an essential guide to understanding various syndromes and their latest treatments. [An] invaluable reference for public and school library collections alike."
— *Library Bookwatch, Apr '03*

Named "Outstanding Reference Book of 1999."
— *New York Public Library, Feb '00*

"An excellent candidate for inclusion in a public library reference section. It's a great source of information. Teachers will also find the book useful. Definitely worth reading."
— *Journal of Adolescent & Adult Literacy, Feb 2000*

"Readable . . . provides a solid base of information regarding successful techniques used with individuals who have learning disabilities, as well as practical suggestions for educators and family members. Clear language, concise descriptions, and pertinent information for contacting multiple resources add to the strength of this book as a useful tool."
— *Choice, Association of College & Research Libraries, Feb '99*

"Recommended reference source."
— *Booklist, American Library Association, Sep '98*

"A useful resource for libraries and for those who don't have the time to identify and locate the individual publications."
— *Disability Resources Monthly, Sep '98*

■

Leukemia Sourcebook

Basic Consumer Health Information about Adult and Childhood Leukemias, Including Acute Lymphocytic Leukemia (ALL), Chronic Lymphocytic Leukemia (CLL), Acute Myelogenous Leukemia (AML), Chronic Myelogenous Leukemia (CML), and Hairy Cell Leukemia, and Treatments Such as Chemotherapy, Radiation Therapy, Peripheral Blood Stem Cell and Marrow Transplantation, and Immunotherapy

Along with Tips for Life During and After Treatment, a Glossary, and Directories of Additional Resources

Edited by Joyce Brennfleck Shannon. 587 pages. 2003. 978-0-7808-0627-6.

"Unlike other medical books for the layperson, . . . the language does not talk down to the reader. . . . This volume is highly recommended for all libraries."
— *American Reference Books Annual, 2004*

". . . a fine title which ranges from diagnosis to alternative treatments, staging, and tips for life during and after diagnosis."
— *The Bookwatch, Dec '03*

Liver Disorders Sourcebook

Basic Consumer Health Information about the Liver and How It Works; Liver Diseases, Including Cancer, Cirrhosis, Hepatitis, and Toxic and Drug Related Diseases; Tips for Maintaining a Healthy Liver; Laboratory Tests, Radiology Tests, and Facts about Liver Transplantation

Along with a Section on Support Groups, a Glossary, and Resource Listings

Edited by Joyce Brennfleck Shannon. 591 pages. 2000. 978-0-7808-0383-1.

"A valuable resource."
—*American Reference Books Annual, 2001*

"This title is recommended for health sciences and public libraries with consumer health collections."
—*E-Streams, Oct '00*

"Recommended reference source."
—*Booklist, American Library Association, Jun '00*

■

Lung Disorders Sourcebook

Basic Consumer Health Information about Emphysema, Pneumonia, Tuberculosis, Asthma, Cystic Fibrosis, and Other Lung Disorders, Including Facts about Diagnostic Procedures, Treatment Strategies, Disease Prevention Efforts, and Such Risk Factors as Smoking, Air Pollution, and Exposure to Asbestos, Radon, and Other Agents

Along with a Glossary and Resources for Additional Help and Information

Edited by Dawn D. Matthews. 678 pages. 2002. 978-0-7808-0339-8.

"This title is a great addition for public and school libraries because it provides concise health information on the lungs."
—*American Reference Books Annual, 2003*

"Highly recommended for academic and medical reference collections." —*Library Bookwatch, Sep '02*

SEE ALSO Respiratory Diseases & Disorders Sourcebook

■

Medical Tests Sourcebook, 2nd Edition

Basic Consumer Health Information about Medical Tests, Including Age-Specific Health Tests, Important Health Screenings and Exams, Home-Use Tests, Blood and Specimen Tests, Electrical Tests, Scope Tests, Genetic Testing, and Imaging Tests, Such as X-Rays, Ultrasound, Computed Tomography, Magnetic Resonance Imaging, Angiography, and Nuclear Medicine

Along with a Glossary and Directory of Additional Resources

Edited by Joyce Brennfleck Shannon. 654 pages. 2004. 978-0-7808-0670-2.

"Recommended for hospital and health sciences libraries with consumer health collections."
—*E-Streams, Mar '00*

"This is an overall excellent reference with a wealth of general knowledge that may aid those who are reluctant to get vital tests performed."
—*Today's Librarian, Jan '00*

"A valuable reference guide."
—*American Reference Books Annual, 2000*

■

Men's Health Concerns Sourcebook, 2nd Edition

Basic Consumer Health Information about the Medical and Mental Concerns of Men, Including Theories about the Shorter Male Lifespan, the Leading Causes of Death and Disability, Physical Concerns of Special Significance to Men, Reproductive and Sexual Concerns, Sexually Transmitted Diseases, Men's Mental and Emotional Health, and Lifestyle Choices That Affect Wellness, Such as Nutrition, Fitness, and Substance Use

Along with a Glossary of Related Terms and a Directory of Organizational Resources in Men's Health

Edited by Robert Aquinas McNally. 644 pages. 2004. 978-0-7808-0671-9.

"A very accessible reference for non-specialist general readers and consumers." —*The Bookwatch, Jun '04*

"This comprehensive resource and the series are highly recommended."
—*American Reference Books Annual, 2000*

"Recommended reference source."
—*Booklist, American Library Association, Dec '98*

■

Mental Health Disorders Sourcebook, 3rd Edition

Basic Consumer Health Information about Mental and Emotional Health and Mental Illness, Including Facts about Depression, Bipolar Disorder, and Other Mood Disorders, Phobias, Post-Traumatic Stress Disorder (PTSD), Obsessive-Compulsive Disorder, and Other Anxiety Disorders, Impulse Control Disorders, Eating Disorders, Personality Disorders, and Psychotic Disorders, Including Schizophrenia and Dissociative Disorders

Along with Statistical Information, a Special Section Concerning Mental Health Issues in Children and Adolescents, a Glossary, and Directories of Resources for Additional Help and Information

Edited by Karen Bellenir. 661 pages. 2005. 978-0-7808-0747-1.

"Recommended for public libraries and academic libraries with an undergraduate program in psychology."
—*American Reference Books Annual, 2006*

"Recommended reference source."
—*Booklist, American Library Association, Jun '00*

Mental Retardation Sourcebook

Basic Consumer Health Information about Mental Retardation and Its Causes, Including Down Syndrome, Fetal Alcohol Syndrome, Fragile X Syndrome, Genetic Conditions, Injury, and Environmental Sources

Along with Preventive Strategies, Parenting Issues, Educational Implications, Health Care Needs, Employment and Economic Matters, Legal Issues, a Glossary, and a Resource Listing for Additional Help and Information

Edited by Joyce Brennfleck Shannon. 642 pages. 2000. 978-0-7808-0377-0.

"Public libraries will find the book useful for reference and as a beginning research point for students, parents, and caregivers."
— American Reference Books Annual, 2001

"The strength of this work is that it compiles many basic fact sheets and addresses for further information in one volume. It is intended and suitable for the general public. This sourcebook is relevant to any collection providing health information to the general public."
— E-Streams, Nov '00

"From preventing retardation to parenting and family challenges, this covers health, social and legal issues and will prove an invaluable overview."
— Reviewer's Bookwatch, Jul '00

■

Movement Disorders Sourcebook

Basic Consumer Health Information about Neurological Movement Disorders, Including Essential Tremor, Parkinson's Disease, Dystonia, Cerebral Palsy, Huntington's Disease, Myasthenia Gravis, Multiple Sclerosis, and Other Early-Onset and Adult-Onset Movement Disorders, Their Symptoms and Causes, Diagnostic Tests, and Treatments

Along with Mobility and Assistive Technology Information, a Glossary, and a Directory of Additional Resources

Edited by Joyce Brennfleck Shannon. 655 pages. 2003. 978-0-7808-0628-3.

". . . a good resource for consumers and recommended for public, community college and undergraduate libraries." *— American Reference Books Annual, 2004*

■

Muscular Dystrophy Sourcebook

Basic Consumer Health Information about Congenital, Childhood-Onset, and Adult-Onset Forms of Muscular Dystrophy, Such as Duchenne, Becker, Emery-Dreifuss, Distal, Limb-Girdle, Facioscapulohumeral (FSHD), Myotonic, and Ophthalmoplegic Muscular Dystrophies, Including Facts about Diagnostic Tests, Medical and Physical Therapies, Management of Co-Occurring Conditions, and Parenting Guidelines

Along with Practical Tips for Home Care, a Glossary, and Directories of Additional Resources

Edited by Joyce Brennfleck Shannon. 577 pages. 2004. 978-0-7808-0676-4.

"This book is highly recommended for public and academic libraries as well as health care offices that support the information needs of patients and their families."
— E-Streams, Apr '05

"Excellent reference." *— The Bookwatch, Jan '05*

■

Obesity Sourcebook

Basic Consumer Health Information about Diseases and Other Problems Associated with Obesity, and Including Facts about Risk Factors, Prevention Issues, and Management Approaches

Along with Statistical and Demographic Data, Information about Special Populations, Research Updates, a Glossary, and Source Listings for Further Help and Information

Edited by Wilma Caldwell and Chad T. Kimball. 376 pages. 2001. 978-0-7808-0333-6.

"The book synthesizes the reliable medical literature on obesity into one easy-to-read and useful resource for the general public."
— American Reference Books Annual, 2002

"This is a very useful resource book for the lay public."
— Doody's Review Service, Nov '01

"Well suited for the health reference collection of a public library or an academic health science library that serves the general population." *— E-Streams, Sep '01*

"Recommended reference source."
— Booklist, American Library Association, Apr '01

"Recommended pick both for specialty health library collections and any general consumer health reference collection." *— The Bookwatch, Apr '01*

■

Oral Health Sourcebook

SEE Dental Care & Oral Health Sourcebook

■

Osteoporosis Sourcebook

Basic Consumer Health Information about Primary and Secondary Osteoporosis and Juvenile Osteoporosis and Related Conditions, Including Fibrous Dysplasia, Gaucher Disease, Hyperthyroidism, Hypophosphatasia, Myeloma, Osteopetrosis, Osteogenesis Imperfecta, and Paget's Disease

Along with Information about Risk Factors, Treatments, Traditional and Non-Traditional Pain Management, a Glossary of Related Terms, and a Directory of Resources

Edited by Allan R. Cook. 584 pages. 2001. 978-0-7808-0239-1.

"This would be a book to be kept in a staff or patient library. The targeted audience is the layperson, but the therapist who needs a quick bit of information on a particular topic will also find the book useful."
— Physical Therapy, Jan '02

"This resource is recommended as a great reference source for public, health, and academic libraries, and is another triumph for the editors of Omnigraphics."
— *American Reference Books Annual, 2002*

"Recommended for all public libraries and general health collections, especially those supporting patient education or consumer health programs."
— *E-Streams, Nov '01*

"Will prove valuable to any library seeking to maintain a current, comprehensive reference collection of health resources. . . . From prevention to treatment and associated conditions, this provides an excellent survey."
— *The Bookwatch, Aug '01*

"Recommended reference source."
— *Booklist, American Library Association, Jul '01*

SEE ALSO *Healthy Aging Sourcebook, Physical & Mental Issues in Aging Sourcebook, Women's Health Concerns Sourcebook*

■

Pain Sourcebook, 2nd Edition

Basic Consumer Health Information about Specific Forms of Acute and Chronic Pain, Including Muscle and Skeletal Pain, Nerve Pain, Cancer Pain, and Disorders Characterized by Pain, Such as Fibromyalgia, Shingles, Angina, Arthritis, and Headaches

Along with Information about Pain Medications and Management Techniques, Complementary and Alternative Pain Relief Options, Tips for People Living with Chronic Pain, a Glossary, and a Directory of Sources for Further Information

Edited by Karen Bellenir. 670 pages. 2002. 978-0-7808-0612-2.

"A source of valuable information. . . . This book offers help to nonmedical people who need information about pain and pain management. It is also an excellent reference for those who participate in patient education."
— *Doody's Review Service, Sep '02*

"Highly recommended for academic and medical reference collections." — *Library Bookwatch, Sep '02*

"The text is readable, easily understood, and well indexed. This excellent volume belongs in all patient education libraries, consumer health sections of public libraries, and many personal collections."
— *American Reference Books Annual, 1999*

"The information is basic in terms of scholarship and is appropriate for general readers. Written in journalistic style . . . intended for non-professionals. Quite thorough in its coverage of different pain conditions and summarizes the latest clinical information regarding pain treatment." — *Choice, Association of College and Research Libraries, Jun '98*

"Recommended reference source."
— *Booklist, American Library Association, Mar '98*

■

Pediatric Cancer Sourcebook

Basic Consumer Health Information about Leukemias, Brain Tumors, Sarcomas, Lymphomas, and Other Cancers in Infants, Children, and Adolescents, Including Descriptions of Cancers, Treatments, and Coping Strategies

Along with Suggestions for Parents, Caregivers, and Concerned Relatives, a Glossary of Cancer Terms, and Resource Listings

Edited by Edward J. Prucha. 587 pages. 1999. 978-0-7808-0245-2.

"An excellent source of information. Recommended for public, hospital, and health science libraries with consumer health collections." — *E-Streams, Jun '00*

"Recommended reference source."
— *Booklist, American Library Association, Feb '00*

"A valuable addition to all libraries specializing in health services and many public libraries."
— *American Reference Books Annual, 2000*

SEE ALSO *Childhood Diseases & Disorders Sourcebook, Healthy Children Sourcebook*

■

Physical & Mental Issues in Aging Sourcebook

Basic Consumer Health Information on Physical and Mental Disorders Associated with the Aging Process, Including Concerns about Cardiovascular Disease, Pulmonary Disease, Oral Health, Digestive Disorders, Musculoskeletal and Skin Disorders, Metabolic Changes, Sexual and Reproductive Issues, and Changes in Vision, Hearing, and Other Senses

Along with Data about Longevity and Causes of Death, Information on Acute and Chronic Pain, Descriptions of Mental Concerns, a Glossary of Terms, and Resource Listings for Additional Help

Edited by Jenifer Swanson. 660 pages. 1999. 978-0-7808-0233-9.

"This is a treasure of health information for the layperson." — *Choice Health Sciences Supplement, Association of College & Research Libraries, May '00*

"Recommended for public libraries."
— *American Reference Books Annual, 2000*

"Recommended reference source."
— *Booklist, American Library Association, Oct '99*

SEE ALSO *Healthy Aging Sourcebook*

■

Podiatry Sourcebook, 2nd Edition

Basic Consumer Health Information about Disorders, Diseases, Deformities, and Injuries that Affect the Foot and Ankle, Including Sprains, Corns, Calluses, Bunions, Plantar Warts, Plantar Fasciitis, Neuromas, Clubfoot, Flat Feet, Achilles Tendonitis, and Much More

Along with Information about Selecting a Foot Care Specialist, Foot Fitness, Shoes and Socks, Diagnostic Tests and Corrective Procedures, Financial Assistance for Corrective Devices, a Glossary of Related Terms, and a Directory of Resources for Additional Help and Information

Edited by Ivy L. Alexander. 543 pages. 2007. 978-0-7808-0944-4.

"Recommended reference source."
    —Booklist, American Library Association, Feb '02

"There is a lot of information presented here on a topic that is usually only covered sparingly in most larger comprehensive medical encyclopedias."
    —American Reference Books Annual, 2002

■

Pregnancy & Birth Sourcebook, 2nd Edition

Basic Consumer Health Information about Conception and Pregnancy, Including Facts about Fertility, Infertility, Pregnancy Symptoms and Complications, Fetal Growth and Development, Labor, Delivery, and the Postpartum Period, as Well as Information about Maintaining Health and Wellness during Pregnancy and Caring for a Newborn

Along with Information about Public Health Assistance for Low-Income Pregnant Women, a Glossary, and Directories of Agencies and Organizations Providing Help and Support

Edited by Amy L. Sutton. 626 pages. 2004. 978-0-7808-0672-6.

"Will appeal to public and school reference collections strong in medicine and women's health. . . . Deserves a spot on any medical reference shelf."
    — The Bookwatch, Jul '04

"A well-organized handbook. Recommended."
    —Choice, Association of College & Research Libraries, Apr '98

"Recommended reference source."
    —Booklist, American Library Association, Mar '98

"Recommended for public libraries."
    —American Reference Books Annual, 1998

SEE ALSO Breastfeeding Sourcebook, Congenital Disorders Sourcebook, Family Planning Sourcebook

■

Prostate & Urological Disorders Sourcebook

Basic Consumer Health Information about Urogenital and Sexual Disorders in Men, Including Prostate and Other Andrological Cancers, Prostatitis, Benign Prostatic Hyperplasia, Testicular and Penile Trauma, Cryptorchidism, Peyronie Disease, Erectile Dysfunction, and Male Factor Infertility, and Facts about Commonly Used Tests and Procedures, Such as Prostatectomy, Vasectomy, Vasectomy Reversal, Penile Implants, and Semen Analysis

Along with a Glossary of Andrological Terms and a Directory of Resources for Additional Information

Edited by Karen Bellenir. 631 pages. 2005. 978-0-7808-0797-6.

Prostate Cancer Sourcebook

Basic Consumer Health Information about Prostate Cancer, Including Information about the Associated Risk Factors, Detection, Diagnosis, and Treatment of Prostate Cancer

Along with Information on Non-Malignant Prostate Conditions, and Featuring a Section Listing Support and Treatment Centers and a Glossary of Related Terms

Edited by Dawn D. Matthews. 358 pages. 2001. 978-0-7808-0324-4.

"Recommended reference source."
    —Booklist, American Library Association, Jan '02

"A valuable resource for health care consumers seeking information on the subject. . . . All text is written in a clear, easy-to-understand language that avoids technical jargon. Any library that collects consumer health resources would strengthen their collection with the addition of the *Prostate Cancer Sourcebook.*"
    —American Reference Books Annual, 2002

SEE ALSO Men's Health Concerns Sourcebook

■

Reconstructive & Cosmetic Surgery Sourcebook

Basic Consumer Health Information on Cosmetic and Reconstructive Plastic Surgery, Including Statistical Information about Different Surgical Procedures, Things to Consider Prior to Surgery, Plastic Surgery Techniques and Tools, Emotional and Psychological Considerations, and Procedure-Specific Information

Along with a Glossary of Terms and a Listing of Resources for Additional Help and Information

Edited by M. Lisa Weatherford. 374 pages. 2001. 978-0-7808-0214-8.

"An excellent reference that addresses cosmetic and medically necessary reconstructive surgeries. . . . The style of the prose is calm and reassuring, discussing the many positive outcomes now available due to advances in surgical techniques."
    —American Reference Books Annual, 2002

"Recommended for health science libraries that are open to the public, as well as hospital libraries that are open to the patients. This book is a good resource for the consumer interested in plastic surgery."
    —E-Streams, Dec '01

"Recommended reference source."
    —Booklist, American Library Association, Jul '01

■

Rehabilitation Sourcebook

Basic Consumer Health Information about Rehabilitation for People Recovering from Heart Surgery, Spinal Cord Injury, Stroke, Orthopedic Impairments, Amputation, Pulmonary Impairments, Traumatic Injury, and More, Including Physical Therapy, Occupational Therapy, Speech/Language Therapy, Massage Therapy, Dance Therapy, Art Therapy, and Recreational Therapy

Along with Information on Assistive and Adaptive Devices, a Glossary, and Resources for Additional Help and Information

Edited by Dawn D. Matthews. 531 pages. 1999. 978-0-7808-0236-0.

"This is an excellent resource for public library reference and health collections."
— *American Reference Books Annual, 2001*

"Recommended reference source."
— *Booklist, American Library Association, May '00*

■

Respiratory Diseases & Disorders Sourcebook

Basic Information about Respiratory Diseases and Disorders, Including Asthma, Cystic Fibrosis, Pneumonia, the Common Cold, Influenza, and Others, Featuring Facts about the Respiratory System, Statistical and Demographic Data, Treatments, Self-Help Management Suggestions, and Current Research Initiatives

Edited by Allan R. Cook and Peter D. Dresser. 771 pages. 1995. 978-0-7808-0037-3.

"Designed for the layperson and for patients and their families coping with respiratory illness. . . . an extensive array of information on diagnosis, treatment, management, and prevention of respiratory illnesses for the general reader." — *Choice, Association of College & Research Libraries, Jun '96*

"A highly recommended text for all collections. It is a comforting reminder of the power of knowledge that good books carry between their covers."
— *Academic Library Book Review, Spring '96*

"A comprehensive collection of authoritative information presented in a nontechnical, humanitarian style for patients, families, and caregivers."
— *Association of Operating Room Nurses, Sep/Oct '95*

SEE ALSO Lung Disorders Sourcebook

■

Sexually Transmitted Diseases Sourcebook, 3rd Edition

Basic Consumer Health Information about Chlamydial Infections, Gonorrhea, Hepatitis, Herpes, HIV/AIDS, Human Papillomavirus, Pubic Lice, Scabies, Syphilis, Trichomoniasis, Vaginal Infections, and Other Sexually Transmitted Diseases, Including Facts about Risk Factors, Symptoms, Diagnosis, Treatment, and the Prevention of Sexually Transmitted Infections

Along with Updates on Current Research Initiatives, a Glossary of Related Terms, and Resources for Additional Help and Information

Edited by Amy L. Sutton. 629 pages. 2006. 978-0-7808-0824-9.

"Recommended for consumer health collections in public libraries, and secondary school and community college libraries."
— *American Reference Books Annual, 2002*

"Every school and public library should have a copy of this comprehensive and user-friendly reference book."
— *Choice, Association of College & Research Libraries, Sep '01*

"This is a highly recommended book. This is an especially important book for all school and public libraries."
— *AIDS Book Review Journal, Jul-Aug '01*

"Recommended reference source."
— *Booklist, American Library Association, Apr '01*

■

Sleep Disorders Sourcebook, 2nd Edition

Basic Consumer Health Information about Sleep and Sleep Disorders, Including Insomnia, Sleep Apnea, Restless Legs Syndrome, Narcolepsy, Parasomnias, and Other Health Problems That Affect Sleep, Plus Facts about Diagnostic Procedures, Treatment Strategies, Sleep Medications, and Tips for Improving Sleep Quality

Along with a Glossary of Related Terms and Resources for Additional Help and Information

Edited by Amy L. Sutton. 567 pages. 2005. 978-0-7808-0743-3.

"This book will be useful for just about everybody, especially the 40 million Americans with sleep disorders."
— *American Reference Books Annual, 2006*

"Recommended for public libraries and libraries supporting health care professionals." — *E-Streams, Sep '05*

". . . key medical library acquisition."
— *The Bookwatch, Jun '05*

■

Smoking Concerns Sourcebook

Basic Consumer Health Information about Nicotine Addiction and Smoking Cessation, Featuring Facts about the Health Effects of Tobacco Use, Including Lung and Other Cancers, Heart Disease, Stroke, and Respiratory Disorders, Such as Emphysema and Chronic Bronchitis

Along with Information about Smoking Prevention Programs, Suggestions for Achieving and Maintaining a Smoke-Free Lifestyle, Statistics about Tobacco Use, Reports on Current Research Initiatives, a Glossary of Related Terms, and Directories of Resources for Additional Help and Information

Edited by Karen Bellenir. 621 pages. 2004. 978-0-7808-0323-7.

"Provides everything needed for the student or general reader seeking practical details on the effects of tobacco use." — *The Bookwatch, Mar '05*

"Public libraries and consumer health care libraries will find this work useful."
— *American Reference Books Annual, 2005*

Sports Injuries Sourcebook, 3rd Edition

Basic Consumer Health Information about Sprains and Strains, Fractures, Growth Plate Injuries, Overtraining Injuries, and Injuries to the Head, Face, Shoulders, Elbows, Hands, Spinal Column, Knees, Ankles, and Feet, and with Facts about Heat-Related Illness, Steroids and Sport Supplements, Protective Equipment, Diagnostic Procedures, Treatment Options, and Rehabilitation

Along with a Glossary of Related Terms and a Directory of Resources for Additional Help and Information

Edited by Sandra J. Judd. 651 pages. 2007. 978-0-7808-0949-9.

"This is an excellent reference for consumers and it is recommended for public, community college, and undergraduate libraries."
— American Reference Books Annual, 2003

"Recommended reference source."
— Booklist, American Library Association, Feb '03

■

Stress-Related Disorders Sourcebook

Basic Consumer Health Information about Stress and Stress-Related Disorders, Including Stress Origins and Signals, Environmental Stress at Work and Home, Mental and Emotional Stress Associated with Depression, Post-Traumatic Stress Disorder, Panic Disorder, Suicide, and the Physical Effects of Stress on the Cardiovascular, Immune, and Nervous Systems

Along with Stress Management Techniques, a Glossary, and a Listing of Additional Resources

Edited by Joyce Brennfleck Shannon. 610 pages. 2002. 978-0-7808-0560-6.

"Well written for a general readership, the *Stress-Related Disorders Sourcebook* is a useful addition to the health reference literature."
— American Reference Books Annual, 2003

"I am impressed by the amount of information. It offers a thorough overview of the causes and consequences of stress for the layperson. . . . A well-done and thorough reference guide for professionals and nonprofessionals alike." *— Doody's Review Service, Dec '02*

■

Stroke Sourcebook

Basic Consumer Health Information about Stroke, Including Ischemic, Hemorrhagic, Transient Ischemic Attack (TIA), and Pediatric Stroke, Stroke Triggers and Risks, Diagnostic Tests, Treatments, and Rehabilitation Information

Along with Stroke Prevention Guidelines, Legal and Financial Information, a Glossary, and a Directory of Additional Resources

Edited by Joyce Brennfleck Shannon. 606 pages. 2003. 978-0-7808-0630-6.

"This volume is highly recommended and should be in every medical, hospital, and public library."
— American Reference Books Annual, 2004

"Highly recommended for the amount and variety of topics and information covered." *— Choice, Nov '03*

■

Surgery Sourcebook

Basic Consumer Health Information about Inpatient and Outpatient Surgeries, Including Cardiac, Vascular, Orthopedic, Ocular, Reconstructive, Cosmetic, Gynecologic, and Ear, Nose, and Throat Procedures and More

Along with Information about Operating Room Policies and Instruments, Laser Surgery Techniques, Hospital Errors, Statistical Data, a Glossary, and Listings of Sources for Further Help and Information

Edited by Annemarie S. Muth and Karen Bellenir. 596 pages. 2002. 978-0-7808-0380-0.

"Large public libraries and medical libraries would benefit from this material in their reference collections."
— American Reference Books Annual, 2004

"Invaluable reference for public and school library collections alike." *— Library Bookwatch, Apr '03*

■

Thyroid Disorders Sourcebook

Basic Consumer Health Information about Disorders of the Thyroid and Parathyroid Glands, Including Hypothyroidism, Hyperthyroidism, Graves Disease, Hashimoto Thyroiditis, Thyroid Cancer, and Parathyroid Disorders, Featuring Facts about Symptoms, Risk Factors, Tests, and Treatments

Along with Information about the Effects of Thyroid Imbalance on Other Body Systems, Environmental Factors That Affect the Thyroid Gland, a Glossary, and a Directory of Additional Resources

Edited by Joyce Brennfleck Shannon. 599 pages. 2005. 978-0-7808-0745-7.

"Recommended for consumer health collections."
— American Reference Books Annual, 2006

"Highly recommended pick for basic consumer health reference holdings at all levels."
— The Bookwatch, Aug '05

■

Transplantation Sourcebook

Basic Consumer Health Information about Organ and Tissue Transplantation, Including Physical and Financial Preparations, Procedures and Issues Relating to Specific Solid Organ and Tissue Transplants, Rehabilitation, Pediatric Transplant Information, the Future of Transplantation, and Organ and Tissue Donation

Along with a Glossary and Listings of Additional Resources

Edited by Joyce Brennfleck Shannon. 628 pages. 2002. 978-0-7808-0322-0.

"Along with these advances [in transplantation technology] have come a number of daunting questions for potential transplant patients, their families, and their health care providers. This reference text is the best single tool to address many of these questions. . . . It will be a much-needed addition to the reference collections in health care, academic, and large public libraries."
— *American Reference Books Annual, 2003*

"Recommended for libraries with an interest in offering consumer health information." — *E-Streams, Jul '02*

"This is a unique and valuable resource for patients facing transplantation and their families."
— *Doody's Review Service, Jun '02*

■

Traveler's Health Sourcebook

Basic Consumer Health Information for Travelers, Including Physical and Medical Preparations, Transportation Health and Safety, Essential Information about Food and Water, Sun Exposure, Insect and Snake Bites, Camping and Wilderness Medicine, and Travel with Physical or Medical Disabilities

Along with International Travel Tips, Vaccination Recommendations, Geographical Health Issues, Disease Risks, a Glossary, and a Listing of Additional Resources

Edited by Joyce Brennfleck Shannon. 613 pages. 2000. 978-0-7808-0384-8.

"Recommended reference source."
— *Booklist, American Library Association, Feb '01*

"This book is recommended for any public library, any travel collection, and especially any collection for the physically disabled."
— *American Reference Books Annual, 2001*

SEE ALSO *Worldwide Health Sourcebook*

■

Urinary Tract & Kidney Diseases & Disorders Sourcebook, 2nd Edition

Basic Consumer Health Information about the Urinary System, Including the Bladder, Urethra, Ureters, and Kidneys, with Facts about Urinary Tract Infections, Incontinence, Congenital Disorders, Kidney Stones, Cancers of the Urinary Tract and Kidneys, Kidney Failure, Dialysis, and Kidney Transplantation

Along with Statistical and Demographic Information, Reports on Current Research in Kidney and Urologic Health, a Summary of Commonly Used Diagnostic Tests, a Glossary of Related Terms, and a Directory of Resources for Additional Help and Information

Edited by Ivy L. Alexander. 649 pages. 2005. 978-0-7808-0750-1.

"A good choice for a consumer health information library or for a medical library needing information to refer to their patients."
— *American Reference Books Annual, 2006*

Vegetarian Sourcebook

Basic Consumer Health Information about Vegetarian Diets, Lifestyle, and Philosophy, Including Definitions of Vegetarianism and Veganism, Tips about Adopting Vegetarianism, Creating a Vegetarian Pantry, and Meeting Nutritional Needs of Vegetarians, with Facts Regarding Vegetarianism's Effect on Pregnant and Lactating Women, Children, Athletes, and Senior Citizens

Along with a Glossary of Commonly Used Vegetarian Terms and Resources for Additional Help and Information

Edited by Chad T. Kimball. 360 pages. 2002. 978-0-7808-0439-5.

"Organizes into one concise volume the answers to the most common questions concerning vegetarian diets and lifestyles. This title is recommended for public and secondary school libraries." — *E-Streams, Apr '03*

"Invaluable reference for public and school library collections alike." — *Library Bookwatch, Apr '03*

"The articles in this volume are easy to read and come from authoritative sources. The book does not necessarily support the vegetarian diet but instead provides the pros and cons of this important decision. The Vegetarian Sourcebook is recommended for public libraries and consumer health libraries."
— *American Reference Books Annual, 2003*

SEE ALSO *Diet & Nutrition Sourcebook*

■

Women's Health Concerns Sourcebook, 2nd Edition

Basic Consumer Health Information about the Medical and Mental Concerns of Women, Including Maintaining Health and Wellness, Gynecological Concerns, Breast Health, Sexuality and Reproductive Issues, Menopause, Cancer in Women, Leading Causes of Death and Disability among Women, Physical Concerns of Special Significance to Women, and Women's Mental and Emotional Health

Along with a Glossary of Related Terms and Directories of Resources for Additional Help and Information

Edited by Amy L. Sutton. 746 pages. 2004. 978-0-7808-0673-3.

"This is a useful reference book, which makes the reader knowledgeable about several issues that concern women's health. It is recommended for public libraries and home library collections." — *E-Streams, May '05*

"A useful addition to public and consumer health library collections."
— *American Reference Books Annual, 2005*

"A highly recommended title."
— *The Bookwatch, May '04*

"Handy compilation. There is an impressive range of diseases, devices, disorders, procedures, and other physical and emotional issues covered . . . well organized, illustrated, and indexed." — *Choice, Association of College & Research Libraries, Jan '98*

SEE ALSO *Breast Cancer Sourcebook, Cancer Sourcebook for Women, Healthy Heart Sourcebook for Women, Osteoporosis Sourcebook*

Workplace Health & Safety Sourcebook

Basic Consumer Health Information about Workplace Health and Safety, Including the Effect of Workplace Hazards on the Lungs, Skin, Heart, Ears, Eyes, Brain, Reproductive Organs, Musculoskeletal System, and Other Organs and Body Parts

Along with Information about Occupational Cancer, Personal Protective Equipment, Toxic and Hazardous Chemicals, Child Labor, Stress, and Workplace Violence

Edited by Chad T. Kimball. 626 pages. 2000. 978-0-7808-0231-5.

"As a reference for the general public, this would be useful in any library." —*E-Streams, Jun '01*

"Provides helpful information for primary care physicians and other caregivers interested in occupational medicine.... General readers; professionals."
—*Choice, Association of College & Research Libraries, May '01*

"Recommended reference source."
—*Booklist, American Library Association, Feb '01*

"Highly recommended." —*The Bookwatch, Jan '01*

Worldwide Health Sourcebook

Basic Information about Global Health Issues, Including Malnutrition, Reproductive Health, Disease Dispersion and Prevention, Emerging Diseases, Risky Health Behaviors, and the Leading Causes of Death

Along with Global Health Concerns for Children, Women, and the Elderly, Mental Health Issues, Research and Technology Advancements, and Economic, Environmental, and Political Health Implications, a Glossary, and a Resource Listing for Additional Help and Information

Edited by Joyce Brennfleck Shannon. 614 pages. 2001. 978-0-7808-0330-5.

"Named an Outstanding Academic Title."
—*Choice, Association of College & Research Libraries, Jan '02*

"Yet another handy but also unique compilation in the extensive *Health Reference Series*, this is a useful work because many of the international publications reprinted or excerpted are not readily available. Highly recommended." —*Choice, Association of College & Research Libraries, Nov '01*

"Recommended reference source."
—*Booklist, American Library Association, Oct '01*

SEE ALSO *Traveler's Health Sourcebook*

649

Teen Health Series
Helping Young Adults Understand, Manage, and Avoid Serious Illness

List price $65 per volume. **School and library price $58 per volume.**

Alcohol Information for Teens
Health Tips about Alcohol and Alcoholism

Including Facts about Underage Drinking, Preventing Teen Alcohol Use, Alcohol's Effects on the Brain and the Body, Alcohol Abuse Treatment, Help for Children of Alcoholics, and More

Edited by Joyce Brennfleck Shannon. 370 pages. 2005. 978-0-7808-0741-9.

"Boxed facts and tips add visual interest to the well-researched and clearly written text."
— *Curriculum Connection, Apr '06*

Allergy Information for Teens
Health Tips about Allergic Reactions Such as Anaphylaxis, Respiratory Problems, and Rashes

Including Facts about Identifying and Managing Allergies to Food, Pollen, Mold, Animals, Chemicals, Drugs, and Other Substances

Edited by Karen Bellenir. 410 pages. 2006. 978-0-7808-0799-0.

Asthma Information for Teens
Health Tips about Managing Asthma and Related Concerns

Including Facts about Asthma Causes, Triggers, Symptoms, Diagnosis, and Treatment

Edited by Karen Bellenir. 386 pages. 2005. 978-0-7808-0770-9.

"Highly recommended for medical libraries, public school libraries, and public libraries."
— *American Reference Books Annual, 2006*

"It is so clearly written and well organized that even hesitant readers will be able to find the facts they need, whether for reports or personal information. . . . A succinct but complete resource."
— *School Library Journal, Sep '05*

Body Information for Teens
Health Tips about Maintaining Well-Being for a Lifetime

Including Facts about the Development and Functioning of the Body's Systems, Organs, and Structures and the Health Impact of Lifestyle Choices

Edited by Sandra Augustyn Lawton. 458 pages. 2007. 978-0-7808-0443-2.

Cancer Information for Teens
Health Tips about Cancer Awareness, Prevention, Diagnosis, and Treatment

Including Facts about Frequently Occurring Cancers, Cancer Risk Factors, and Coping Strategies for Teens Fighting Cancer or Dealing with Cancer in Friends or Family Members

Edited by Wilma R. Caldwell. 428 pages. 2004. 978-0-7808-0678-8.

"Recommended for school libraries, or consumer libraries that see a lot of use by teens."
— *E-Streams, May '05*

"A valuable educational tool."
— *American Reference Books Annual, 2005*

"Young adults and their parents alike will find this new addition to the *Teen Health Series* an important reference to cancer in teens."
— *Children's Bookwatch, Feb '05*

Complementary and Alternative Medicine Information for Teens
Health Tips about Non-Traditional and Non-Western Medical Practices

Including Information about Acupuncture, Chiropractic Medicine, Dietary and Herbal Supplements, Hypnosis, Massage Therapy, Prayer and Spirituality, Reflexology, Yoga, and More

Edited by Sandra Augustyn Lawton. 405 pages. 2006. 978-0-7808-0966-6.

Diabetes Information for Teens
Health Tips about Managing Diabetes and Preventing Related Complications

Including Information about Insulin, Glucose Control, Healthy Eating, Physical Activity, and Learning to Live with Diabetes

Edited by Sandra Augustyn Lawton. 410 pages. 2006. 978-0-7808-0811-9.

Diet Information for Teens, 2nd Edition

Health Tips about Diet and Nutrition

Including Facts about Dietary Guidelines, Food Groups, Nutrients, Healthy Meals, Snacks, Weight Control, Medical Concerns Related to Diet, and More

Edited by Karen Bellenir. 432 pages. 2006. 978-0-7808-0820-1.

"Full of helpful insights and facts throughout the book. . . . An excellent resource to be placed in public libraries or even in personal collections."
— *American Reference Books Annual, 2002*

"Recommended for middle and high school libraries and media centers as well as academic libraries that educate future teachers of teenagers. It is also a suitable addition to health science libraries that serve patrons who are interested in teen health promotion and education."
— *E-Streams, Oct '01*

"This comprehensive book would be beneficial to collections that need information about nutrition, dietary guidelines, meal planning, and weight control. . . . This reference is so easy to use that its purchase is recommended."
— *The Book Report, Sep-Oct '01*

"This book is written in an easy to understand format describing issues that many teens face every day, and then provides thoughtful explanations so that teens can make informed decisions. This is an interesting book that provides important facts and information for today's teens."
— *Doody's Health Sciences Book Review Journal, Jul-Aug '01*

"A comprehensive compendium of diet and nutrition. The information is presented in a straightforward, plain-spoken manner. This title will be useful to those working on reports on a variety of topics, as well as to general readers concerned about their dietary health."
— *School Library Journal, Jun '01*

Drug Information for Teens, 2nd Edition

Health Tips about the Physical and Mental Effects of Substance Abuse

Including Information about Marijuana, Inhalants, Club Drugs, Stimulants, Hallucinogens, Opiates, Prescription and Over-the-Counter Drugs, Herbal Products, Tobacco, Alcohol, and More

Edited by Sandra Augustyn Lawton. 468 pages. 2006. 978-0-7808-0862-1.

"A clearly written resource for general readers and researchers alike."
— *School Library Journal*

"This book is well-balanced. . . . a must for public and school libraries."
— *VOYA: Voice of Youth Advocates, Dec '03*

"The chapters are quick to make a connection to their teenage reading audience. The prose is straightforward and the book lends itself to spot reading. It should be useful both for practical information and for research, and it is suitable for public and school libraries."
— *American Reference Books Annual, 2003*

"Recommended reference source."
— *Booklist, American Library Association, Feb '03*

"This is an excellent resource for teens and their parents. Education about drugs and substances is key to discouraging teen drug abuse and this book provides this much needed information in a way that is interesting and factual."
— *Doody's Review Service, Dec '02*

Eating Disorders Information for Teens

Health Tips about Anorexia, Bulimia, Binge Eating, and Other Eating Disorders

Including Information on the Causes, Prevention, and Treatment of Eating Disorders, and Such Other Issues as Maintaining Healthy Eating and Exercise Habits

Edited by Sandra Augustyn Lawton. 337 pages. 2005. 978-0-7808-0783-9.

"An excellent resource for teens and those who work with them."
— *VOYA: Voice of Youth Advocates, Apr '06*

"A welcome addition to high school and undergraduate libraries." — *American Reference Books Annual, 2006*

"This book covers the topic in a lucid manner but delves deeper into every aspect of an eating disorder. A solid addition for any nonfiction or reference collection."
— *School Library Journal, Dec '05*

Fitness Information for Teens

Health Tips about Exercise, Physical Well-Being, and Health Maintenance

Including Facts about Aerobic and Anaerobic Conditioning, Stretching, Body Shape and Body Image, Sports Training, Nutrition, and Activities for Non-Athletes

Edited by Karen Bellenir. 425 pages. 2004. 978-0-7808-0679-5.

"Another excellent offering from Omnigraphics in their *Teen Health Series*. . . . This book will be a great addition to any public, junior high, senior high, or secondary school library."
— *American Reference Books Annual, 2005*

Learning Disabilities Information for Teens

Health Tips about Academic Skills Disorders and Other Disabilities That Affect Learning

Including Information about Common Signs of Learning Disabilities, School Issues, Learning to Live with a Learning Disability, and Other Related Issues

Edited by Sandra Augustyn Lawton. 337 pages. 2005. 978-0-7808-0796-9.

"This book provides a wealth of information for any reader interested in the signs, causes, and consequences

of learning disabilities, as well as related legal rights and educational interventions. . . . Public and academic libraries should want this title for both students and general readers."
— *American Reference Books Annual, 2006*

Mental Health Information for Teens, 2nd Edition
Health Tips about Mental Wellness and Mental Illness

Including Facts about Mental and Emotional Health, Depression and Other Mood Disorders, Anxiety Disorders, Behavior Disorders, Self-Injury, Psychosis, Schizophrenia, and More

Edited by Karen Bellenir. 400 pages. 2006. 978-0-7808-0863-8.

"In both language and approach, this user-friendly entry in the *Teen Health Series* is on target for teens needing information on mental health concerns."
— *Booklist, American Library Association, Jan '02*

"Readers will find the material accessible and informative, with the shaded notes, facts, and embedded glossary insets adding appropriately to the already interesting and succinct presentation."
— *School Library Journal, Jan '02*

"This title is highly recommended for any library that serves adolescents and parents/caregivers of adolescents."
— *E-Streams, Jan '02*

"Recommended for high school libraries and young adult collections in public libraries. Both health professionals and teenagers will find this book useful."
— *American Reference Books Annual, 2002*

"This is a nice book written to enlighten the society, primarily teenagers, about common teen mental health issues. It is highly recommended to teachers and parents as well as adolescents."
— *Doody's Review Service, Dec '01*

Sexual Health Information for Teens
Health Tips about Sexual Development, Human Reproduction, and Sexually Transmitted Diseases

Including Facts about Puberty, Reproductive Health, Chlamydia, Human Papillomavirus, Pelvic Inflammatory Disease, Herpes, AIDS, Contraception, Pregnancy, and More

Edited by Deborah A. Stanley. 391 pages. 2003. 978-0-7808-0445-6.

"This work should be included in all high school libraries and many larger public libraries. . . . highly recommended."
— *American Reference Books Annual, 2004*

"*Sexual Health* approaches its subject with appropriate seriousness and offers easily accessible advice and information."
— *School Library Journal, Feb '04*

Skin Health Information for Teens
Health Tips about Dermatological Concerns and Skin Cancer Risks

Including Facts about Acne, Warts, Hives, and Other Conditions and Lifestyle Choices, Such as Tanning, Tattooing, and Piercing, That Affect the Skin, Nails, Scalp, and Hair

Edited by Robert Aquinas McNally. 429 pages. 2003. 978-0-7808-0446-3.

"This volume, as with others in the series, will be a useful addition to school and public library collections."
— *American Reference Books Annual, 2004*

"There is no doubt that this reference tool is valuable."
— *VOYA: Voice of Youth Advocates, Feb '04*

"This volume serves as a one-stop source and should be a necessity for any health collection."
— *Library Media Connection*

Sports Injuries Information for Teens
Health Tips about Sports Injuries and Injury Protection

Including Facts about Specific Injuries, Emergency Treatment, Rehabilitation, Sports Safety, Competition Stress, Fitness, Sports Nutrition, Steroid Risks, and More

Edited by Joyce Brennfleck Shannon. 405 pages. 2003. 978-0-7808-0447-0.

"This work will be useful in the young adult collections of public libraries as well as high school libraries."
— *American Reference Books Annual, 2004*

Suicide Information for Teens
Health Tips about Suicide Causes and Prevention

Including Facts about Depression, Risk Factors, Getting Help, Survivor Support, and More

Edited by Joyce Brennfleck Shannon. 368 pages. 2005. 978-0-7808-0737-2.

Tobacco Information for Teens
Health Tips about the Hazards of Using Cigarettes, Smokeless Tobacco, and Other Nicotine Products

Including Facts about Nicotine Addiction, Immediate and Long-Term Health Effects of Tobacco Use, Related Cancers, Smoking Cessation, Tobacco Use Prevention, and Tobacco Use Statistics

Edited by Karen Bellenir. 440 pages. 2007. 978-0-7808-0976-5.

Health Reference Series

Adolescent Health Sourcebook, 2nd Edition

Adult Health Concerns Sourcebook

AIDS Sourcebook, 4th Edition

Alcoholism Sourcebook, 2nd Edition

Allergies Sourcebook, 3rd Edition

Alzheimer Disease Sourcebook, 4th Edition

Arthritis Sourcebook, 2nd Edition

Asthma Sourcebook, 2nd Edition

Attention Deficit Disorder Sourcebook

Autism & Pervasive Developmental Disorders Sourcebook

Back & Neck Sourcebook, 2nd Edition

Blood & Circulatory Disorders Sourcebook, 2nd Edition

Brain Disorders Sourcebook, 2nd Edition

Breast Cancer Sourcebook, 2nd Edition

Breastfeeding Sourcebook

Burns Sourcebook

Cancer Sourcebook, 5th Edition

Cancer Sourcebook for Women, 3rd Edition

Cancer Survivorship Sourcebook

Cardiovascular Diseases & Disorders Sourcebook, 3rd Edition

Caregiving Sourcebook

Child Abuse Sourcebook

Childhood Diseases & Disorders Sourcebook

Colds, Flu & Other Common Ailments Sourcebook

Communication Disorders Sourcebook

Complementary & Alternative Medicine Sourcebook, 3rd Edition

Congenital Disorders Sourcebook, 2nd Edition

Contagious Diseases Sourcebook

Cosmetic & Reconstructive Surgery Sourcebook, 2nd Edition

Death & Dying Sourcebook, 2nd Edition

Dental Care and Oral Health Sourcebook, 3rd Edition

Depression Sourcebook, 2nd Edition

Dermatological Disorders Sourcebook, 2nd Edition

Diabetes Sourcebook, 4th Edition

Diet & Nutrition Sourcebook, 3rd Edition

Digestive Diseases & Disorder Sourcebook

Disabilities Sourcebook

Disease Management Sourcebook

Domestic Violence Sourcebook, 2nd Edition

Drug Abuse Sourcebook, 2nd Edition

Ear, Nose & Throat Disorders Sourcebook, 2nd Edition

Eating Disorders Sourcebook, 2nd Edition

Emergency Medical Services Sourcebook

Endocrine & Metabolic Disorders Sourcebook, 2nd Edition

EnvironmentalHealth Sourcebook, 2nd Edition

Ethnic Diseases Sourcebook

Eye Care Sourcebook, 3rd Edition

Family Planning Sourcebook

Fitness & Exercise Sourcebook, 3rd Edition

Food Safety Sourcebook

Forensic Medicine Sourcebook

Gastrointestinal Diseases & Disorders Sourcebook, 2nd Edition

Genetic Disorders Sourcebook, 3rd Edition

Head Trauma Sourcebook

Headache Sourcebook

Health Insurance Sourcebook

Healthy Aging Sourcebook

Healthy Children Sourcebook

Healthy Heart Sourcebook for Women

Hepatitis Sourcebook

Household Safety Sourcebook

Hypertension Sourcebook

Immune System Disorders Sourcebook, 2nd Edition

Infant & Toddler Health Sourcebook

Infectious Diseases Sourcebook